USMLE STEP 3 RECALL

VOLUME EDITOR

MICHAEL W. RYAN, MD, MS
Resident Physician
Department of Internal Medicine
St. Louis University Hospital
St. Louis, Missouri

RECALL SERIES EDITOR

LORNE H. BLACKBOURNE, MD, FACS
Fellow, Trauma/Critical Care
Department of Surgery
Miami School of Medicine
Miami, Florida

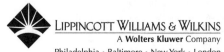

LIPPINCOTT WILLIAMS & WILKINS
A **Wolters Kluwer** Company

Philadelphia • Baltimore • New York • London
Buenos Aires • Hong Kong • Sydney • Tokyo

Editor: Neil Marquardt
Managing Editor: Beth Goldner
Marketing Manager: Scott Lavine
Production Editor: Bill Cady
Cover/text Designer: Karen Klinedinst
Compositor: TECHBOOKS
Printer: R.R.Donnelley & Sons

Copyright © 2003 Lippincott Williams & Wilkins

351 West Camden Street
Baltimore, MD 21201

530 Walnut Street
Philadelphia, PA 19106

Printed in the United States of America

Library of Congress Cataloging-in-Publication Data

USMLE step 3 recall / volume editor, Michael W. Ryan.
   p. ; cm.—(Recall series)
   Includes index.
   ISBN 0-7817-3617-X
   1. Medicine—Examinations, questions, etc. 2. Medicine—Outlines, syllabi, etc.
3. Medicine—Computer-assisted instruction. I. Title: USMLE step three recall.
II. Ryan, Michael W. III. Series.
   [DNLM: 1. Medicine—Examination Questions. W 18.2 U862 2003]
   R834.5 .U855 2003
   610'.76—dc21   2002030004

The publishers have made every effort to trace the copyright holders for borrowed material. If they have inadvertently overlooked any, they will be pleased to make the necessary arrangements at the first opportunity.

To purchase additional copies of this book, call our customer service department at **(800) 638-3030** or fax orders to **(301) 824-7390**. International customers should call **(301) 714-2324.**

Visit Lippincott Williams & Wilkins on the Internet: http://www.LWW.com. Lippincott Williams & Wilkins customer service representatives are available from 8:30 am to 6:00 pm, EST.

04 05 06
2 3 4 5 6 7 8 9 10

Dedication

This book is dedicated to my good friend Dave Peck, who passed away last year from complications of colon cancer.

Preface

If you are a busy resident looking for a highly effective, interactive review resource covering only the most relevant material in both paper and digital book format to study for the USMLE Step 3 exam, then purchase this product.

The active-learning question-and-answer format was chosen to ensure rapid comprehension of essential material. This book goes beyond covering the material like standard texts—it reinforces the critical points necessary to do well on the Step 3 exam. Your confidence and mastery of the material will increase dramatically with each interactive review session.

The content was chosen after comparing the official USMLE Step 3 study outline to the key points stressed in over 2000 review questions and by residents with high scores on the exam. Only the essential information is covered here. And it can be read on paper or your personal digital assistant. This will ensure easy access to the material without the necessity of carrying the book.

Congratulations on purchasing the only active-learning USMLE Step 3 review resource available that can be read on your personal digital assistant.

Associate Editors

Michele A. Brother, MD
Clinical Instructor
Department of Internal Medicine
St. Louis University School of
  Medicine
Physician
Departments of Pediatrics and
  Internal Medicine
SSM Medical Group
St. Louis, Missouri
Chapter 10, Pediatrics

Patricia D. Brown, MD
Associate Professor
Division of Infectious Diseases
Wayne State University School of
  Medicine
Detroit, Michigan
Chapter 7, Infectious Disease

Edwin B. George, MD, PhD
Assistant Professor
Department of Neurology
Wayne State University School of
  Medicine
John D. Dingell VA Medical
  Center
Detroit, Michigan
Chapter 8, Neurology

**John Gilroy, MD, FRCP (CAN),
FACP**
Clinical Professor
Department of Neurology
Wayne State University
Detroit, Michigan
Chairman, Neurology
Department of Medicine
William Beaumont Hospital
Royal Oak, Michigan
Chapter 8, Neurology

Kenneth A. Ginsburg, MD
Associate Professor
Department of Obstetrics and
  Gynecology
Assistant Dean for Clinical Education
Office of Academic and Student
  Programs
Wayne State University School of
  Medicine
Detroit, Michigan
Chapter 9, Obstetrics and Gynecology

**Stuart C. Gordon, MD, FACP,
FACG**
Director, Division of
  Gastroenterology-Hepatology
William Beaumont Hospital
Royal Oak, Michigan
Clinical Associate Professor of
  Medicine
Wayne State University School of
  Medicine
Detroit, Michigan
Chapter 5, Gastroenterology

Michael J. Haas, PhD
Assistant Research Professor
Division of Endocrinology
Department of Internal Medicine
St. Louis University School of
  Medicine
St. Louis, Missouri
Chapter 3, Endocrine Disorders

Terry Kowalenko, MD
Assistant Clinical Professor
Department of Emergency Medicine
Wayne State University School of
  Medicine
Detroit, Michigan
Chapter 4, Emergency Medicine

Marc D. Meissner, MD, CM, FACC, FACP
Associate Professor
Department of Internal Medicine
Wayne State University School of Medicine
Staff Cardiologist and Electrophysiologist
Division of Cardiology
Department of Medicine
Sinai-Grace Hospital
Detroit, Michigan
Chapter 1, Cardiology

Robert Gene Moore, MD
Associate Professor
Department of Urology
Baylor College of Medicine
Methodist Hospital
Houston, Texas
Chapter 15, Surgery

Michael John Quinn, MD
Assistant Professor
Department of Psychiatry
St. Louis University School of Medicine
St. Louis, Missouri
Chapter 11, Psychiatry

James A. Rowley, MD
Assistant Professor
Department of Medicine
Wayne State University School of Medicine
Attending Staff
Department of Medicine
Detroit Medical Center
Detroit, Michigan
Chapter 12, Pulmonary Disorders

James H. Sondheimer, MD, FACP
Associate Professor
Department of Medicine
Wayne State University School of Medicine
Medical Director, Hemodialysis Unit
Department of Nephrology
Harper University Hospital
Detroit, Michigan
Chapter 13, Nephrology

Contributors

Ibrahim Abdulhamid, MD
Assistant Professor
Department of Pediatrics
Wayne State University School of
    Medicine
Director, Pediatric Pulmonary
    Medicine
Department of Pediatrics
Children's Hospital of Michigan
Detroit, Michigan
Chapter 10, Pediatrics
Chapter 12, Pulmonary
    Disorders

Loutfi Sami Aboussouan, MD
Assistant Professor
Department of Internal Medicine
Wayne State University School of
    Medicine
Assistant Professor
Department of Pulmonary/Critical
    Care
Harper University Hospital
Detroit, Michigan
Chapter 12, Pulmonary
    Disorders

Jocelyn Y. Ang, MD
Assistant Professor
Department of Pediatrics
Wayne State University School of
    Medicine
Attending Physician
Division of Infectious Diseases
Department of Pediatrics
Children's Hospital of Michigan
Detroit, Michigan
Chapter 10, Pediatrics

Peter Baumann, MD
Division of Gynecology
Department of Obstetrics and
    Gynecology
Wayne State University School of
    Medicine
Detroit, Michigan
Chapter 9, Obstetrics and Gynecology

Stanley M. Berry, MD
Associate Professor
Division of Maternal-Fetal Medicine
Department of Obstetrics and
    Gynecology
Wayne State University School of
    Medicine
Detroit, Michigan
Chapter 9, Obstetrics and Gynecology

Patricia D. Brown, MD
Associate Professor of Medicine
Division of Infectious Disease
Wayne State University School of
    Medicine
Detroit, Michigan
Chapter 7, Infectious Disease
Chapter 8, Neurology

Lavoisier Cardozo, MD, FACP
Professor of Medicine
Department of Internal Medicine
Wayne State University School of
    Medicine
Chief of Medicine
Department of Medicine
Detroit Receiving Hospital
Detroit, Michigan
Chapter 11, Psychiatry

Arthur M. Carlin, MD, FACS
Assistant Professor
Department of Surgery
Wayne State University School of
    Medicine
General Surgeon
Department of Surgery
Detroit Medical Center
Detroit, Michigan
Chapter 15, Surgery

**Subodh Chauhan, MD,
MRCOG**
Fellow
Division of Reproductive
    Endocrinology
Department of Obstetrics and
    Gynecology
Wayne State University School of
    Medicine
Detroit, Michigan
*Chapter 9, Obstetrics and
    Gynecology*

Carl Christensen, MD
Associate Professor
Division of Gynecology
Department of Obstetrics and
    Gynecology
Wayne State University School of
    Medicine
Detroit, Michigan
*Chapter 9, Obstetrics and
    Gynecology*

Jean Marie Elwing, MD
Chief Resident Physician,
    Internal Medicine
Department of Internal
    Medicine/Pediatrics
St. Louis University Hospital
St. Louis, Missouri
Chapter 10, Pediatrics

Jayson B. Field, MD
Resident Physician
Department of Obstetrics and
    Gynecology
Wayne State University School of
    Medicine
Detroit, Michigan
Chapter 9, Obstetrics and Gynecology

John M. Flack, MD, MPH
Professor and Associate Chairman
    for Academic Affairs and Chief
    Quality Officer
Department of Internal Medicine
Wayne State University School of
    Medicine
Director, Cardiovascular and
    Epidemiology and Clinical
    Applications
Department of Internal Medicine
Harper University Hospital
Detroit, Michigan
Chapter 1, Cardiology

**Daniel A. C. Frattarelli, MD,
FAAP**
Fellow, Pediatric Clinical
    Pharmacology
Wayne State University School of
    Medicine
Division of Clinical Pharmacology
Children's Hospital of Michigan
Detroit, Michigan
Chapter 4, Emergency Medicine
Chapter 10, Pediatrics

Edwin B. George, MD, PhD
Assistant Professor
Department of Neurology
Wayne State University School of
    Medicine
John D. Dingell VA Medical Center
Detroit, Michigan
Chapter 4, Emergency Medicine
Chapter 8, Neurology

John Gilroy, MD, FRCP (CAN), FACP
Clinical Professor
Department of Neurology
Wayne State University School of
    Medicine
Detroit, Michigan
Chairman, Neurology
Department of Medicine
William Beaumont Hospital
Royal Oak, Michigan
Chapter 4, Emergency Medicine
Chapter 8, Neurology

Kenneth A. Ginsburg, MD
Associate Professor
Department of Obstetrics and
    Gynecology
Assistant Dean for Clinical
    Education
Office of Academic and Student
    Programs
Wayne State University School of
    Medicine
Detroit, Michigan
*Chapter 9, Obstetrics and
    Gynecology*

Kirsten A. Guenther, MD
Staff Physician
Department of Emergency
    Medicine
William Beaumont Hospital
Royal Oak, Michigan
Chapter 4, Emergency Medicine

Tiffany T. Hall, MD
Resident Physician
Departments of Internal Medicine
    and Pediatrics
St. Louis University Hospital/
    Cardinal Glennon Children's
    Hospital
St. Louis, Missouri
Chapter 10, Pediatrics

Melanie Hanna-Johnson, MD
Assistant Professor
Department of Internal Medicine
Wayne State University School of
    Medicine
Assistant Professor
Department of Internal Medicine
Detroit Receiving Hospital/
    University Health Center
Detroit, Michigan
*Chapter 9, Obstetrics and
    Gynecology*
Chapter 11, Psychiatry
Chapter 12, Pulmonary Disorders

Mohamad Ammar Hatahet, MD, FACP
Assistant Professor
Department of Medicine
Wayne State University School of
    Medicine
Detroit, Michigan
Chapter 1, Cardiology
Chapter 3, Endocrine Disorders

Jill Hechtman, MD
Resident Physician
Department of Obstetrics and
    Gynecology
Wayne State University School of
    Medicine
Detroit, Michigan
*Chapter 9, Obstetrics and
    Gynecology*

John A. Hopper, MD
Assistant Professor
Departments of Internal Medicine,
    Pediatrics, and Psychiatry
Wayne State University School of
    Medicine
Detroit, Michigan
Chapter 7, Infectious Disease
Chapter 10, Pediatrics

Jeff Hugus, MD
Senior Resident Physician
Department of Emergency Medicine
Sinai-Grace Hospital/Detroit
 Medical Center
Detroit, Michigan
Chapter 4, Emergency Medicine

Nahla Khalek, MD
Resident Physician
Department of Obstetrics and
 Gynecology
Wayne State University School of
 Medicine
Detroit, Michigan
Chapter 9, Obstetrics and Gynecology

Carole Kowalczyk, MD
Assistant Professor
Division of Reproductive
 Endocrinology
Department of Obstetrics and
 Gynecology
Wayne State University School of
 Medicine
Detroit, Michigan
Chapter 9, Obstetrics and Gynecology

Leilani E. LaBianco, MD
Resident Physician
Department of Emergency Medicine
Sinai-Grace Hospital
Wayne State University School of
 Medicine
Detroit, Michigan
Chapter 4, Emergency Medicine

Paul Makela, MD
Assistant Professor
Division of Gynecology
Department of Obstetrics and
 Gynecology
Wayne State University School of
 Medicine
Detroit, Michigan
Chapter 9, Obstetrics and Gynecology

Kochurani Maliekel, MD
Assistant Professor
Department of
 Hematology/Oncology
St. Louis University School of
 Medicine
St. Louis, Missouri
*Chapter 6, Hematology and
 Oncology*

**Patrick Joseph McLaughlin,
MD**
Assistant Professor
Department of Medicine
Wayne State University School of
 Medicine
Medical Director, Coronary Care
 Unit
Department of Cardiology
Harper University Hospital
Detroit, Michigan
Chapter 1, Cardiology

**Marc D. Meissner, MD, CM,
FACC, FACP**
Associate Professor
Department of Internal Medicine
Wayne State University School of
 Medicine
Staff Cardiologist and
 Electrophysiologist
Division of Cardiology
Department of Medicine
Sinai-Grace Hospital
Detroit, Michigan
Chapter 1, Cardiology

Jodi L. Ralston, MD
Physician
Department of Emergency
 Medicine
William Beaumont Hospital
Royal Oak, Michigan
Chapter 4, Emergency Medicine

Jerrie S. Refuerzo, MD
Fellow
Division of Maternal-Fetal
  Medicine
Department of Obstetrics and
  Gynecology
Wayne State University School of
  Medicine
*Chapter 9, Obstetrics and
  Gynecology*

Randall Lee Reher, MD
Assistant Professor
Division of Cardiology
Department of Internal Medicine
Wayne State University School of
  Medicine
Detroit, Michigan
Chapter 1, Cardiology

James A. Rowley, MD
Assistant Professor
Department of Medicine
Attending Staff
Detroit Medical Center
Detroit, Michigan
Chapter 1, Cardiology
Chapter 12, Pulmonary Disorders

Firdous A. Siddiqui, MD
Assistant Professor
Department of Gastroenterology
Wayne State University School of
  Medicine
Detroit, Michigan
Chapter 5, Gastroenterology

**James H. Sondheimer, MD,
FACP**
Associate Professor
Department of Medicine
Wayne State University School of
  Medicine
Medical Director, Hemodialysis
  Unit
Department of Nephrology
Harper University Hospital
Detroit, Michigan
Chapter 13, Nephrology

Anne Tintinalli, MD
Attending Physician
Department of Emergency
  Medicine
Detroit Receiving Hospital
Detroit, Michigan
Chapter 4, Emergency Medicine

The Test

USMLE Step 3 is a two-day computerized test consisting of multiple-choice questions and case simulations.

The first day of testing includes roughly 350 multiple-choice questions divided into blocks of 25 to 50 items with 30 to 60 minutes given to complete each block. Forty-five minutes of break time are allowed. However, if question blocks are finished early, this time is added to your break time.

The second day is divided into approximately 150 multiple-choice questions divided into blocks of 25 to 50 items, as in day one. The second day also includes 9 computer-based case simulations over 3 hours and 45 minutes. Break time is provided as in day one.

Multiple-choice questions are single-best-answer formats. Questions may be stand-alone or be sequenced together in sets of 2 to 5. Test items present detailed clinical situations and may involve one or more figures. It is recommended that all examinees take the testing tutorial provided on the USMLE CD provided within the registration packet.

Computer-based simulations provide the examinee with the clinical setting and introductory patient information. Free text entry of orders based on the information provided is the primary means of interacting with the format. With each order entered, an update on the patient's condition is available. No photographs or sounds will be provided. It is recommended that the examinee become familiar with the Primum CCS software provided on the CD from the USMLE.

The "rapid-fire" questions and answers in *USMLE Step 3 Recall* will provide you with the necessary fund of knowledge needed to excel on this exam.

Acknowledgments

I would like to thank my parents for being strong advocates of education through-out my life. Without their support and encouragement, an accomplishment such as this would not have been possible.

I would also like to thank Dr. Ricardo Brown for being my mentor during my Masters in Physiology. His teachings were transferable to many of my life pursuits, including this courageous project.

I especially wish to thank all the contributors and associate editors at Wayne State University and St. Louis University for their valuable input and dedication to this endeavor.

And I want to thank Krista Ryan, my wife, for being such a strong supporter of my dreams and aspirations.

Contents

Preface.. vii
Associate Editors ix
Contributors xi
The Test xvii
Acknowledgments.. xix

1   Cardiology...1
2   Dermatology 44
3   Endocrine Disorders...55
4   Emergency Medicine..74
5   Gastroenterology...113
6   Hematology and Oncology 159
7   Infectious Disease...176
8   Neurology..187
9   Obstetrics and Gynecology 239
10 Pediatrics...288
11 Psychiatry...329
12 Pulmonary Disorders...351
13 Nephrology..384
14 Rheumatology 414
15 Surgery 434
    Index 451

1   Cardiology

HYPERTENSION

COARCTATION OF THE AORTA

What is coarctation of the aorta?	A localized narrowing of the aortic arch, most commonly just distal to the origin of the left subclavian artery near the insertion of the ligamentum arteriosum
What are the symptoms?	Children and young adults usually asymptomatic; may have hypertension, murmurs, headache, and epistaxis
What are the associated conditions?	Bicuspid aortic valve and gonadal dysgenesis
What signs are found on physical exam?	Upper extremity hypertension; asymmetric pulses in upper extremities with absent, weak, or delayed pulses in lower extremities; harsh systolic murmur, sometimes heard between the scapulae
What does the electrocardiogram (ECG) reveal?	Left ventricular hypertrophy
What radiographic finding suggests the diagnosis?	Rib notching on chest x-ray, indentation of aorta at site of coarctation, and prestenotic and poststenotic dilatation (the "3" sign) along the left paramediastinal shadow
How is the diagnosis confirmed?	Arteriogram and/or Doppler echocardiogram and/or MRI
What is the treatment?	Surgery
What are the dreaded complications for older untreated patients?	Left ventricular failure, cerebral aneurysm and hemorrhage, infective endocarditis

CUSHING SYNDROME

What causes Cushing syndrome?	Adrenal overproduction [adrenal tumors or ectopic adrenocorticotropic hormone (ACTH) stimulation from an oat-cell (small cell) lung cancer], and exogenously administered steroid (most common)
When does Cushing syndrome become Cushing disease?	When the excess cortisol is caused by abnormally increased ACTH secreted by the pituitary (pituitary adenoma)
What are the symptoms?	Weakness, fatigue, moodiness, and easy bruising
What are the signs?	Hypertension and cushingoid appearance (truncal obesity, striae, impaired glucose tolerance, hirsutism, easy bruising, acne, osteoporosis); not present in every case, other signs may be present
What are the associated lab values?	Increased serum, urinary cortisol, and cortisol metabolites; hypokalemia and mild hyperglycemia (effects of cortisol)
How is it diagnosed?	1 mg overnight dexamethasone suppression test and 24-hour urinary free cortisol
What is the treatment for pituitary tumors?	Transsphenoidal microadenomectomy
What is the treatment for adrenal tumors?	Surgical resection, if possible

ESSENTIAL HYPERTENSION

What is essential hypertension?	Most common (~95% of cases) form of hypertension in unselected populations not attributable to secondary or surgically curable causes (e.g., mineralocorticoid excess, pheochromocytoma, or critical renal artery stenosis)

Which is more important as a cause of cardiovascular disease: systolic or diastolic blood pressure (BP)?

Both are important, but systolic confers greater risk than diastolic BP.

Are there reversible, nonsurgical causes of hypertension?

Hypothyroidism can cause isolated diastolic BP elevations; anemia, beriberi, Paget disease, aortic insufficiency, and hyperthyroidism can cause disproportionate elevations of systolic compared to diastolic BP.

How does hypertension affect the cardiovascular system?

Long-term effects: damage to arterial vasculature and target organs (e.g., brain, kidney, heart), and peripheral vasculature, potential for stroke, kidney insufficiency or failure, left ventricular hypertrophy, heart failure, MI, peripheral arterial disease

Who is at risk?

Hypertension is more common among persons who are older, have kidney disease, diabetes mellitus, are physically inactive, consume excessive amounts of alcohol, or are overweight.

Are African Americans at higher risk for hypertension than other racial or ethnic groups?

Yes. African Americans, particularly women, have a greater burden of environmental risk factors (e.g., obesity, physical inactivity) than whites; however, there is no credible evidence that genetic factors explain the excess hypertension incidence and prevalence in African Americans.

How does hypertension present?

May be no symptoms; or may be one or more of the constellation of weakness, fatigue, exercise intolerance, sleep disturbance, headache, and chest pain linked to the height of BP elevation.

How is the diagnosis made?

Confirmation of BP levels:
$\geq 125/75$ mm Hg with <1 g/day of proteinuria
$130/85$ mm Hg with kidney disease, diabetes mellitus, or heart failure
$\geq 140/90$ mm Hg in all other persons

What is the workup?

Detailed history, physical exam, serum creatinine/estimated glomerular filtration rate, electrolytes, blood urea nitrogen, glucose, cholesterol, urinalysis, and electrocardiogram (ECG)

Are there other potentially useful tests?

Echocardiograms when systolic heart function is a concern; spot urine albumin:creatinine ratios

What are the common physical findings?

Hypertensive retinopathy—arteriolar narrowing, arteriovenous nicking, and, in severe cases, segmental arteriolar spasm, hemorrhages, and exudates; laterally displaced point of maximal impulse; S_4 gallop

What is the treatment?

Lifestyle modifications: alcohol <2 drinks per day, aerobic exercise, weight loss if overweight, dietary sodium restriction
Antihypertensive drugs: diuretics, angiotensin-converting enzyme (ACE) inhibitors, β-blockers, angiotensin-receptor antagonists, α-blockers, calcium antagonists; in a few cases, sympatholytic and direct vasodilator drugs

Are there other lifestyle modifications that may lower BP?

Reducing saturated fat intake or increasing potassium, magnesium, and/or calcium intake

How aggressive should treatment be?

Gradually attain blood pressure <125/75 mm Hg if >1 g/24 hours of proteinuria is present; <130/80–85 mm Hg in persons with diabetes mellitus, heart failure, or kidney insufficiency; or <140/90 mm Hg in all others.

What role does race or ethnicity play in optimal drug selection for hypertensives?

Very little. Choose drugs based on best available evidence with virtually no consideration of race/ethnicity, particularly since highest risk patients (i.e., diabetes, kidney disease) typically require three or more drugs to attain goal BP levels.

Are there any potentially serious side effects with commonly used antihypertensive drugs?

Angioedema occurs with ACE inhibitors in ~3/1000 individuals; can occur, though less frequently, with angiotensin-receptor blockers. African Americans appear to be at higher risk for this complication.

Do some patients require immediate or emergent treatment of their BP levels?

Yes.

What are the criteria for immediate treatment of BP elevations?

Hypertensive urgencies occur when target-organ damage is thought to be imminent if BP is not reduced over ensuing hours to days. Optimally, oral medications (e.g., clonidine) are used at BP levels >220 mm Hg systolic and >115 mm Hg diastolic.

What are the criteria for in-patient, emergent hypertension treatment?

New or worsening target-organ damage (e.g., heart failure, kidney insufficiency, cerebrovascular insufficiency); treatment in such situations should occur in hospital setting suitable for administration of drugs that can be titrated for immediate BP effect (e.g., nitroglycerin or nitroprusside).

HYPERALDOSTERONISM

What is primary hyperaldosteronism?

Autonomous secretion of aldosterone from the adrenal gland as a consequence of either a solitary adenoma (most common) or hyperplasia of both adrenal glands (less common)

How does hyperaldosteronism present?

Virtually all affected are hypertensive and often, though not always, manifest hypokalemia with renal potassium wasting, hypomagnesemia, metabolic alkalosis, and hypernatremia.

What are the clinical clues that hyperaldosteronism is present?

Early-onset hypertension; hypertension associated with severe target-organ injury; refractory hypertension or hypertensive urgencies or emergencies, especially with metabolic manifestations

Who is at risk?

Typically, persons between ages 30–50 years; women affected more often than men

What is the workup for hyperaldosteronism?

To screen, obtain a morning plasma aldosterone:renin ratio; results are useful irrespective of medication status.

What is a positive screening test?

About half of persons with a ratio >25 and with elevated plasma aldosterone level ultimately will have primary hyperaldosteronism.

What is the approach to diagnosis?

Confirmed by inability of intravenous or oral salt-loading to suppress 24-hour urinary excretion of aldosterone to <14 μg, or inability of plasma aldosterone ratio to suppress to <30 after 50 mg oral captopril

What other tests are helpful in making the diagnosis?

Computed tomography (CT) or magnetic resonance imaging (MRI) are preferred to localize and determine adrenal pathology; adrenal vein sampling and adrenal NP-59 scans can help localize site of autonomous production.

What must primary hyperaldosteronism be differentiated from?

Glucocorticoid remedial aldosteronism (GRA)

How is primary aldosteronism differentiated from GRA?

Persons with GRA are typically normotensive but can be hypertensive; electrolytes are usually normal; family history of premature stroke, particularly hemorrhagic variety

What is GRA?	A genetic, autosomal-dominant condition that predisposes to hypertension as a consequence of an abnormal 11-β hydroxylase gene causing 18-hydroxysteroids beyond the zona glomerulosa of the adrenal gland
How is GRA diagnosed?	Genetic analysis for abnormal chimeric 11-β hydroxylase gene; documentation of elevated 18-hydroxylated steroid secretion in urine; or dexamethasone suppression of excess urinary steroids
How is GRA treated?	Oral steroids in doses adequate to suppress excessive production of 18-hydroxylated steroids
How is primary hyperaldosteronism treated?	Medical or surgical (unilateral adrenalectomy) therapies
What are the indications for surgical therapy?	Unilateral adenoma in a good surgical candidate
What are the indications for medical therapy?	Unilateral adenoma in a poor surgical candidate and bilateral adrenal hyperplasia
What medical therapies are useful?	Thiazide- and potassium-sparing diuretics (especially spironolactone), potassium supplements, and calcium antagonists are especially useful along with other antihypertensive agents and dietary sodium restriction.

PHEOCHROMOCYTOMA

What is pheochromocytoma?	A paraganglioma tumor arising from chromaffin cells in the adrenal medulla that secretes catecholamines (norepinephrine, epinephrine, dopamine) either continuously or episodically

Anatomically, where are most pheochromocytomas found?

10–20% are multiple; 90% in adrenal medulla; most common sites for extra-adrenal paragangliomas (in descending order of frequency)—para-aortic region, urinary bladder, thorax, head and neck, and pelvis

How does pheochromocytoma present clinically?

Majority have sustained hypertension: half of those with sustained hypertension also have paroxysmal BP elevations and symptoms of catecholamine excess; slightly fewer than half have BP elevations only during paroxysmal attacks

What is the effect of catecholamine hypersecretion on the cardiovascular system?

Orthostatic hypotension (attributable to downregulation of catecholamine receptors) is very common; less common is heart failure attributable to catecholamine cardiomyopathy.

Are there any special clinical presentations suggestive of pheochromocytoma?

Paroxysms of symptoms/BP elevations triggered by exercise, urination, defecation, anesthesia, or surgery; also, consider pheochromocytoma in refractory, malignant, or accelerated hypertension

What are the symptoms of pheochromocytoma?

Sweating, tachycardia/palpitations, anxiety, neurosis, headache, pallor, weight loss; but may be asymptomatic

With what relatively common conditions might pheochromocytoma be confused?

Labile hypertension with hyperdynamic circulation, thyrotoxicosis, ingestion of sympathomimetic drugs, and abrupt discontinuation of sympatholytic drugs causing rebound hypertension

Is pheochromocytoma associated with other diseases?

Von Hippel-Lindau, neurofibromatosis, multiple endocrine neoplasia (MEN) types 2A and 2B

Are pheochromocytomas inherited?

Some, particularly bilateral or multifocal, pheochromocytomas are inherited in an autosomal dominant fashion with or without associated disease conditions.

Can pheochromocytoma tumors be malignant?	Yes; approximately 1 in 10 in adults and 1 in 50 among children; half of malignant pheochromocytomas are located in extra-adrenal locations
What are the best screening tests?	Plasma metanephrine:creatinine ratio, plasma catecholamines, timed urine collections for metanephrine, metanephrine:creatinine urine catecholamines, and 3-methoxy-4-hydroxymandelic acid [vanillylmandelic acid (**VMA**)]
Are there differences among the screening tests?	24-hour urinary metanephrine:creatinine ratio is more specific than urinary metanephrine (fewer false positives); plasma metanephrine:creatinine ratio is more sensitive than plasma catecholamines.
Are any other tests useful?	Chromogranin A is elevated in 90% and chromogranin B in 80% of pheochromocytomas.
What is the diagnostic workup?	After demonstration of catecholamine hypersecretion, anatomic localization is the logical next step.
What imaging studies may be useful?	MRI and CT scans (most readily available); however, CT scans are of limited value for extra-adrenal tumor localization.
What other tests are useful in localizing pheochromocytoma?	^{123}I- or ^{131}I-metaiodobenzylguanidine (MIBG) scintigraphy can localize ectopic, functioning pheochromocytoma; ^{111}In-octreotide scintigraphy is less sensitive than MIBG scanning, but can help localize head and neck chemodectomas.
What is the surgical treatment for pheochromocytoma?	Surgical excision of solitary tumors after BP control. Avoid neuromuscular relaxants because of hypotension risk.

Are there other special considerations before surgery?	Yes. Many patients with pheochromocytoma manifest intravascular volume depletion.
What is the medical treatment for pheochromocytoma?	Intravenous (IV) phentolamine, an α-adrenergic blocker, in hypertensive crises; nonselective α-blocker phenoxybenzamine, selective $α_1$-antagonists, β-blockers (only after α-blocker), and calcium antagonists

RENAL PARENCHYMAL HYPERTENSION

What is renal parenchymal hypertension?	A reduction in functioning kidney mass or major renal vessels that may impair salt and water excretion, expand intravascular volume, attenuate vasodilatory responses, and activate sympathetic nervous system activity, causing hypertension or worsening existing hypertension
What are the most common causes of renal parenchymal hypertension?	Diabetes mellitus, glomerulonephritis, infections, ischemia, autoimmune diseases, hereditary conditions, and drug exposures (e.g., chronic analgesics or cyclosporine post-transplantation)
How does renal parenchymal hypertension present?	With hypertension typically requiring multiple drugs (3 or more) to achieve BP control (<130/80–85 mm Hg) and evidence of reduced kidney function and/or disease
What are the laboratory clues to renal parenchymal disease?	Typically, though not invariably, elevated serum creatinine, reduced estimated glomerular filtration rate (not always), dipstick positive proteinuria, hematuria (usually microscopic), anemia (when glomerular filtration rate is <60 mL/min per 1.73 m^2), low serum albumin

What are the clinical clues to renal parenchymal disease?

Nocturia, lower extremity edema, periorbital edema, urinary tract symptoms, flank pain, urinary tract infections, incidental findings of reduced or asymmetrical kidney size or function, or anatomic abnormalities

Who is at risk for renal parenchymal disease?

Older persons; also, those with long-standing and typically poorly controlled diabetes mellitus or hypertension, lupus, human immunodeficiency virus (HIV) infection, atherosclerotic kidney disease, family history of end-stage kidney disease, analgesic abusers, overweight persons, and smokers

What is the workup for renal parenchymal hypertension?

Serum creatinine, estimated glomerular filtration rate (GFR), spot urinary albumin:creatinine ratio, dipstick urine protein measurement, microscopic exam of urine sediment, renal artery duplex scanning or captopril scintigraphy or renal ultrasonography (kidney size/echogenicity/obstruction)

What is the approach to diagnosis?

Confirm reduced kidney function with reduced estimated GFR (<60 mL/min per 1.73 m^2) and absence of hypertension before onset of kidney disease

What other tests are helpful in making the diagnosis?

Serum cystatin C is a more sensitive marker of GFR than creatinine; magnetic resonance angiography, helical CT scanning, and CO_2 renal angiography can identify critical renal artery stenoses; CT scanning and intravenous pyelography (IVP) have also been used.

What must renal parenchymal hypertension be differentiated from?

Hypertension-induced kidney insufficiency; however, whether hypertension or kidney disease came first, their coexistence leads to a more rapid loss of kidney function and more difficulty in controlling BP.

How is hypertension-induced kidney insufficiency treated?

Aggressive BP control to <130/80–85 mm Hg with combined lifestyle modifications (salt restriction, smoking cessation, weight loss) and multiple antihypertensive drugs; use of ACE inhibitors, angiotensin-receptor blockers, or both; periodic monitoring of GFR and proteinuria.

How is renal parenchymal hypertension treated?

Similarly to hypertension-induced kidney insufficiency, though a search for reversible causes of kidney disease may lead to treatment of an underlying systemic condition or elimination of a toxic exposure

RENOVASCULAR DISEASE

What is renovascular hypertension?

The most common form of secondary or surgically curable hypertension; a consequence of critical stenosis of one or both renal arteries

What are the most common causes of renovascular hypertension?

Atherosclerosis in late middle-aged and older persons; fibromuscular dysplasia in younger women

How does it present?

Refractory hypertension, hypertension with renal insufficiency, or renal insufficiency without hypertension (ischemic nephropathy); kidney insufficiency is uncommon in fibromuscular dysplasia.

What are the clinical clues that renovascular hypertension is present?

Precipitous rise in creatinine after initiating ACE inhibitors or angiotensin-receptor blockers and flash pulmonary edema are clinical clues, but neither is highly sensitive or specific.

Who is at risk?

Persons at risk for, or with clinical manifestations of, atherosclerotic disease, smokers, persons with diabetes mellitus, older persons, including those with long-standing essential hypertension

What are the physical findings?

Abdominal upper quadrant bruit; most relevant are biphasic ones, bruits in other locations, and hypertensive retinopathy and other signs of blood pressure-related target-organ injury (e.g., left ventricular enlargement)

What are the indications to initiate a workup?

Refractory hypertension, kidney insufficiency, or both; an incidental finding of kidney size disparity; flash pulmonary edema with preserved systolic function; rise in creatinine >30% after starting ACE inhibitor or angiotensin-receptor blocker treatment

What is the workup for renovascular hypertension?

Two major screening tests—renal artery duplex scan and captopril renograms

Are there special considerations regarding the renal artery duplex scan?

Renal artery duplex scans are highly operator dependent; in very overweight persons, obtaining technically satisfactory scans is more difficult.

Are there special considerations regarding the captopril renogram?

Not as useful for detecting bilateral renal artery stenosis; use the MAG-3 isotope in those with renal insufficiency because the more commonly used DTPA gives poor images in this setting.

What are the major diagnostic tests for renovascular hypertension?

Renal angiography is the gold standard; except in the most high probability cases, is most useful after obtaining an abnormal functional screening test.

What other renal artery imaging tests are useful in defining renal artery anatomy?

Magnetic resonance angiography, CO_2 angiography, and helical CT scanning

Are there special considerations when defining kidney anatomy in persons with kidney insufficiency?

The risk of kidney injury can be lessened, but not eliminated, by using non-ionic contrast agents, ensuring adequate hydration before the procedure, and possibly by pretreatment with oral N-acetylcysteine. CO_2 or magnetic resonance angiography, the latter with gadolinium enhancement, are minimally to non-nephrotoxic ways to image renal arteries.

Are any tests absolutely unhelpful?

Plasma renin activity is not useful; selective renal vein renin values are not indicated because persons with essential hypertension can lateralize renin production to one side and persons with renovascular hypertension that responds to revascularization may not lateralize.

What is the treatment for renovascular hypertension?

Medical therapy with lifestyle changes and drugs; renal angioplasty with stent placement or surgical revascularization

What is the indication for revascularization?

Inability to control blood pressure, progressive loss of kidney function even if blood pressure is controlled, unilateral small kidney, ischemic nephropathy

What are the risks of revascularization?

Death, loss of kidney function, and coronary ischemia in patients with atheromatous disease affecting several vascular territories; in patients with creatinine >2.0, risk of dialysis appears to be greater with angioplasty than surgery; however, risk of death is greater with surgery.

CONGESTIVE HEART FAILURE (CHF)

AORTIC REGURGITATION

What is aortic regurgitation (AR)?

Regurgitation of the blood flow back into the left ventricle due to a structural abnormality of the aortic valve, the wall of the aortic root, or both

What are some causes of AR?

Rheumatic (most common), bicuspid aortic valve, infective endocarditis, trauma, collagen vascular diseases, ventricular septal defects, senile degenerative disease, any disease that dilates the aorta

(e.g., severe hypertension, Marfan, dissection, aneurysm, connective tissue diseases, syphilis)

How does AR classically present?

Acute: severe dyspnea, palpitations, hypotension

Chronic: begins asymptomatically, then gradual exertional dyspnea, orthopnea, paroxysmal nocturnal dyspnea, and symptoms of left ventricular dysfunction late in disease

How does AR affect the left ventricle (LV)?

Acute AR: Abrupt introduction of a large volume of blood into the left ventricle increases left ventricular end-diastolic pressure (LVEDP), leading to acute dyspnea or pulmonary edema.

Chronic AR: Initially, cardiac output increases (Frank-Starling mechanism) and the left ventricle remains normal in size but hypertrophies and mass increases. Later, the ventricle begins to dilate and cardiac output falls. When the left ventricle can dilate no farther, LVEDP increases and dyspnea results.

What may the physical exam show in chronic or advanced AR?

High-pitched diastolic decrescendo murmur early after A_2 at the left sternal border. Severity of AR correlates better with duration of murmur than with its intensity. S_3 is heard with LV dysfunction; S_1 may be decreased or absent. May be an apical diastolic rumble (Austin Flint murmur) and/or an enlarged and displaced apical pulse.

What are some other physical exam findings in chronic or advanced AR?

De Musset sign: nodding of the head

Quincke sign: visible pulsations in capillaries with gentle compression of nailbed or lip

Widened pulse pressure: systolic BP elevated, diastolic BP <60 mm Hg

Corrigan pulse: visualizing a rapid rise and sudden collapse of pulse ("water-hammer pulse")

Traube sign: "pistol-shot" sound heard over the femoral artery

Duroziez sign: "to-and-fro" murmur heard during mild compression of femoral artery

Austin Flint murmur: soft, low-pitched, rumbling mid-diastolic murmur caused by displacement of anterior leaflet of mitral valve by AR stream

What are the associated ECG findings?

May be normal; may have findings of left ventricular hypertrophy with strain pattern

What are the associated chest x-ray findings?

Increased cardiothoracic ratio in chronic AR

How is AR diagnosed?

Physical exam and echocardiogram

What is the management approach for AR?

Antibiotic prophylaxis against endocarditis is advised. Medical therapy includes vasodilator therapy (e.g., ACE inhibitors, hydralazine, or calcium channel blocker).

What are some class 1 indications for aortic valve replacement?

Acute AR with symptoms or pulmonary edema

Chronic severe AR with symptoms or patients undergoing CABG or surgery on the aorta or other heart valves

New York Heart Association (NYHA) functional class III or IV

Mild to moderate left ventricular dysfunction (ejection fraction <50%)

Progressive or severe left ventricular dilatation (end-systolic dimension >55 mm) or declining exercise tolerance

Do current guidelines support valve replacement solely because of a decline in ejection fraction during exercise?

No

Is there a reference on guidelines for management of valvular heart disease?	Yes. Bonow R, Carabello B, deLeon Jr A, et al: ACC/AHA guidelines. *Circulation* 1998;98:1949–1984; *Journal of the American College of Cardiology* 1998;32:1486–1588.

AORTIC STENOSIS

What is aortic stenosis (AS)?	Narrowing of the aortic valve orifice with progressive obstruction of left ventricular outflow
How does AS affect the left ventricle?	Concentric pressure hypertrophy of left ventricle with preserved systolic function. Left ventricular function declines and the ventricle dilates late in the disease.
What are some causes of AS?	Senile degenerative (most common; older patients; valve calcified and sclerosed), unicuspid or bicuspid valve (younger patients), rheumatic heart disease
What is the classic presentation?	Minimal symptoms early; more symptoms may occur with greater degree of stenosis; exertional dyspnea; angina; syncope; CHF may occur with more significant degrees of stenosis
What causes the symptoms?	Increased afterload leads to hypertrophy and wall stress. Obstruction causes decreased systemic and coronary blood flow. Oxygen supply/demand mismatch occurs.
What may the physical exam show?	Depends on degree of stenosis: delayed sustained dampened carotid upstroke (pulsus parvus et tardus); sustained left ventricular impulse; soft or absent A_2 and a late-peaking crescendo-decrescendo systolic ejection murmur at the left sternal boarder radiating to the carotid arteries; soft S_4

What are the associated ECG findings?

Left ventricular hypertrophy with T-wave inversion (especially I, aVL, and left precordial leads)

What are the chest x-ray findings?

Calcifications in the area of the aortic valve; often dilatation of ascending aorta; rounding of cardiac apex and cardiac enlargement if left ventricle dilatation has occurred

How is it diagnosed?

Characteristic physical exam with confirmation by echocardiogram; cardiac catheterization advised in certain situations

What is the treatment for mild AS?

There is no good medical treatment. Avoid dehydration and vasodilatation (e.g., diuretics and nitrates). Antibiotic prophylaxis against endocarditis is recommended.

What is severe AS?

Aortic valve orifice of about $0.8–0.9$ cm^2 or $<0.5–0.6$ cm^2/m^2 BSA; aortic valve gradient of >50 mm Hg in presence of normal cardiac output

What is the main treatment of severe AS?

Surgical valve replacement. Valvuloplasty is used in some situations (e.g., some children and young adults with congenital noncalcified AS, or patients too ill or frail to undergo surgery).

When is aortic valve replacement surgery indicated?

Severe AS with symptoms (dyspnea, CHF, syncope, or angina)
Asymptomatic severe AS with declining left ventricle function or exertional hypotension
Open-heart surgery required for other reasons (e.g., coronary artery bypass grafting)

What testing is required before surgical intervention?

Echocardiogram (all) and cardiac catheterization (if possibility of coronary artery disease)

What are some special considerations in AS?	Patients are advised to have antibiotic prophylaxis against infective endocarditis. Class 1 indications for surgical valve replacement include symptoms with severe AS. Surgery may be helpful in patients with severe AS, declining left ventricular function, or both. Rheumatic AS rarely occurs without associated mitral valve involvement.
Is there a reference on guidelines for management of valvular heart disease?	Yes. Bonow R, Carabello B, deLeon Jr A, et al: ACC/AHA guidelines. *Circulation* 1998;98:1949–1984; *Journal of the American College of Cardiology* 1998;32:1486–1588.

HYPERTROPHIC CARDIOMYOPATHY

What is hypertrophic cardiomyopathy (HCM)?	Left or right ventricular hypertrophy, or both, usually asymmetric and classically involving the interventricular septum. A variant with predominant apical involvement is common in Japanese HCM patients.
What other terms have been used to describe this condition?	Idiopathic hypertrophic subaortic stenosis (IHSS); muscular subaortic stenosis
What are the causes of HCM?	Not known, but genetics likely play a key role. Stimulus for its development is unknown. HCM is frequently a hereditary disorder (>50% of the time). Hereditary form is autosomal dominant, with transmission to first-degree relatives in 50% of familial cases.
How does HCM present?	There is great variability. Many are asymptomatic, or only mildly symptomatic. The presenting symptom may be sudden death. Dyspnea on exertion, angina, and syncope/presyncope may be present.

How does HCM cause syncope?

Arrhythmias, hemodynamic factors (e.g., outflow tract obstruction), and/or abnormal autonomic function (vasodepressor syncope)

What may be found on physical exam?

May be normal in asymptomatic patients without gradients; others may have left ventricular lift and forceful diffuse apical impulse. S_4 and sometimes S_3. Typical murmur is harsh and systolic; may occur later in systole; crescendo decrescendo; radiates to the base and apex (but not the neck). Murmur increases with Valsalva maneuver (during strain) or standing; decreases with squatting, Müller maneuver, or isometric handgrip. Carotid upstroke may have a bifid quality. Apical impulse exhibiting a three-component "triple-ripple" character is classic in this disorder, but rare.

What may be seen on ECG?

Left ventricular hypertrophy with deep, prominent Q-waves that simulate MI (inferior, precordial, or both)

What are the associated chest x-ray findings?

May be fairly normal

How is HCM diagnosed?

Echocardiogram can determine the diagnosis and degree of outflow tract obstruction.

What may be part of management of patients with HCM?

Avoidance of competitive sports, strenuous activity
Avoidance of digitalis, diuretics, nitrates, and β-adrenergic agonists
Antibiotic prophylaxis for endocarditis
β-Adrenergic blockers
Verapamil or diltiazem
Disopyramide (in some patients)
Dual-chamber pacing relieves symptoms in some patients
Implantable cardioverter defibrillator (ICD) in patients at high risk for sudden death

Myotomy/myectomy in symptomatic HCM refractory to medical/device treatment

Some patients have benefitted from deliberate septal ablation (e.g., with alcohol)

Check first-degree relatives with echocardiography

Genetic counseling recommended for affected progeny

What are some of the strongest risk factors for sudden death?

Young agent (<30 years) at diagnosis, cardiac arrest, sustained ventricular tachycardia, family history of sudden death, bad genotype, recurrent syncope, massive left ventricular hypertrophy, repetitive nonsustained ventricular tachycardia

What treatments have been used in high-risk patients?

Implantable cardioverter-defibrillators (preferred); amiodarone

MITRAL REGURGITATION

What is mitral regurgitation (MR)?

Reverse (regurgitant) blood flow across the mitral valve from the left ventricle into the left atrium

What are some causes of MR?

Rheumatic heart disease (33% of cases), mitral valve prolapse, mitral annular calcification (age related), infective endocarditis, congenital, papillary muscle dysfunction (ischemia/MI), trauma, degenerative (e.g., myxomatous), and any disease that enlarges the left ventricle (cardiomyopathies)

How does acute MR classically present?

Dyspnea and acute pulmonary congestion, secondary to sudden increase in left ventricular end-diastolic pressure and left atrial pressure

How does chronic MR classically present?

Asymptomatic until later in disease progression; then fatigue, exertional dyspnea, orthopnea, and weakness. Right-sided heart failure can occur in patients with associated pulmonary vascular disease and pulmonary hypertension; finding of low output state may be more prominent.

What is the general pathophysiology of MR?

The left ventricle decompresses into the left atrium and also expels blood out of the aorta. As severity of MR increases, left ventricular volume increases and function progressively declines, left ventricle dilates, left atrial compliance and size often increase, and forward cardiac output decreases. In patients with severe MR, ejection fraction of 50–60% is still consistent with left ventricular dysfunction.

What may the physical exam show in chronic MR?

Hyperdynamic left ventricle, displaced apex, holosystolic murmur radiating to axilla or base of heart (depends on lesion). If patient is in heart failure, an S_3 and pulmonary rales may be heard. If pulmonary hypertension is present, findings are consistent with this.

What are the ECG findings?

No specific findings. May be left or right atrial enlargement or a left ventricular hypertrophy pattern. Atrial fibrillation may be present as the atrium enlarges.

What are the chest x-ray findings?

Straightening of the left heart border, an atrial double density, or elevation of left mainstem bronchus. Mitral valve calcifications, cardiomegaly, and pulmonary congestion may be present.

How is MR diagnosed?

Physical exam and echocardiogram to determine cause and severity

What is the medical treatment of MR?

Acute MR: IV vasodilators (e.g., nitroprusside), IV inotropes, and possibly intra-aortic balloon counterpulsation. Mitral valve replacement usually required urgently.

Chronic MR: Evaluate and treat underlying cause (e.g., ischemia). Antibiotic prophylaxis of infective endocarditis is advised. Afterload-reducing agents, especially ACE inhibitors, are the initial treatment. All patients with severe MR should be considered for mitral valve repair, if possible, or replacement surgery.

What are some class 1 indications for mitral valve surgery in nonischemic severe MR?

NYHA functional class II, III, or IV; left ventricular ejection fraction >60%; end-systolic dimension <45 mm
Symptomatic or asymptomatic; left ventricular ejection fraction 50–60%; end-systolic dimension 45–50 mm
Symptomatic or asymptomatic; left ventricular ejection fraction 30–50%; and/or end-systolic dimension 50–55 mm

Is there a reference on guidelines for management of valvular heart disease?

Yes. Bonow R, Carabello B, deLeon Jr A, et al: ACC/AHA guidelines. *Circulation* 1998;98:1949–1984; *Journal of the American College of Cardiology* 1998;32:1486–1588.

PULMONARY EDEMA

What is pulmonary edema?

Congested lung tissue with fluid in the interstitial spaces and alveoli

What classifications may be used?

Based on mechanism: cardiogenic (increased pulmonary capillary pressure) vs. noncardiogenic (altered alveolar-capillary membrane permeability); lymphatic insufficiency; unknown or incompletely understood

What are some causes of cardiogenic pulmonary edema?

Mitral stenosis and other valvular heart disease; left ventricular failure

What are some causes of noncardiogenic pulmonary edema?

Adult respiratory distress syndrome, infections, toxins, neurogenic, and high altitude

How may pulmonary edema present?

Dyspnea, tachypnea, anxiety, restlessness

What can be found on physical exam?

Rales, rhonchi, wheezing, use of accessory respiratory muscles; pink frothy expectorate in cardiogenic edema

What should generally be included in the workup?

Good history, physical exam, chest x-ray, arterial blood gas (ABG), and ECG

What are the usual chest x-ray findings?

Diffuse bilateral interstitial and perihilar vascular engorgement, alveolar infiltrates

What other chest x-ray findings are more likely in cardiogenic edema?

Kerley B lines, pleural effusions, possibly enlarged heart

Do the findings on chest x-ray always correlate well with the clinical findings?

No; it can take hours for chest x-ray findings to appear once symptoms develop, and it may take days for the chest x-ray to return to normal once therapy is initiated.

How can cardiogenic and noncardiogenic edema be differentiated?

Clinical history is most important. If needed, measure pulmonary artery occlusion pressure (PAOP); a value of <18 mm Hg suggests noncardiogenic edema.

What is the treatment?

Correct underlying cause(s); oxygen; diuretics (furosemide) in cardiogenic edema; other measures and medications for treatment of CHF

What additional pharmacologic agents may be used in cardiogenic edema if above therapy is inadequate?

Morphine sulfate, nitroglycerin, nitroprusside, and inotropic agents (e.g., dobutamine or phosphodiesterase inhibitors) can be helpful.

When is mechanical ventilation indicated?

Coexisting hypercapnia or inadequate oxygenation (PaO_2 <60 mm Hg on FIO_2 100% by mask)

| Name a good reference on evaluation and management of CHF in the adult. | Hunt SA, Baker DW, Chin MH, et al: ACC/AMA guidelines for the evaluation and management of chronic heart failure in the adult: executive summary. *Journal of the American College of Cardiology* 2001;38(7):2101–2113. |

CHEST PAIN

ACUTE PERICARDITIS

What are the symptoms of acute pericarditis?	Most commonly, chest pain: usually substernal, may worsen with inspiration and recumbent position, may lessen with sitting up or leaning forward (cough may be present)
Name physical signs of acute pericarditis.	Pericardial friction rub, which may be present, absent, intermittent, or changing over time; fever sometimes
Are there lab abnormalities associated with acute pericarditis?	Erythrocyte sedimentation rate may be elevated, possibly pericardial effusion, mild leukocytosis, and ECG abnormalities
What are the phases of the pericardial friction rub?	Presystolic (or atrial systolic), systolic, and early diastolic. Rubs may be heard best with patient upright and leaning forward.
What are some causes of pericarditis?	Infectious (e.g., Coxsackie A and B, echovirus), uremic, neoplastic, post-traumatic, post-MI, post-irradiation, idiopathic, drug-induced, related to collagen vascular disease
What drugs can cause pericarditis?	Procainamide, hydralazine, methysergide, anticoagulants, phenytoin
What are some ECG differences between acute pericarditis and acute ischemia?	Acute pericarditis: PR depression (atrial involvement), diffuse ST elevation (usually concave), T waves inverted after J points return to baseline, arrhythmias and conduction abnormalities rare

Acute ischemia: localized ST elevation, Q waves (with Q wave infarcts), T inversion while ST still up, arrhythmias and conduction abnormalities more common

What condition may relate to acute pericarditis?

Pericardial effusion and tamponade

How is pericardial fluid diagnosed?

Echocardiography. Other imaging modalities may be helpful in certain circumstances (e.g., MRI).

What is the treatment for acute pericarditis?

Treat underlying cause. Nonsteroidal anti-inflammatory drugs (NSAIDs); in certain situations, corticosteroids; in some cases, pericardiocentesis. In purulent pericarditis, a pericardial window with drainage may be necessary.

Name a potentially tragic consequence of mistaking acute pericarditis for acute MI.

Administration of a thrombolytic agent to a patient with acute pericarditis might result in a hemorrhagic pericardial effusion and cardiac tamponade.

ACUTE PNEUMOTHORAX

What is a pneumothorax?

Accumulation of air in the pleural space with secondary lung collapse

What are some causes of pneumothorax?

Idiopathic (primary), chronic obstructive pulmonary disease (COPD), cystic fibrosis, HIV/AIDS, trauma, invasive procedures (central line placement, thoracentesis), mechanical ventilation

What are risk factors for primary spontaneous pneumothorax?

Male gender, tobacco use, tall and thin body habitus

What infection is associated with pneumothorax in AIDS?

Pneumocystis carinii pneumonia (PCP); highest risk if receiving pentamidine for prophylaxis

What are the clinical features of pneumothorax?	Acute onset of chest pain: acute, localized to one side, usually pleuritic; acute dyspnea
What are the physical signs of pneumothorax?	Tachycardia, tachypnea; absent tactile fremitus, hyperresonance, and decreased breath sounds on affected side
What tests should be ordered?	Chest x-ray and ABG
What does the ABG typically show?	Hypoxemia and hypocapnia
What is the usual treatment of pneumothorax?	Aspiration of air (catheter connected to chest tube or one-way valve device); 100% oxygen
When is pleurodesis indicated?	Recurrent primary spontaneous pneumothorax. Consider use in patients with COPD and HIV.
When is surgery indicated?	Persistent air leak, incomplete re-expansion of lung
What is the rate of recurrence in primary spontaneous pneumothorax?	25%, most within 2 years of first episode
What is a tension pneumothorax?	A pneumothorax in which the pleural pressure is greater than atmospheric pressure throughout expiration
When is a tension pneumothorax most likely to occur?	After trauma or during mechanical ventilation
Why is a tension pneumothorax feared?	Because it is associated with severe respiratory distress and hypotension
What signs and symptoms may be observed with a tension pneumothorax?	Labored breathing, diaphoresis, cyanosis, distended neck veins, tracheal deviations, subcutaneous emphysema, hypotension

What is the treatment?	Prompt aspiration of air with a large-bore needle

AORTIC DISSECTION

How are aortic dissections anatomically classified?	Type A (proximal) originating in the ascending aorta and extending at least to the aortic arch (formerly, DeBakey type I), or originating in and confined to the ascending aorta (formerly, DeBakey type II) Type B (distal) originating in the descending thoracic aorta (formerly, DeBakey type III)
Why this classification?	For prognostic and therapeutic reasons: in general, surgery is indicated for dissection involving the ascending aorta; in absence of ascending aortic involvement, generally medical management.
List some causes of aortic dissection.	Cystic medial degeneration associated with hypertension and advanced age; congenital cystic medial degeneration (e.g., Marfan and Ehlers-Danlos syndromes); blunt chest trauma; rare complication of cardiac catheterization or cardiac surgery
What other conditions have been associated with aortic dissection?	Bicuspid aortic valve, coarctation of aorta, arteritis (especially giant cell), pregnancy (3rd trimester to several months postpartum), Noonan and Turner syndromes
How do aortic dissections present?	The vast majority present with excruciating "tearing" chest, jaw, or back pain of sudden onset associated with the acute dissection. A small minority are chronic dissections discovered incidentally on an imaging study. Less common symptoms with acute dissection: CHF, syncope, and cerebrovascular accident (CVA).

What are the physical findings?	Variable; reflect location of dissection. Hypertension (70% in distal, 30% in proximal), pulse deficits, aortic regurgitation murmur, neurologic manifestations.
What are the cardiac complications of ascending aorta dissection?	Extension into sinus of Valsalva, causing acute aortic regurgitation and/or closure of (usually the right) coronary artery, resulting in acute MI. Extension into the pericardial sac, causing hemopericardium and usually cardiac tamponade.
What are the neurologic complications of aortic dissection?	CVA when the innominate or left carotid arteries are compromised. Paraparesis or paralysis when spinal arteries are compromised.
What are the major imaging modalities to evaluate suspected aortic dissection?	MRI, CT scan, contrast aortography, transesophageal echocardiography
What are the advantages of transesophageal echocardiography in diagnosing aortic dissection?	Bedside procedure that can be performed quickly; noninvasive and requires no contrast dye; metal valvular prostheses and pacemakers do not interfere with visualization; highly sensitive for ascending arch dissections and cardiac complications
What are the limitations of transesophageal echocardiography in visualizing aortic dissections?	The limited ability to visualize the aortic arch, the proximal descending thoracic aorta, and the abdominal aorta below the diaphragm
What is the medical treatment for acute aortic dissection?	Place patients in acute care setting for close monitoring of multiple parameters. Aim to stop progression of the dissecting hematoma. Decrease shear force of cardiac contraction on the aorta by decreasing left ventricular contractility with β-blocker (if contraindicated, use negative inotropic calcium-channel

blocker, e.g., verapamil, diltiazem); additional blood pressure control with vasodilator (e.g., IV nitroprusside). Initiate β-blocker first; vasodilator alone increases shear force in the aorta. IV infusion of labetalol, a combined α- and β-blocker, is a good alternative.

What are the indications for surgical management of aortic dissection?

Acute proximal dissection; acute distal dissection complicated by progression with vital organ compromise; rupture or impending rupture (saccular aneurysm formation); retrograde extension into the ascending arch; patient with Marfan syndrome

COSTOCHONDRAL PAIN

What is costochondral pain?

Pain originating from the rib bones or rib cartilage

What may cause costochondral pain?

Recent chest trauma (e.g., falls, motor vehicle accident), inflammation, or costochondritis

How does costochondral pain present?

Sharp localized pain that may be reproducible with palpation

How is it diagnosed?

History, presentation with pain on palpation

What treatment may be tried?

NSAIDs

GASTROESOPHAGEAL REFLUX DISEASE AND ESOPHAGEAL DYSMOTILITY

What are the characteristics of gastroesophageal reflux disease (GERD)?

A retrosternal burning sensation that radiates upward; typically precipitated by big meals or recumbency, and often relieved by antacids or milk

Name some atypical symptoms of GERD.

Sore throat, hoarse voice, chest pain, cough, and asthma-like dyspnea

Can GERD be asymptomatic?	Yes
What pathophysiologic changes precipitate GERD?	Inappropriate transient lower esophageal sphincter relaxation, increased intra-abdominal pressure, hiatal hernia, and diaphragmatic disease
What are the complications of GERD?	Erosive esophagitis, dental erosions, stricture formation, dysphagia, and Barrett esophagus
What diagnostic studies may be helpful early in suspected gastrointestinal causes of chest pain?	Upper GI endoscopy and ambulatory 24-hour pH monitoring
What conservative measures should be taken, preferably before starting medical therapy?	Avoid provocative foods, avoid alcoholic beverages, avoid recumbency for 3 hours after a meal, elevate head of the bed using a wedge, and lose weight if obese
What is the treatment for GERD?	Mild cases: H_2-receptor antagonist or prokinetic agent Severe or persistent cases, advanced erosive esophagitis, and Barrett esophagus: proton pump inhibitors If medical therapy fails: surgical fundoplication is effective in many patients.
What symptoms may be present in patients with esophageal motility disorders?	Retrosternal chest pain, dysphagia
Which studies may be helpful in diagnosis?	Barium studies, esophageal manometry, provocative pharmacologic studies (e.g., with methacholine)

MEDIASTINAL EMPHYSEMA

What is mediastinal emphysema?	Air within the mediastinum

What can cause mediastinal emphysema?	Rupture of an emphysematous bleb, pneumomediastinum, pneumoperitoneum, or esophageal rupture
How does mediastinal emphysema present?	Severe pain with audible crepitus in the mediastinum; severe retching often precedes esophageal rupture.
How is mediastinal emphysema diagnosed?	Chest x-ray with or without esophagram (suspected esophageal rupture); other tests may be required.
What is the treatment?	IV antibiotics and prompt surgical consultation

ACUTE MYOCARDIAL INFARCTION

What ECG leads correspond to the locations of acute ST-segment elevation in myocardial infarction (MI)?	Left ventricular wall segments: septal—V_{1-2}; anterior—V_{2-4}; lateral—I, aVL, V_{5-6}; inferior—II, III, aVF; posterior—V_{1-2} (ST segment depression). Right ventricle: RV_{3-4}.
What are the minimum ST elevation criteria for diagnosing an acute MI?	ST elevation in two contiguous leads: 0.1 mV in limb leads; 0.2 mV in precordial leads; 0.05 mV in leads RV_3 and RV_4
What mechanism is responsible for most MIs?	Disruption of atherosclerotic plaque, leading to platelet aggregation, thrombus formation, and occlusion of an epicardial coronary artery
What are major risk factors for atherosclerotic coronary artery disease and acute MI?	Cigarette smoking, diabetes mellitus, hypertension, hypercholesterolemia, history of premature atherosclerotic coronary artery disease in a primary relative (parent, sibling, offspring)
When a patient presents with severe chest pain and nonspecific ST segment changes, what potentially catastrophic conditions are included in the differential diagnosis?	Acute MI, pulmonary embolus, dissecting thoracic aortic aneurysm

During the first 72 hours after presentation with an acute MI, what serious complications can occur?

Malignant ventricular arrhythmias, complete heart block, cardiogenic shock, papillary muscle dysfunction or rupture with sudden severe mitral regurgitation, rupture of the interventricular septum or free wall of the left ventricle

Describe the mechanism of shock due to left ventricular infarction.

A weakened left ventricle is unable to provide adequate stroke volume (and cardiac output), so hypotension and shock can result. Furthermore, the weakened left ventricle cannot handle the blood flow from the pulmonary vasculature (preload), so pulmonary capillary pressure increases and pulmonary edema develops.

Describe the mechanism of shock due to right ventricular infarction.

When the right ventricle fails, an inadequate volume of blood is delivered through the pulmonary vasculature to the left ventricle (inadequate preload) so that stroke volume and cardiac output fall, leading to hypotension.

What is the most effective way to treat shock due to left ventricular infarction?

Efforts to establish flow in the culprit vessel(s), inotropic support (dobutamine or dopamine), and preload reduction (venodilation with nitroglycerin and diuresis); may need intra-aortic balloon support

What is the most effective way to treat shock due to right ventricular infarction?

Vigorous administration of IV fluid. The right ventricle becomes a passive conduit for fluid delivery through the pulmonary vasculature to the left ventricle, providing it with adequate preload.

What single drug has proven effective in both primary and secondary prevention of MI?

Aspirin

What types of medication have been shown to improve long-term prognosis after an acute MI?

Aspirin, β-blockers, statins, and, in patients with reduced left ventricular ejection fraction, ACE inhibitors

What is the treatment for acute ST-segment elevation MI?	In the absence of contraindications, IV administration of a thrombolytic (fibrinolytic) agent. In hospitals with a cardiac catheterization laboratory and cardiac surgery, primary percutaneous transluminal coronary angioplasty is an alternative if it can be performed in a timely fashion.
What is the most devastating complication of administering a thrombolytic agent?	Major and minor bleeding complications. In 0.1% of cases, intracranial bleed occurs, resulting in hemorrhagic stroke.
What are some of the gender differences in the clinical syndromes of coronary artery disease (CAD)?	Women are more likely than men to present with angina rather than MI as first manifestation of CAD. Women are on average 5–10 years older at time of presentation.
Where can I learn more about the current approach to acute MI?	In the *AHA 2000 Handbook of Emergency Cardiovascular Care for Healthcare Providers* and in Braunwald E, Antman EM, Beasley JW, et al: ACC/AHA guidelines for the management of patients with unstable angina and non-ST segment elevation MI: executive summary and recommendations. *Circulation* 2000;102:1193–1209.

PLEURISY

What is pleurisy?	Inflammation of the pleura (of the lungs)
What are some types of pleurisy?	Wet (i.e., with effusion), dry (i.e., fibrinous), encysted hemorrhagic, purulent, suppurative
What are some possible causes of pleurisy?	Connective tissue disease (e.g., lupus, rheumatoid arthritis), viral illness, lung/chest wall abscess, pneumonia, malignancy (bronchial carcinoma), pulmonary infarction, and pneumothorax

How may pleurisy present?	Dyspnea with a sharp stabbing, unilateral, pleuritic chest pain
What may be appreciated on physical exam?	Restricted breathing on affected side and friction rub on auscultation
What may the chest x-ray reveal?	Depends on type and cause; pleural effusion may be present.
How is it diagnosed?	History, physical examination, and presentation
What is the treatment?	Correct underlying cause, administer NSAIDs and aspirin

PRINZMETAL ANGINA

What is Prinzmetal angina?	A syndrome of chest pain and ST-segment elevations on ECG; results from spasm of an epicardial coronary artery; also known as variant angina
Is Prinzmetal angina associated with atherosclerotic disease?	The first cases described were patients who *angiographically* appeared to have no coronary stenosis. Later, Prinzmetal syndrome was observed in some patients to be secondary to spasm at or near the site of an atherosclerotic lesion. Recent observations using intravascular ultrasound suggest that Prinzmetal patients with "clean coronaries" actually had mild atherosclerosis at the site(s) of spasm.
What are symptoms and possible consequences of the coronary spasm in Prinzmetal angina?	Most patients suffer varying periods of chest pain, usually at rest, and recover spontaneously or after medical treatment. Complications include serious ventricular tachyarrhythmias, atrioventricular (AV) block, MI, and (rarely) sudden death.
Are the risk factors for Prinzmetal angina similar to those for atherosclerotic coronary disease?	Prinzmetal patients tend to be younger than those with atherosclerotic disease. Many are heavy cigarette smokers.

How do patients with Prinzmetal angina respond to the medications usually given for angina pectoris?

Direct coronary vasodilators—nitrates and calcium channel blockers—are the drugs of choice. Response to β-blockers is variable. β-Blockers may decrease frequency of angina in patients with fixed obstructive coronary lesions. However, β-blockers may not be effective because of some degree of β_2-blocking activity, which potentially can promote vasospasm. Aspirin, because it blocks the synthesis of the vasodilator prostacyclin, may worsen vasospasm. Prazosin, an α-adrenoreceptor blocker, may be of value in some patients.

Is there a role for angioplasty in Prinzmetal angina?

When coronary spasm is associated with a fixed atherosclerotic lesion, symptoms may be diminished or eliminated with angioplasty of the lesion.

What is the value of exercise testing in Prinzmetal angina?

Limited, because response is variable (no ST changes, ST depression, ST elevation all can be seen).

What tests can provoke coronary artery vasospasm in patients with Prinzmetal angina?

Ergonovine, hyperventilation, acetylcholine, and cold pressor test

PULMONARY EMBOLISM

Where do pulmonary emboli embolize from?

Mostly from pelvic veins or deep veins of legs; occasionally from an arm vein or right-sided heart chamber

What are the most common coagulopathies known to predispose to deep venous thrombosis?

Activated protein C resistance (factor V Leiden), protein C deficiency, protein S deficiency, antithrombin III deficiency, plasminogen deficiency

Name some situations that increase risk for deep venous thrombosis.

Surgery, trauma, stroke, spinal cord injury, immobilization; indwelling central venous catheter

Name some risk factors for deep venous thrombosis.

Obesity, increased age, cigarette smoking, oral contraceptives, pregnancy, postpartum, certain malignancies

What are some signs and symptoms of pulmonary embolus?

Dyspnea, tachypnea, tachycardia, chest pain, cough, syncope, hemoptysis

How does ECG help in the differential diagnosis of a patient suspected of having a pulmonary embolus?

Many nonspecific ECG changes are seen with pulmonary embolus, but are not helpful. When an acute ST-segment elevation MI is ruled in, ECG helps rule out pulmonary embolus. When new ECG changes of right ventricular strain appear (right axis deviation, complete or incomplete right bundle branch block, large S waves in leads I and aVL, QS waves in leads III and aVF, T-wave inversions in leads III and aVF or V_1–V_4), they are suggestive of a large pulmonary embolus.

What is the usefulness of plasma D-dimer in the diagnosis of pulmonary embolus?

A useful screening tool that is positive whenever endogenous fibrinolysis is occurring. It is, therefore, not specific for pulmonary embolus but is positive in 90% of patients who have a pulmonary embolus.

What is the usefulness of ABG analysis in the diagnosis of pulmonary embolus?

Minor abnormalities, especially in PaO_2, are common, but rarely helpful in distinguishing from other pulmonary or cardiac conditions.

What is the usefulness of the chest x-ray in diagnosing pulmonary embolus?

Chest x-ray abnormalities are rare, nonspecific, and often subtle. The peripheral wedge-shaped density (Hampton hump) that delineates pulmonary infarction from pulmonary embolus is very uncommon and almost never seen at presentation.

How is the definitive diagnosis of pulmonary embolus made?

Traditionally, pulmonary angiogram was the gold standard while ventilation-perfusion scintigraphy studies of the lung demonstrating a high probability due to mismatched defects were considered adequate evidence to treat pulmonary embolus. Increasingly, chest CT scan (especially spiral CT) is replacing scintigraphy and angiography.

What is the medical treatment of pulmonary embolus?

Unless there is evidence of massive pulmonary embolus, hospitalize until acute symptoms resolve; give heparin for immediate anticoagulation; as discharge is anticipated, convert to warfarin, which is typically continued for 3 to 6 months; supplemental oxygen and pain medication as needed in hospital.

What is the role of the inferior vena cava filter in the management of patients with pulmonary embolus?

Indications include patients at high risk for bleeding with prolonged anticoagulation; recurrent pulmonary emboli; extensive or progressive deep venous thrombosis.

What is the hemodynamic effect of repeated pulmonary emboli?

Over years, chronic pulmonary hypertension

What are the hemodynamic effects of acute pulmonary emboli?

Severity varies; in the acute setting, either multiple simultaneous emboli or one or two large emboli may lead to severe acute pulmonary hypertension, right ventricular failure with systemic venous congestion, and decreased flow of blood to the left heart, resulting in hypotension and shock.

What is the treatment for massive pulmonary embolus?

IV thrombolytic (e.g., TPA); if contraindicated, surgical embolectomy

ARRHYTHMIAS AND CONDUCTION DISORDERS

ATRIAL FIBRILLATION

What is atrial fibrillation?

The most common sustained arrhythmia, characterized electrographically by variable, generally low-amplitude voltage, with baseline undulation corresponding to atrial rates >300 beats/min. Ventricular rate is generally irregularly irregular.

What conditions can be associated with atrial fibrillation?

Hypertension, drugs (cocaine, ethanol, theophylline, caffeine), hyperthyroidism, pericarditis, ischemia, or valvular heart disease

What symptoms may be present?

A wide range: none (asymptomatic), palpitations, "skipped" beats, light-headedness, breathlessness, angina, syncope, systemic embolism; or cardiac arrest (if rapid pre-excited atrial fibrillation)

What are patients at risk for?

Cardiac thromboembolic events (e.g., stroke)

How is atrial fibrillation diagnosed?

Characteristic ECG, generally with irregularly irregular ventricular response

What is the initial treatment if hemodynamic status is compromised (myocardial ischemia, MI, hypotension, or CHF)?

Prompt electrical cardioversion

What is the initial treatment goal in mild well-tolerated cases?

Control ventricular rate with calcium-channel blockers, β-blockers, provide anticoagulation (in absence of contraindication)

What are possible therapeutic approaches if atrial fibrillation has been present for >48 hours?

1. Rate control, and anticoagulation for at least 3 weeks before, and at least several weeks after, cardioversion
2. Rate control and transesophageal echocardiography to exclude left atrial thrombus, then cardioversion if no clot visualized. This approach requires anticoagulation with and after cardioversion.

What purpose does anticoagulation serve? Decreases risk of thromboembolic event

When is cardioversion without anticoagulation acceptable? There is no guaranteed safe period, but many feel that duration of <24 hours is safe for cardioversion.

What are the choices for cardioversion? Pharmacologic and electrical. Choice of pharmacologic agent should be guided in part by left ventricular function.

What are some of the risk factors for stroke? Hypertension, CHF, age >60 years, left ventricular dysfunction, diabetes mellitus, and previous systemic emboli

Name a good reference for management of patients with atrial fibrillation. Fuster V, Ryden LE, Asinger RW, et al: ACC/AHA/ESC guidelines for the management of patients with atrial fibrillation: executive summary. *Circulation* 2001;104:2118–2150.

ATRIAL FLUTTER

In what situations is atrial flutter generally seen? Patients with organic heart disease

What symptoms may be present? A wide range: none (asymptomatic), palpitations, skipped beats, light-headedness, breathlessness, angina, syncope, systemic embolism

How is atrial flutter diagnosed? ECG shows regular undulation (sawtooth pattern) that is best appreciated in the inferior leads, with an atrial rate of 250–350 per minute. Other patterns and types exist.

What is the usual ventricular rate on ECG? Depends on degree of AV block (e.g., 2:1, 3:1), but if 2:1 AV block is present, rate will be 150 if atrial rate is 300.

What is the treatment? Similar to that for atrial fibrillation. Use of type I agents (e.g., flecainide), if not used with an AV nodal blocking agent, may result in a more rapid ventricular rate. AV nodal blocking agent is important.

AV NODAL RE-ENTRANT TACHYCARDIA

What is AV nodal re-entrant tachycardia?

The most common paroxysmal supraventricular tachycardia (PSVT) that originates above the ventricles in the AV junction

How does AV nodal re-entrant tachycardia present?

Often with sudden transient episodes of increased heart rate (150–250 beats/min) without or with symptoms (palpitations, light-headedness, angina, and syncope)

How is AV nodal re-entrant tachycardia diagnosed?

Several ECG patterns possible:
1. P within QRS or barely at end of QRS (most typical)
2. P farther from QRS (uncommon variant)

What is the initial acute therapy?

Vagal maneuvers (carotid sinus massage and Valsalva maneuver)

What is the next step if vagal maneuvers fail?

Adenosine, or IV diltiazem to slow or block AV node

What treatments are available for AV nodal re-entrant tachycardia?

Radiofrequency ablation or pharmacologic therapy [calcium-channel blockers (e.g., verapamil), β-blockers, digoxin, or membrane active agents (e.g., propafenone)]

TORSADES DE POINTES

What is torsades de pointes?

A wide-complex polymorphic ventricular tachycardia with QRS complexes that progressively change direction (axis) in setting of prolonged QT interval

What are some risk factors?

History of ventricular tachycardia or ventricular fibrillation, poor ventricular

	function, CHF, female gender, metabolic abnormalities (e.g., low potassium or calcium), bradycardia/pauses
Name some drugs that can cause torsades de pointes.	Antiarrhythmic drugs (e.g., quinidine, procainamide), erythromycin, terfenadine, tricyclic antidepressants, and loratadine (Claritin)
What is the treatment?	Treat underlying cause. Discontinue offending agents; give IV bolus of magnesium sulfate; increase heart rate (in pause-dependent torsades) to 90–120 beats/min using either isoproterenol or temporary pacing.
When should electrical cardioversion be considered?	In cases of sustained torsades de pointes despite above measures, or with any hemodynamic instability

VENTRICULAR FIBRILLATION

Define ventricular fibrillation.	A cardiac arrhythmia characterized by uncoordinated ventricular depolarizations and contractions that can result in absence of cardiac output; major cause of sudden cardiac death (SCD) syndrome
What is the main risk factor for ventricular fibrillation?	Left ventricular dysfunction secondary to CAD
What are the main presentations of ventricular fibrillation?	SCD, syncope
How is ventricular fibrillation diagnosed?	ECG showing undulating baseline with no identifiable P waves or discrete QRS complexes
What is the treatment, and what should every physician know?	Basic and advanced cardiac life support (BCLS and ACLS) guidelines, beginning with immediate unsynchronized electric cardioversion

What should be done if ventricular fibrillation persists or recurs?	Follow ACLS guidelines, reassess ABCDs, give epinephrine, consider antiarrhythmic agents (e.g., amiodarone, lidocaine)
What should you think of when ventricular fibrillation occurs?	Acute ischemia, MI and, much less commonly, hypothermia or severe electrolyte abnormalities with underlying predisposition

VENTRICULAR TACHYCARDIA

Define ventricular tachycardia.	Tachyarrhythmia consisting of three or more consecutive complexes of ventricular origin at ≥ 100 beats/min
What are some underlying causes?	Ischemia (coronary artery disease), MI, electrolyte imbalance, drugs, cardiomyopathy, long QT syndromes
What are the symptoms of ventricular tachycardia?	May be asymptomatic, or may experience palpitations, breathlessness, light-headedness, angina, and syncope.
What is the treatment if the patient is hemodynamically unstable?	Synchronized electric cardioversion
What is the treatment in clinically stable patients?	Depends on type of ventricular tachycardia and context. Follow ACLS protocols.
What are management approaches to ventricular tachycardia?	Radiofrequency ablation (higher success rates for certain kinds, e.g., in structurally normal hearts) and implantable cardioverter-defibrillator; pharmacologic therapy (e.g., antiarrhythmic drugs) may be helpful in certain situations

2 ___

Dermatology

SKIN ERUPTIONS

ACNE VULGARIS

Define acne vulgaris.
Common form of acne affecting the hair follicle and associated sebaceous gland

Who is at greatest risk?
Adolescents and young adults (e.g., women in their 20s and 30s, in whom acne is due to hormonal shifts)

Name four causes of hair follicle plugging leading to acne.
1. Excess sebum production
2. Overgrowth of *Propionibacterium acnes*
3. Inflammation
4. Abnormal keratin production

Excess of what hormone is associated with acne?
Androgens

How does acne vulgaris present?
Most often in adolescents with mild disease (open and closed comedones) or more severe disease (papules, pustules, nodules and cysts) on the face and trunk

How is the diagnosis made?
History and physical exam

What first-line topical treatments are available, and how do they work?
Benzoyl peroxide (decreases *P. acne*), retinoic acid (decreases abnormal keratin production), and the topical antibiotics erythromycin and clindamycin (decrease microbial irritants that cause local inflammation)

When should systemic treatment be considered?
If papules, pustules, or nodules are found on physical exam

What systemic agents are commonly used?	Erythromycin and tetracycline
When is tetracycline contraindicated?	Pregnancy and young children
What medical treatment is available for severe nodular cystic acne with scarring?	Isotretinoin (Accutane)
What is an absolute contraindication to Accutane?	Pregnancy
What should be ordered before prescribing Accutane or tetracycline for a female patient?	Pregnancy test
What two additional measures are suggested for female patients receiving Accutane?	1. Use oral contraception or the most effective available contraception from 1 month prior until 1 month after discontinuation of therapy 2. Avoid systemic antibiotics (owing to possible risk of oral contraception failure)

ACTINIC KERATOSIS

What is actinic keratosis?	A precancerous lesion characterized by clonal proliferation of atypical keratinocytes
What are the two risk factors?	Sun-exposed skin; immunocompromise
How does it present?	Firm, well-marginated, reddish papule, diameter <1 cm, with rough feel (like sandpaper); typically changes to yellow-brown color when exposed to ultraviolet light
How is the diagnosis made?	Biopsy

What treatment is available?	Cryosurgery
What are two alternative treatments?	Topical 5-fluorouracil cream Electrocautery
What are untreated patients at risk for?	Squamous cell carcinoma (1 : 1000 risk)

CANDIDIASIS

What organism causes candidiasis?	*Candida albicans*
Who is at risk?	Immunosuppressed patients, persons with diabetes, and obese patients
How does it present on the skin?	Itching and burning sensation; beefy-red lesions of varying sizes on warm, moist areas of the body (e.g., inner thigh, axillae, beneath breasts)
How does oral candidiasis present?	White plaques on oral mucosa and tongue
How are oral and skin candidiasis diagnosed?	Microscopic visualization of yeast and pseudohyphae using 10% potassium hydroxide
What is the treatment for skin lesions?	Nystatin cream or ketoconazole cream
What is the treatment for oral candidiasis?	Nystatin liquid ("swish and swallow")

CELLULITIS

What is cellulitis?	An acute bacterial infection of the skin
What causes it?	Group A β-hemolytic streptococci (GABHS) and *Staphylococcus aureus*

What are the risk factors?	Diabetes, immunosuppression, skin trauma, lymphatic and venous obstruction
How does cellulitis present?	Localized tender, warm, red skin lesions with diffuse border
Where does it commonly appear?	Lower extremities
What should be included in the workup?	CBC, Gram stain and cultures of skin lesions, blood cultures, possibly skin biopsy
What is the treatment?	Antibiotics (oxacillin or a cephazolin), bed rest, elevate affected area, and treat underlying conditions if present.
What additional treatment may be required in persons with diabetes?	Anaerobic antibiotics (e.g., metronidazole or clindamycin) due to increased risk of polymicrobial infection

CONTACT DERMATITIS

Define contact dermatitis.	An acute or chronic condition resulting from direct skin contact with chemicals or allergens
Name some common irritants.	Soaps, detergents, dyes, solvents, drugs, cosmetics, poison ivy, poison oak, rubber, latex, and metals
How do mild cases present?	Erythema, edema, and pruritus in area of irritant contact
How do severe cases present?	Severe swelling and blistering in area of irritant contact
How is the diagnosis made?	History and patch testing
What is the treatment?	Remove and avoid irritant, wash affected area with soap and water, administer antihistamine (for pruritus) and topical corticosteroids

What is added to therapy in severe cases (especially if face is affected)?	Systemic steroids (i.e., prednisone)

HERPES ZOSTER ("SHINGLES")

What causes herpes zoster?	A latent reaction to the varicella-zoster virus
What disease did the virus cause when it first infected the patient?	Herpes varicella (chickenpox)
Where does the virus lie dormant in the body?	Sensory nerve ganglia
Who is at risk for reactivation of the dormant virus?	Elderly persons and immunocompromised patients
How does it present?	Usually with a 3-day prodrome of fever, malaise, and pain distributed unilaterally along one or a few dermatomes, followed by vesicular eruptions in the affected dermatomes
Can the vesicles transmit the virus by direct contact?	Yes
How is the diagnosis often made?	History and presentation
How is the diagnosis confirmed?	Positive Tzanck smear demonstrating multinucleated giant cells
What is the initial treatment?	Analgesics
What additional treatment is used in immunocompromised patients?	Acyclovir

If pain persists in the affected dermatome, what additional medication should be considered?	Corticosteroids

PSORIASIS

Define psoriasis.	A dermatologic disorder characterized by an increased proliferation of epidermal cells
Name an associated risk factor.	Family history
Name four factors that can precipitate an attack.	Trauma, stress, drugs (e.g., β-blockers), and infection
How does psoriasis present?	Silvery scales on bright red, well-demarcated plaques, most often on the knees, elbows, and scalp
What nail findings may be appreciated on physical exam?	Pitting or onycholysis
How is the diagnosis made?	History and presentation
What confirms the diagnosis?	Skin biopsy
What is the treatment?	Ultraviolet light, topical corticosteroids, and topical tar

SCABIES

What causes scabies?	Female *Sarcoptes scabiei* ("itch mite") lays eggs in the skin, releasing larvae that irritate the hair follicles
How does it present?	Excoriations from scratching intensely pruritic erythematous papular skin lesions. Commonly presents on the hands, axillary folds, trunk, buttocks, and genitalia. Lesions are often 2–3 mm long and the width of a hair.

Is it contagious?	Yes, by direct contact or fomites
How is it diagnosed?	Microscopic visualization of scabies mites, eggs, or feces
What is the treatment?	Permethrin 5% cream or lindane 1% cream
What additional measure can minimize reinfection?	Wash all clothing, sheets, and linens in hot water and detergent

SYPHILIS

What causes syphilis?	The spirochete *Treponema pallidum*
How is it transmitted?	Sexual contact (most common), blood transfusions, and vertical transmission from mother to infant
How does primary syphilis present?	One or more painless, indurated, superficial ulcerations (chancre) 3 weeks after exposure to the organism
Without treatment, how long will it take the chancre to heal?	6–8 weeks
How does secondary syphilis present?	Flu-like illness (malaise, headache, anorexia), generalized nontender lymphadenopathy, and a maculopapular rash (especially on palms and soles)
How does tertiary syphilis present on the skin?	Cutaneous gumma
With what additional features can tertiary syphilis present?	Cardiovascular (aortic aneurysms) and neurologic disease (general paresis, tabes dorsalis, or meningitis)
How are primary, secondary, and tertiary syphilis diagnosed?	History, presentation, and positive serologic studies

What histologic test is helpful in diagnosing primary syphilis?	Dark-field microscopy of lesion exudates visualizes treponemes
What nontreponemal serologic tests are helpful in diagnosing primary syphilis?	Venereal Disease Research Laboratory (VDRL) and rapid plasma reagin (RPR)
What treponemal serologic tests are helpful in diagnosing primary syphilis?	Fluorescent treponemal antibody absorption test (FTA-ABS) and microhemagglutination-*Treponema pallidum* (MHA-TP)
What is the treatment for all three types?	Benzathine penicillin G, 2.4 million units in a single IM dose

LUMPS AND TUMORS OF THE SKIN

BASAL CELL CARCINOMA (BCC)

What is basal cell carcinoma?	The most common malignant skin cancer
BCC is derived from what cell line?	Epidermal basal keratinocytes
What is the number one risk factor?	Excessive exposure to sunlight
Who is at increased risk?	Light-skinned persons
Where does BCC commonly present?	Face or nose
How does BCC commonly present?	It begins as a pale "pearly" papule with dilated blood vessels (telangiectasia), then enlarges peripherally and develops a central depression or ulceration that crusts and bleeds.
How is the diagnosis made?	Biopsy
What is the treatment?	Surgical excision

MALIGNANT MELANOMA

Malignant melanoma is derived from what cell line?	Melanocytes
What is the most common type?	Superficial spreading (70%)
What are the risk factors?	Sun exposure (severe burn in childhood), dysplastic nevi, prior melanoma, family history (first-degree relative), and xeroderma pigmentosum
Which body regions are at increased risk of developing superficial spreading melanoma in men and women?	Trunk in men; lower extremities in women
How does superficial spreading melanoma present?	Pigmented skin lesion. Think ABCD: **A**symmetry; **B**order irregularity; **C**olor variation; **D**iameter >6 mm. Bleeding and ulceration may occur.
How is the diagnosis made?	Excisional biopsy
What is the treatment?	Wide excision
What additional treatment is required if regional lymph nodes are affected?	Regional lymph node excision
What is the most important prognostic factor?	Thickness (depth of tumor invasion)
What are the 10-year survival rates for the following:	
Lesions <0.76 mm thick?	96%
Lesions >3.6 mm thick?	31%

What depth of invasion is correlated with a high risk of metastasis?	0.76 mm
Where does melanoma metastasize?	Almost anywhere in the body, but most commonly to regional lymph nodes, liver, lungs, skin, bone, and small intestine
What additional therapy is required if it has metastasized?	Chemotherapy, radiation, and immunotherapy

SQUAMOUS CELL CARCINOMA (SCC)

What is squamous cell carcinoma?	A malignant skin cancer that arises from keratinocytes
What are the risk factors for SCC?	Actinic keratosis, sun-exposed skin, immunosuppression, and light-skinned individuals who sunburn easily and tan poorly
How does it present?	Crusted red papule that becomes nodular and occasionally ulcerates
Do skin metastases occur in SCC lesions?	Uncommon (<7%); however, SCC may invade underlying tissue and has a higher risk of metastasis in oral cavity lesions (up to 30%).
How is the diagnosis made?	Biopsy
What is the treatment?	Surgical excision

VIRAL WARTS

What causes viral warts?	Human papillomavirus (HPV)
What are the risk factors?	Local irritation or trauma
How do viral warts present?	Sharply demarcated firm nodules with a cornified epithelium; shape varies; <1 cm in size. Commonly affected areas include fingers, knees, elbows, and feet.

What is the treatment?	Although most warts disappear spontaneously (50%), chemicals (salicylic and lactic acid) and cryotherapy (liquid nitrogen) are often used. Recurrences are frequent despite therapy.

OTHER SKIN LESIONS

KELOIDS

What causes keloids?	Irregular organization of fibroblasts following skin injury
What are the risk factors?	Dark skin and recent skin trauma or inflammation
How does it present?	Enlarging, well-demarcated scar following skin trauma
What is the treatment?	Local steroid injections

3   Endocrine Disorders

DIABETES MELLITUS

What is diabetes mellitus?

A chronic disorder that is primarily the result either of a relative or complete lack of insulin secretion by the β-cells of the pancreas, or of defects in insulin receptors

Name the three classifications of diabetes mellitus (DM).

Insulin-dependent (type 1), non-insulin-dependent (type 2), and secondary causes

What are some common secondary causes of DM?

Medications (e.g., steroids, thiazide diuretics) and pancreatic insufficiency

Which type of DM has a stronger genetic predisposition?

Type 2 greater than type 1 due to 90% concordance rate in monozygotic twins

How does type 1 DM present?

Often before the age of 30, with abrupt onset of weight loss, polydipsia, polyphagia, and polyuria

How does type 2 DM present?

Often in obese persons after the age of 40, with gradual onset of weight loss, polydipsia, polyphagia, and polyuria or with an abnormal lab test

What additional signs may be found in chronic diabetes?

End-organ complications (retinopathy, neuropathy, peripheral vascular disease, macrovascular disease, nephropathy, foot disease, and depression)

How is the diagnosis made in asymptomatic patients?

1. By a fasting plasma glucose level >126 mg/dL on two separate occasions, or
2. By a positive 2-hour oral glucose tolerance test (two values at 2 hours exceeding 200 mg/dL)

How is the diagnosis made in symptomatic patients?

Presence of symptoms (e.g., weight loss, polyuria) with a random plasma glucose level of >200 mg/dL

What is the initial treatment for both type 1 and type 2 diabetes mellitus?

Diabetic diet (60% carbohydrates, 15% protein, and 25% fat, not exceeding 35 kcal/kg per day) and physical activity to attain ideal body weight

How are treatment regimens for DM monitored?

Numerous daily capillary blood glucose measurements

What are the recommended fasting, preprandial, and postprandial glucose levels?

Fasting and preprandial of
  70–120 mg/dL
Postprandial of <160 mg/dL

What lab test is used to assess glycemic control over the last 4 weeks?

Glycosylated hemoglobin A_{Ic}

What is the next therapy in type 1 DM when initial treatment with diet and exercise fails?

Insulin therapy

Describe in detail how to develop an insulin regimen that simulates normal insulin secretion.

Treat with insulin using a regimen to simulate normal insulin secretion patterns:
1. Begin with 10 units of intermediate-acting insulin 30–60 minutes before breakfast and 5 units at bedtime. Monitor blood glucose levels before meals and at bedtime.
2. Increase intermediate-acting insulin every 3–5 days to attain blood glucose goals (70–120 mg/dL premeal, 70–160 mg/dL at bedtime).
3. Add 2–5 units (depending on patient size) of short-acting insulin 30–60 minutes before breakfast and/or the evening meal.

4. Intensify regimen with multiple intermediate and short-acting insulin preparations given before meals until a satisfactory response in blood glucose levels is obtained.

What is the next therapy in type 2 DM when initial treatment with diet and exercise fails?

Oral hypoglycemic agents, e.g., sulfonylureas, metformin (Glucophage), acarbose (Precose), insulin sensitizers (rosiglitazone and pioglitazone)
Follow with insulin if needed

What medication should be avoided in patients taking insulin?

β-Blockers, because they mask the autonomic sequelae of hypoglycemia

What are some commonly used insulin preparations?

See Table 3-1.

DIABETIC KETOACIDOSIS (DKA)

What is diabetic ketoacidosis?

An acute life-threatening complication of uncontrolled diabetes resulting in hyperglycemia, hyperglucagonemia, increased stress hormones, and ketone body production

Is DKA more common in type 1 or type 2 diabetes?

Type 1

Table 3-1. Commonly Used Insulin Preparations

Type and Preparation	Onset (h)	Peak (h)	Duration (h)
Ultra-rapid-acting (human)	0.2–0.5	0.5–2	3–4
Short-acting			
Regular (human)	0.5–1	2–3	6–8
U-500 (pork)	1–3	6–12	12–18
Intermediate-acting			
NPH (human)	1.5	4–10	16–24
Lente (human)	3	7–15	16–24
Long-acting			
Ultralente (human)	3–4	9–15	22–28
Mixtures (human)			
70/30 (NPH/regular)	0.5–1	3–12	16–24
50/50 (NPH/regular)	0.5–1	2–12	16–24

What can cause it?

Stress (often infection), myocardial infarction (MI), cerebrovascular accident (CVA), or noncompliance with insulin treatment regimen

How do mild cases present?

Polyuria, polydipsia, unexplained weight loss, vomiting, and vague abdominal pain

How does it appear in severe cases?

Hyperventilation (Kussmaul sign), shock, and coma

What comprises the workup?

Serum electrolytes, serum ketones, arterial blood gas, electrocardiogram to evaluate possible MI or hyperkalemia, complete blood cell count, chest radiograph, and bacterial cultures if infection is suspected

How is DKA diagnosed?

Hyperglycemia, hyperketonemia, and metabolic acidosis with an elevated anion gap

What is the treatment?

Hospitalize. Begin fluid resuscitation using isotonic 0.9% saline and a bolus of 10–15 units of insulin followed by IV insulin at 5–10 units per hour; begin empiric antibiotics if infection (stress) is suspected.

What should be used if sodium levels are >155 mmol/L?

0.45% saline

What lab tests are ordered hourly to monitor progress?

Serum glucose, electrolytes, and anion gap

When is saline changed to 5% dextrose?

When serum glucose decreases to between 250 and 300 mg/dL

Why is this done?

Infusion of dextrose allows continuation of insulin therapy, which helps decrease remaining ketoacidosis.

What electrolyte abnormality are patients at risk for during insulin therapy?	Hypokalemia
Which patients are at increased risk of hypokalemia?	Patients with renal insufficiency, oliguria, or both
What is the treatment for hyperkalemia?	Potassium supplementation (use potassium phosphate if hypophosphatemia is present)
When is bicarbonate therapy considered?	Shock or coma, when pH falls below 7.1, or if severe hyperkalemia is present
What is the treatment?	2 amps (80–100 mEq) of sodium bicarbonate per liter of 0.45% saline

NONKETOTIC HYPEROSMOLAR COMA

What causes nonketotic hyperosmolar coma?	Hyperglycemia, dehydration, and hyperosmolality
What is the main risk factor?	Type 2 DM
What can precipitate it?	Stress, stroke, or excessive carbohydrate intake
How does the patient present?	Lethargic, obtunded, or coma with severe hyperglycemia and dehydration in the absence of ketoacidosis
What is the treatment?	Isotonic (0.9%) saline followed by 0.45% saline (if hypernatremia is present) and small doses of parenteral insulin with rigorous blood glucose monitoring
What electrolyte abnormality are patients at risk for when insulin is given?	Hypokalemia

What is the treatment?	Potassium supplementation
When is bicarbonate therapy considered?	If pH is <7.1
What tests are ordered to monitor therapy?	Blood glucose and serum electrolyte levels

HYPOGLYCEMIA

Name the two main risk factors for hypoglycemia.	Diabetes mellitus and postgastrectomy patients
Name the two common types and the risk factor for each.	Postprandial (postgastrectomy) Fasting (diabetes mellitus)
Which drugs most commonly cause fasting hypoglycemia?	Insulin and sulfonylureas
How does it present in mild cases?	Anxiety, diaphoresis, tachycardia, lethargy, confusion, and headache
How do severe cases present?	Seizure, stupor, coma, or focal neurologic findings
How is the diagnosis made?	Hypoglycemic symptoms with a low glucose level, relieved with treatment
What is the treatment for mild hypoglycemia?	Oral carbohydrates (e.g., fruit, fruit juice, crackers)
What is the treatment for severe hypoglycemia?	Intravenous (IV) D_5 solution; subcutaneous (SC) or intramuscular (IM) glucagon if IV access is not available
What test is used to evaluate therapy?	Plasma glucose level every 15–30 minutes
What is the long-term treatment?	Adjust drug therapy, diet, and physical activity

DISEASES OF THE THYROID AND PARATHYROID GLAND

HYPOTHYROIDISM

What is hypothyroidism?	A hypometabolic condition resulting from a decrease in thyroid hormone at the cellular level
What are the risk factors?	Hashimoto thyroiditis, neck radiation or surgery (history of thyrotoxicosis or cancer), drugs (iodine, lithium, interferon alfa, and interleukin-2), and pituitary disease
How does it present?	Often nonspecific symptoms including cold intolerance, fatigue, weight gain, paresthesias (hand and feet), constipation, and hoarseness
What might be found on physical exam?	Bradycardia, hypothermia, periorbital edema, dry skin, nonpitting edema, and decreased tendon reflexes (prolonged relaxation)
How is primary hypothyroidism diagnosed?	High plasma levels of thyroid-stimulating hormone (TSH)
How is secondary hypothyroidism (pituitary disease) diagnosed?	Normal TSH with a decreased T_4 index
What is the treatment?	Thyroxine (T_4); start at 50–100 μg/day (start with 25 μg/day in elderly patients or patients with heart disease) and slowly taper up until TSH level is normalized
What is a possible complication of hypothyroidism?	Myxedema crisis
What can cause it?	Infection (common), trauma, and cold exposure

How does it present?	Hypothermia, hyporeflexia, bradycardia, hypotension, hyponatremia, and hypoventilation
What is the treatment?	IV thyroxine
What additional treatment is suggested in secondary hypothyroidism?	Hydrocortisone (decreases risk of concomitant adrenal insufficiency)

HYPERTHYROIDISM

What is hyperthyroidism?	A disease characterized by excess free-thyroid hormone in the body due to a hyperfunctioning thyroid gland
What is the most common cause?	Graves disease (gamma immunoglobin binding to TSH receptors)
Who is at increased risk of Graves disease?	Middle-aged women (30 to 60 years of age)
Name four other less common causes.	Excess medication (T_4, Amiodarone) Toxic nodular goiter (often older patients with autonomously functioning nodules) Thyroiditis (painful tender goiter, viral illness, and transient hyperthyroidism) Cancer (papillary type most common in the thyroid gland, as well as TSH-secreting pituitary tumors)
Name some common symptoms.	Palpitations, anxiety, nervousness, insomnia, heat intolerance, increased sweating, weight loss, hair loss, and frequent bowel movements
What signs may be apparent on physical exam?	Goiter, tachycardia, fine tremor, stare, eyelid lag, atrial fibrillation, warm skin, and brisk tendon reflexes
Name two signs that are specific to Graves disease.	Exophthalmos and pretibial myxedema (pretibial nonpitting edema)

How might Graves disease present in the elderly patient?	Atrial fibrillation, heart failure, weakness, or weight loss
How is it diagnosed?	Low TSH ($<$0.1 μU/mL) and high T_4 or free thyroxine index
What diagnostic tests are ordered if cancer is suspected?	Fine needle aspiration and thyroid scans
What is the pharmacologic therapy for hyperthyroidism?	Long-term therapy with antithyroid drugs methimazole and propylthiouracil (PTU)
What is their mechanism of action?	Both inhibit thyroid hormone synthesis, but PTU also inhibits conversion of T_4 to T_3.
Name four serious side effects of methimazole and PTU.	Agranulocytosis, drug-induced lupus syndrome, hepatitis, and vasculitis
What concomitant medical therapy is useful to decrease hyperthyroid symptoms?	β-Blockers
What nuclear medicine therapy is available?	One or two doses of radioactive iodine (RAI) to impair thyroid hormone synthesis over the next several months
Name a contraindication to RAI treatment.	Pregnancy
What is a common risk of RAI therapy and how is it treated?	Hypothyroidism, which is treated with thyroxine
What surgical treatment is available when medical therapy fails or the patient refuses RAI therapy?	Subtotal thyroidectomy

What are the potential side effects?	Hypothyroidism (more common) and hypoparathyroidism (less common)
What is the dreaded complication of Graves disease?	Thyroid storm (often triggered by stress or infection), which is a medical emergency
How does thyroid storm present?	Fever, tachycardia, weakness, delirium, and shock
What is the treatment?	IV fluids, steroids, PTU, potassium iodide, and a β-blocker

PRIMARY HYPERPARATHYROIDISM

What is primary hyperparathyroidism?	A disease of increased parathyroid hormone (PTH) secretion resulting in hypercalcemia
What causes increased PTH?	Parathyroid adenoma (most common), hyperplasia, or carcinoma (rare)
Who is usually affected?	Women over age 30; elderly women
What is the most common cause of secondary hyperparathyroidism?	Hypocalcemia from chronic renal failure (decreased vitamin D hydroxylation)
How does it present?	Most patients are asymptomatic with an abnormal screening test, but some present with "painful bones, renal stones, abdominal groans, and psychic overtones" if PTH is >13 mg/dL.
How is the diagnosis made?	Hypercalcemia (on at least two occasions), hypophosphatemia, and elevated PTH
What additional laboratory test result may be found?	Elevated alkaline phosphatase (in patients with significant bone disease) and hypercalciuria
What radiographic studies should be performed?	Ultrasound and computed tomography (CT) to reveal parathyroid adenomas

What is the treatment if serum calcium rises above 13–15 mg/dL?

Diuresis with furosemide and hydration with intravenous saline (increases renal calcium excretion), parenteral salmon calcitonin, pamidronate (bisphosphonate with antiresorptive properties), mithramycin (inhibits bone resorption), and phosphate

What is the definitive treatment for patients with serum calcium levels above 11 mg/dL?

Parathyroidectomy

What is the treatment for patients with mildly elevated calcium levels?

Increase fluid intake, administer oral phosphate and exogenous estrogen

OTHER ENDOCRINE DISORDERS

ADRENOCORTICAL INSUFFICIENCY

What is adrenocortical insufficiency?

Insufficient steroid output from the adrenal cortex due to a disease of the adrenal glands (primary failure) or disorders of the pituitary or hypothalamus (secondary failure)

Name four causes of primary adrenal failure.

Autoimmune destruction (Addison disease, most common), infection, hemorrhagic adrenal infarction, metastasis

Name two common causes of secondary adrenal failure.

Glucocorticoid therapy, pituitary failure due to disease or surgery

How does it present?

Anorexia, nausea, vomiting, weakness, weight loss, fatigue

What additional features may occur only in primary adrenal failure?

Hyperpigmentation [due to excess adrenocorticotropic hormone (ACTH)], hypoglycemia, and hyperkalemia and volume depletion (due to aldosterone deficiency)

What presentation should significantly increase your suspicion?

A hypotensive orthostatic patient with hyperpigmentation who fails to respond to fluids and has hyponatremia, hyperkalemia, or hypoglycemia of unknown etiology

Who is at increased risk?

People with AIDS (disseminated infection or ketoconazole treatment) Steroid-dependent patients whose exogenous steroids are abruptly withdrawn

How is it diagnosed?

Inadequate response to cosyntropin (Cortrosyn; ACTH) stimulation test (cortisol level does not increase after administration of ACTH)

What lab results distinguish primary and secondary causes?

Primary causes have elevated ACTH and low aldosterone; secondary causes have low ACTH and normal aldosterone.

What is the treatment?

Hydrocortisone, 20–30 mg/day (increase dose during high stress or infection)

What additional treatment is required if hypoaldosteronism exists?

A mineralocorticoid, fludrocortisone (Florinef) 0.05 to 0.1 mg/day, when symptoms of orthostatic hypotension or hyperkalemia also exist

CUSHING SYNDROME

What is Cushing syndrome?

A syndrome characterized primarily by effects of excess cortisol, although excess mineralocorticoids and androgenic steroids also may be present

What causes it?

Administration of exogenous glucocorticoids (most common) or excess production of cortisol by the adrenal cortex

What lung disease is associated with Cushing syndrome?

Small cell lung cancer can produce ACTH, which stimulates the adrenal cortex to produce excess cortisol

What is Cushing disease?	Excess cortisol production from the adrenal cortex caused by increased ACTH secreted by the pituitary, often from a pituitary microadenoma
What are the symptoms of Cushing syndrome?	Fatigue, weakness, depression, abdominal striae, thin skin, and easy bruising
What are the signs of excess systemic cortisol?	Truncal obesity, rounded face, impaired glucose tolerance, hirsutism, acne, abdominal striae, and osteoporosis
What screening tests are used?	A 24-hour urine free-cortisol level (absent morning cortisol increase) and an overnight 1-mg dexamethasone suppression test
If the screening test is positive, what test is ordered next?	Low-dose dexamethasone suppression test
What diagnostic test strongly suggests a secondary cause?	ACTH level high or low; dexamethasone nonsuppressing
What is the treatment?	Transsphenoidal microadenectomy
What treatment is available for nonsurgical candidates?	Pituitary irradiation

ANTERIOR PITUITARY DISEASES

What can cause anterior pituitary diseases?	Benign pituitary adenoma, infiltrative disease, autoimmune phenomena, hypothalamic disease
Which hormones are usually affected by functioning pituitary tumors?	ACTH, growth hormone (GH), and prolactin (PRL, most common)
Which hormones are rarely affected?	TSH, follicle-stimulating hormone (FSH), and luteinizing hormone (LH)

How might patients present?	Chronic headache, visual disturbance (bitemporal hemianopsia), pituitary hormone imbalance
How would hyperprolactinemia commonly present?	Galactorrhea and amenorrhea in women; impotence and loss of libido in men
How would GH insufficiency present in children?	Growth retardation and hypoglycemia
How does excess GH present?	Gigantism in children, acromegaly in adults
How does excess ACTH present?	Cushing syndrome
What lab results suggest the diagnosis?	Abnormal level of GH, PRL, or ACTH
What lab test strongly suggests the diagnosis in GH-producing tumors?	Glucose challenge test
How is the diagnosis made?	CT or magnetic resonance (MR) imaging (preferred)
What medical therapy may be used to control small PRL-secreting adenomas?	Treatment with the dopamine agonists bromocriptine or cabergoline
When is transsphenoidal surgery with or without radiation warranted?	In patients with hormone excess or neurologic symptoms
What additional therapy may be required in hypopituitarism?	Hormone replacement

POSTERIOR PITUITARY DISEASES

What two hormones are made in the hypothalamus and released by the posterior pituitary?	Oxytocin and vasopressin (antidiuretic hormone)
What disease results from insufficient release of vasopressin?	Diabetes insipidus (DI)
What disease results from excessive release of vasopressin?	Syndrome of inappropriate antidiuretic hormone secretion (SIADH)
What causes neurogenic DI?	Insufficient release of vasopressin by the pituitary
What causes nephrogenic DI?	Distal nephron does not respond to vasopressin.
What are four risk factors for DI?	Head trauma, neurosurgical procedures, brain tumors, and drugs (ethanol, phenytoin, or lithium)
How does DI present?	Excessive thirst and polyuria
What may be apparent on physical exam?	Dehydration and hypovolemia
How is the diagnosis of DI made?	Dilute urine and increased serum osmolality
What test is ordered to distinguish between central and nephrogenic DI?	Water deprivation test
What is the treatment for symptomatic neurogenic DI?	The intranasal vasopressin analog desamino-8-D-arginine vasopressin (DDAVP, desmopressin)

What is the treatment for nephrogenic DI?	Hydration and thiazide diuretics
What are the risk factors for SIADH?	Small cell lung carcinoma, pulmonary diseases (e.g., pneumonia, tuberculosis), stroke, head injury, and drugs (e.g., chlorpropamide, carbamazepine, and diuretics)
How does SIADH present?	With symptoms of hyponatremia, such as lethargy, muscle cramps, confusion, headache, focal neurologic defects, convulsions, and coma
What are the associated lab findings?	Hyponatremia with a concentrated urine
How is the diagnosis made?	With the associated lab findings after all other causes have been ruled out (e.g., diuretics, dehydration, and anterior pituitary, renal, adrenal, and thyroid disease)
What is the initial treatment?	Correct underlying cause and restrict fluid intake
What medication may be added to inhibit the action of antidiuretic hormone (ADH)?	Demeclocycline
What is the treatment for severely hyponatremic (sodium <120 mmol/L) patients presenting with coma or seizure?	IV infusion of hypertonic saline to raise serum sodium until it reaches 120 mmol/L or until neurologic symptoms subside

OSTEOPOROSIS

What is osteoporosis?	Loss of bone mass
Name some risk factors associated with osteoporosis.	Personal history of adult fracture, adult fracture in a first-degree relative, age, sex, and racial background

Name some causes of secondary osteoporosis.	Hyperthyroidism, hyperparathyroidism, osteomalacia, multiple myeloma, and medications (glucocorticoids most common, and T_4 over-replacement)
How is bone mineral density measured and reported?	Dual-energy x-ray absorptiometry (DXA) at spine and hip. Values are reported as standard deviation from the mean for young, normal controls (T-score), and as standard deviation from the mean for an age- and sex-matched control group (Z-score).
What treatments are available to increase bone mineral density?	Nutritional therapy (calcium and vitamin D supplements), hormone replacement therapy, and bisphosphonate treatment (alendronate and risedronate)

OVERWEIGHT AND OBESITY

Based on the body mass index (BMI), how are the stages of underweight, normal, and obesity defined?	Underweight: <18.5 kg/m^2 Normal: 18.5–24.9 kg/m^2 Overweight: 25.0–29.9 kg/m^2 Obesity stage I: 30.0–34.9 kg/m^2 Obesity stage II: 35.0–39.9 kg/m^2 Extreme obesity III: $\geqslant40$ kg/m^2
What are the sex-specific cutoffs of waist circumference that identify increased relative risk for the development of obesity-associated risk factors in adults with a BMI of 25–34.9 kg/m^2?	Men >102 cm (>40 inches), women >88 cm (>35 inches)
What proportion of the adult American population is estimated to be overweight or obese?	About half
What comorbidities are associated with obesity?	Type 2 diabetes mellitus, hypertension, coronary artery disease, hyperlipidemia, sleep apnea, biliary tract disease, osteoarthritis of the knees, and certain cancers

What proportion of obese adults has associated comorbidities?

About two thirds

In addition to overeating and not enough physical activity, what factors possibly play a role in causing obesity?

Hereditary predisposition, viruses (particularly adenovirus), hormones (particularly leptin), metabolic abnormalities (hypothyroidism and Cushing syndrome)

Before treating obesity, what medical conditions must be ruled out?

Hypothyroidism and Cushing syndrome

What metabolic abnormalities can be ascribed to obese patients with type 2 diabetes?

Degree of insulin resistance, hyperglycemia, and plasma free-fatty acid levels

To lose weight, people in the typical BMI range of 27–35 kg/m² should achieve how much caloric deficit?

A decrease of 300 to 500 kcal/day will result in weight loss of about 0.5–1 lb/week and a 10% loss in 6 months.

What specific behavioral strategies should be used in managing obese patients?

Self-monitoring of eating habits and physical activity, stress management, stimulus control, problem solving, contingency management, cognitive restructuring, and social support

What is the optimal exercise regimen the obese person should follow to lose weight?

All adults should set a long-term goal to accumulate 30 minutes or more of moderate-intensity physical activity on most, and preferably all, days of the week.

What two drugs have the Food and Drug Administration approved for the treatment of obesity?

Sibutramine 10–15 mg/day and orlistat 120 mg 3 times a day with meals

What are the contraindications to using sibutramine?

During or within 2 weeks of taking monoamine oxidase inhibitors (MAOs) or concomitant centrally acting appetite suppressants, anorexia, poorly controlled hypertension or coronary artery disease, congestive heart failure, arrhythmia, or stroke

Name three common side effects of orlistat.

Oily flatus, oily discharge, fecal urgency and incontinence

What is the treatment of last resort?

For a select group of patients, surgical intervention (gastric bypass or gastroplasty) can be recommended.

4

Emergency Medicine

CRITICAL CARE

What are the principles of critical care management of the acutely injured patient?	Primary survey, resuscitation, secondary survey, continued resuscitation, and, finally, definitive care
Describe the primary survey.	Identify and treat life-threatening conditions in the order they are likely to cause death or disability. Remember the ABCs of patient management: **A**irway maintenance with cervical spine control; **B**reathing and ventilation; **C**irculation with hemorrhage control; **D**isability (neurologic status); **E**xposure, environmental control. Assess patient's vital functions in that order; do not move on until each function is stabilized.
How does one assess the airway?	Look for foreign bodies or signs of facial, mandibular, or tracheal/laryngeal fractures that may cause obstruction. Based on mechanism of injury, maintain a strong suspicion for cervical spine injury; avoid excessive movement of the neck, using manual in-line immobilization if necessary. Suspect cervical spine injury in any patient with altered consciousness, blunt injury above the clavicles, or multisystem trauma.
How does one assess breathing and ventilation?	Breathing and ventilation involve the lungs, chest wall, diaphragm, and nervous system. Decreased consciousness, pneumothorax (open or tension), flail chest, pulmonary contusion, hemothorax, and rib fractures may impair ventilation. Visually inspect and auscultate the chest to reveal any injury that acutely impairs ventilation.

How does one assess circulation and control hemorrhage?

Identify acute, massive hemorrhage rapidly by assessing level of consciousness, skin color, and pulse. A decrease in circulating blood volume may result in altered consciousness, although this sign is neither sensitive nor specific. Ashen or white skin may indicate blood loss of at least 30%. Rapid, diminished, or absent peripheral pulses are often a sign of acute hypovolemia. Absent central pulses indicate massive volume loss and the need for immediate fluid resuscitation. Life-threatening hemorrhage may occur into the thoracic or abdominal cavities, into muscles secondary to fractures, or externally secondary to penetrating trauma. Control external bleeding by direct manual pressure; do not use tourniquets and hemostats.

How is disability assessed?

Perform a rapid neurologic assessment (if possible) before administering paralytic or sedative agents. Assess pupil size and reactivity. Describe level of consciousness using one of two methods. (1) The mnemonic **AVPU**: **A**lert; responds to **V**ocal stimuli; responds to **P**ainful stimuli; **U**nresponsive. (2) The more detailed and quantitative Glasgow Coma Scale (GCS): the sum of points for the best response in each of three areas. Eye opening: 4—spontaneous, 3—to verbal stimuli, 2—to painful stimuli, 1—none. Verbal response: 5—oriented, 4—confused, 3—inappropriate words, 2—incomprehensible sounds, 1—none. Motor response: 6—obeys commands, 5—localizes pain, 4—withdraws to pain, 3—decorticate posturing, 2—decerebrate posturing, 1—none. Signs of severe intracranial injury: GCS <8, deteriorating GCS score, unequal pupils, unequal motor exam, open head injury, or depressed skull fracture.

What does "exposure and environmental control" stand for?

The patient must be completely undressed and examined front and back to identify all signs of injury. Afterward, cover the patient and protect from hypothermia, a grave complication in the trauma victim.

What are the components of resuscitation?

Perform resuscitation with the primary survey, addressing each problem as it is identified. Airway resuscitative maneuvers include jaw thrust, chin lift, and placement of a nasopharyngeal airway. Endotracheal intubation may be required to maintain airway patency. Give appropriate treatment for injuries impairing ventilation and breathing, including supplemental oxygen (ideally by face mask). Concurrent with circulation assessment, establish at least two large-bore peripheral IV catheters. Use central venous catheters and venous cutdowns as necessary. Draw blood for basic studies, and type and crossmatch. Initiate immediate fluid resuscitation with 2 L of IV crystalloid solution (Ringer lactate or normal saline) for patients with signs of hemorrhage. Failure to respond to initial fluid resuscitation indicates need for urgent administration of packed red blood cells (type specific or O negative).

What does the secondary survey consist of?

Only after completing the primary survey does one proceed to the secondary survey, which is a complete, more thorough head-to-toe re-exam of the patient. Obtain x-rays, generally including views of lateral cervical spine, chest, and pelvis; order x-rays of extremities as indicated. Place a urinary catheter to decompress the bladder and monitor urine output, and a gastric catheter to empty the stomach and prevent aspiration. Maintain continuous cardiac, blood pressure, and pulse oximetry monitoring to assess the patient's response to resuscitation.

What happens after the secondary survey?

Consult with other appropriate services (e.g., trauma, orthopaedics, neurosurgery) about further diagnostic testing and definitive treatment. Diagnostic tests include CT scans of head, abdomen, and pelvis, and diagnostic peritoneal lavage.

HEAD TRAUMA

In what two ways are head injuries classified?

Open: skull fracture, often with cerebrospinal fluid (CSF) leakage; requires prompt neurosurgical intervention. Mechanical forces can directly damage brain tissue.

Closed: cranial vault remains intact, but associated intracranial hemorrhage or significant brain edema may require neurosurgical intervention.

What is the mechanism of brain injury in closed head trauma?

Normally, the brain is protected from mechanical shock because it floats in CSF. Sudden acceleration or deceleration causes contact with the inside of the skull and deformation of the brain. Contusion results from deformation sufficient to rupture small blood vessels, usually in cortex near the brain surface, and may be associated with tearing of vessels in the pia arachnoid (subarachnoid blood), or tearing of the bridging veins (subdural hemorrhage). Diffuse axonal injury occurs when deformation causes axons to stretch.

What are "coup" and "contrecoup" injuries?

As the brain moves in the cranial vault, the area of maximum deformation, and therefore injury, often occurs directly beneath an external impact (i.e., coup injury), but may also occur at the opposite pole of the brain [i.e., contrecoup ("opposite the blow") injury].

What is a "brain concussion"?	Occurs when mechanical trauma to the head results in transient neurologic deficit, usually loss of consciousness (also transient vertigo or visual disturbance). Associated with increased risk of delayed complications secondary to brain edema or intracranial hemorrhage.
What are the significant signs and symptoms in closed head injuries?	Skull depressions, Battle sign, hemotympanum, CSF rhinorrhea, anisocoria, and anosmia. History of altered consciousness or other neurologic deficit immediately after injury, even if transient, indicates brain concussion and possibility of delayed symptoms.

What is the significance of the following?

Battle sign	Ecchymosis behind the ear; suggests basilar skull fracture
Hemotympanum	Visualization of blood behind eardrum on otoscopic exam; suggests basilar skull fracture
CSF rhinorrhea	Leakage of CSF through nose; suggests basilar skull fracture
Anisocoria	Asymmetry of pupils and their reaction to light; sign of impending brain herniation due to mass effects from intracranial hemorrhage or brain edema compressing the ipsilateral third cranial nerve
Anosmia	Loss of sense of smell; occurs when olfactory bulbs undergo traction as the brain moves in the cranial vault, often shearing loose from the cribriform plate; reflects increased severity of injury

What is the significance of seizure activity immediately after a closed head injury?	Infrequently, brain contusions can give rise to immediate seizure activity. Often difficult to tell if the seizure caused or resulted from the head trauma, especially after falls or single-vehicle accidents. Evaluate patient for causes of seizure other than the

immediate head trauma. Seizures that occur early (minutes to days) after head injury are less likely to result in chronic seizures than those that occur later (>1 week).

How should head injuries be evaluated?

All significant head trauma has potential for cervical spine injury; stabilize cervical spine until cleared by x-ray. For unconscious or multiple trauma patients, promptly assess and stabilize **A**irway, **B**reathing, and **C**irculation (trauma ABCs). Once stable, assess disability via neurologic history and exam; determine need for further evaluation and management. The Glasgow Coma Scale is useful to evaluate prognosis but cannot substitute for a more complete neurologic exam.

What radiographic studies are often performed in patients with brain concussion or residual neurologic deficits?

Brain imaging, preferably computed tomography (CT) scan (sensitive for skull fractures and intracranial hemorrhage). Magnetic resonance imaging (MRI) has greater sensitivity for contusions and edema, but these do not alter immediate management if too mild to appear on CT. Opacification of the mastoid air cells by blood on CT scan is sign of occult basilar skull fracture; epidural hemorrhages can be associated with skull fractures.

What monitoring is helpful?

Frequent neurologic checks, especially if risk of significant brain edema. Consider intracranial pressure monitor when brain edema is significant.

How is a closed head injury treated?

Primarily supportive care. Neurosurgical intervention usually needed for depressed skull fracture, CSF leakage, significant intracranial hemorrhage, or brain edema. Giving antibiotics to all patients with basilar skull fracture or CSF leakage has not been proven to prevent meningitis; monitor those at risk for occult skull fracture for signs of meningitis. Monitor all patients with significant brain injury for brain edema, adult respiratory distress syndrome (ARDS), electrolyte disturbances [syndrome of inappropriate antidiuretic hormone (SIADH), central salt wasting syndrome], and seizures.

What is the overall prognosis?

Worst prognosis: patients who present in coma; may evolve into persistent vegetative state. Patients who recover from coma may have persistent neurologic deficits depending on injury location and severity; however, may continue to improve for 1 year or more after injury, especially with rehabilitation therapy for cognitive deficits.

Good prognosis: patients with only minor head trauma, with or without brief loss of consciousness (LOC). Patients with seizures that occur immediately after head trauma, or within several days, generally have lower incidence of chronic seizures than those with seizures that occur >1 week after trauma. Secondary seizure disorders may develop as late as several years after injury.

CHEST TRAUMA

CARDIAC TAMPONADE

What is cardiac tamponade?

Accumulation of intrapericardial fluid causes an increase in intrapericardial pressure. When pressure exceeds the right atrial (RA) filling pressure, the amount of blood delivered to the ventricles decreases. The resultant decreased stroke volume may lead to hemodynamic compromise.

What is the most common cause of cardiac tamponade?

Penetrating trauma to the anterior chest

What are the causes of cardiac tamponade in the nontrauma patient?

Metastatic malignancy (most commonly, lung and breast), uremia, bacterial or tubercular pericarditis, anticoagulant hemorrhage, systemic lupus erythematosus, post-radiation

What are the clinical features of cardiac tamponade?

Classically, pulsus paradoxus >15 mm Hg, with hypotension, jugular venous distention (JVD), and diminished heart sounds (Beck triad)

What is pulsus paradoxus?

An abnormal drop in systolic blood pressure during inspiration, due to the increase in afterload caused by negative intrapleural pressure (normal drop <10 mm Hg)

How does the electrocardiogram (ECG) appear?

May show low QRS voltage and T-wave flattening; may demonstrate electrical alternans (beat-to-beat variation in P- and R-wave amplitude).

How does the chest x-ray appear?

Normal or enlarged cardiac silhouette, with clear lung fields

How should the diagnosis of cardiac tamponade be made?

Based on clinical findings

What other studies may be used to diagnose tamponade?

Transthoracic echocardiogram—a rapid, noninvasive bedside test—may demonstrate as little as 15 mL of intrapericardial fluid, and right atrial (RA) compression and right ventricular (RV) diastolic collapse.

What other conditions may present with hypotension and JVD?

Tension pneumothorax, air embolism, and myocardial dysfunction

What is the therapy of cardiac tamponade?

Fluid resuscitation via two large-bore peripheral intravenous (IV) lines, followed by pericardiocentesis (diagnostic and therapeutic) and thoracotomy (definitive therapy)

How do you perform pericardiocentesis?	Use an 18-gauge spinal needle with a stopcock and 20-mL syringe attached, and the V lead of the ECG monitor clipped to the needle. Enter the chest at the left paraxyphoid region at a 45° angle, aiming at the left scapular tip. Advance 4–5 cm, aspirating every 1–2 mm. Stop when fluid is obtained, a cavity or pulsations are felt, or ECG changes occur.
What are the complications of pericardiocentesis?	Penetration of the right ventricle, causing tamponade, dysrhythmias, and false positives

FLAIL CHEST

What is flail chest?	A segmental fracture (fractures in two or more locations on the same rib) of three or more adjacent ribs resulting in an unstable portion of the chest wall. Most often occurs anteriorly or laterally.
How does flail chest occur?	From blunt trauma to the chest
How is it diagnosed?	Visual inspection: palpation of bony crepitus and tenderness; paradoxical motion of chest wall often seen
What is paradoxical chest wall motion?	During inspiration—paradoxical inward movement of the flail segment; during expiration—outward movement of the flail segment
What is the significant complication of flail chest?	Hypoxemia. The main cause is the underlying lung contusion that occurs when the sustained force was great enough to fracture the ribs.
What is the appearance of the chest x-ray in a patient with flail chest?	The fractured rib segments are apparent, with associated hemothorax or pneumothorax. Pulmonary contusion, evident by 6 hours after injury, appears as opacification of lung areas.

What is the worst outcome of a patient with flail chest?	As fluid moves into the area of pulmonary contusion, lung compliance decreases and work of breathing increases. Due to decreasing efficiency of respiration, the patient may fatigue easily and precipitously, and progress to respiratory arrest.
What is the initial treatment of flail chest?	Supplemental oxygen and analgesia, either oral, parenteral, or via intercostal nerve block Incentive spirometry to aid adequate pulmonary toilet Mechanical ventilation if severe hypoxemia or respiratory distress
What are the most important indicators of the respiratory status of a patient with flail chest?	Clinical assessment of respiratory rate and effort, and arterial oxygen saturation. Monitor patient by continuous pulse oximetry or serial arterial blood gas analysis, or both.
When should patients be placed on mechanical ventilation?	If oxygen saturation <90% or pO_2 <80 mm Hg on supplemental oxygen, if patient is in shock, has three or more associated injuries, severe head trauma, previous pulmonary disease, fracture of 8 or more ribs, or age >65 years
Is surgical fixation of the ribs required?	Rarely. Supportive treatment with analgesia, supplemental oxygen, and mechanical ventilation as needed are mainstays of therapy.

HEMOTHORAX

What is a hemothorax?	An accumulation of blood in one or both hemithoraces
What is the cause of hemothorax?	Most often, penetrating chest trauma that disrupts systemic or hilar vessels; also may result from blunt trauma

In an adult, what is a massive hemothorax?

Rapid accumulation of >1500 mL of blood in a hemithorax
Continued accumulation of >200 mL/h per hemithorax

What is the significance of a massive hemothorax?

A life-threatening condition through three mechanisms:
1. Massive hypovolemia decreases preload and left ventricular function.
2. The affected lung collapses, impairing ventilation and perfusion and causing hypoxia.
3. The vena cava is compressed, further impairing preload.

How do you diagnose a hemothorax?

In patient with thoracic trauma, suspect hemothorax if unilateral decreased breath sounds, dullness to chest percussion, or any signs of respiratory distress. Neck veins may be distended or flat, depending on patient's volume status.

What is the role of x-rays and ultrasound in diagnosing hemothorax?

Chest x-ray is used to diagnose hemothorax. An upright or decubitus film may detect as little as 200–300 mL of fluid collection, viewed as blunting of the costophrenic angle (upright) and layered fluid (decubitus); however, as much as 1 L of fluid in the chest may be missed on a supine film. The role of ultrasound is currently controversial.

What is the treatment of a hemothorax?

Decompression of the chest cavity and simultaneous restoration of circulating blood volume. Nearly all hemothoraces require decompression with tube thoracostomy (chest tube); massive hemothoraces generally require thoracotomy in the operating room to repair major vessel injury.

How is a tube thoracostomy performed?

1. With patient prepped and draped sterilely, anesthetize skin, subcutaneous tissue, and intercostal muscles with lidocaine.
2. Make a transverse skin incision 2–3 cm long on top of the fifth or sixth rib, so as to enter chest at the fourth or fifth intercostal space.
3. With a clamp, bluntly dissect the subcutaneous tissue and intercostal muscles superior to the rib. The intercostal muscle fascia and parietal pleura are entered with the clamp. This generally requires a moderate amount of force; keep the clamp open while withdrawing it from the chest cavity to ensure that the hole remains open.
4. Explore the chest cavity with a finger; verify that the opening is in the pleural space, and that there are no loculations or adhesions.
5. Position the tube in the chest cavity in the appropriate location, using a finger or clamp to guide its tip. Use a 38 French or larger tube. Direct the tube posteriorly and medially. Be sure that the last tube fenestration remains within the pleural space.
6. Suture the tube in place with heavy nonabsorbable suture; snugly wrap the ends of the suture around the tube and tie them. Apply a sterile dressing.
7. Attach the open end of the chest tube to a suction and fluid collection device.
8. Order a postprocedure chest x-ray to ensure proper tube placement, re-expansion of lung, and evacuation of fluid.

What are three possible complications of a tube thoracostomy?

Misplacement of the tube below the diaphragm may injure intra-abdominal organs.

The tube may enter the lung parenchyma, causing damage to the airway or blood vessels.

Failure to re-expand the lung or evacuate the blood; this may be corrected by placement of a second tube.

What is autotransfusion? When should it be administered?

Collection of blood retrieved from the chest tube into a sterile, heparinized device that allows for its transfusion back into the patient. Consider in patients with massive hemothorax, hemodynamic instability, and when the blood is unlikely to be contaminated by any concurrent injury below the diaphragm.

Are prophylactic antibiotics indicated after chest tube placement for traumatic hemothorax?

Duration of therapy remains controversial, but early administration of antibiotics reduces the incidence of pneumonia and empyema.

PNEUMOTHORAX

What is a pneumothorax?

The abnormal presence of air in the pleural space, compressing the affected lung

What are the causes of pneumothorax?

Spontaneous—most often due to rupture of emphysematous bullae in chronic obstructive pulmonary disease. Other risk factors: cystic fibrosis, drug use, and infection with *Pneumocystis carinii.*

Secondary—blunt or penetrating chest trauma or barotrauma associated with mechanical ventilation. Also significant incidence of iatrogenic pneumothorax after attempted subclavian and internal jugular vein cannulation.

What is a tension pneumothorax?

A life-threatening condition whereby intrapleural pressure causes complete collapse of the affected lung, with displacement of mediastinal contents. Hypotension occurs when kinking of the inferior vena cava impairs preload.

How does one diagnose a simple pneumothorax?

Signs and symptoms depend on size and rate of accumulation. Acute unilateral chest pain occurs in up to 95% of patients, dyspnea in 80%. Decreased breath sounds, hypertympany, tachypnea, and tachycardia occur less frequently. The 6-foot upright posteroanterior chest x-ray has 83% sensitivity for pneumothorax.

How does the chest x-ray appear in a pneumothorax?

As a radiolucent line separating visceral and parietal pleura. A tension pneumothorax ideally should not be diagnosed radiographically, but appears as lung collapse with mediastinal shift. Attempts to quantify pneumothorax volume are fraught with inaccuracy, although CT is better in this regard. Comparison of inspiratory and expiratory films may aid in diagnosing a small pneumothorax.

How does one diagnose a tension pneumothorax?

It is a true emergency, and should be diagnosed and treated based on physical exam. In a trauma victim or patient on mechanical ventilation, suspect tension pneumothorax in the presence of respiratory distress associated with hypotension, unilateral decreased breath sounds and hypertympany, and a contralaterally deviated trachea. Neck veins may be flat or distended, depending on patient's volume status.

How does one treat a simple pneumothorax?

Options include observation, catheter aspiration, and tube thoracostomy. Always administer supplemental oxygen, both to treat hypoxia and to increase pleural air reabsorption. Some stable patients with small, asymptomatic spontaneous pneumothoraces may be treated as outpatients with oxygen and followed with serial x-rays, although up to 40% ultimately may require thoracostomy. Single or sequential catheter aspiration also may be used, and a one-way Heimlich valve may be attached after failed simple aspiration. Patients not eligible for these re-expansion techniques require hospital admission and tube thoracostomy.

How does one perform catheter aspiration?

Using a small catheter attached to a stopcock and a 60-mL syringe, enter the pleural space at either the second intercostal space in the midclavicular line, or in the fourth or fifth intercostal space in the anterior axillary line. Aspirate until resistance is met, close the stopcock, and obtain a chest x-ray. Aspiration of >4 L suggests a continued air leak. If re-expansion is achieved, observe the patient and discharge home, with tube and Heimlich valve in place, if repeat 6-hour x-ray confirms persistent re-expansion.

How does one treat a tension pneumothorax?

Immediate needle decompression in the second intercostal space in the midclavicular line will convert the tension pneumothorax to a simple pneumothorax. Follow with tube thoracostomy (definitive treatment).

What is an open pneumothorax? How is it treated?

Also known as a "sucking chest wound." Occurs when a large defect of the chest wall causes air to enter the chest preferentially through the defect rather than via the trachea. The defect becomes the path of least resistance for air entry when its size is approximately two-thirds the diameter of the trachea. Treat emergently by placing an overlying dressing taped on three sides, allowing it to function as a flutter valve.

SHOCK

ANAPHYLACTIC SHOCK

What is anaphylaxis?

An acute systemic reaction involving multiple organ systems to an IgE-mediated release of chemical mediators from mast cells and basophils, occurring in previously sensitized individuals, resulting in circulatory and respiratory collapse

Name the four most common causes of fatal anaphylaxis.	Parenteral penicillin, hymenoptera stings, nuts, and shellfish
Name the major preformed vasoactive mediators of anaphylaxis.	Histamine, eosinophilic chemotactic factor of anaphylaxis (ECF-A), neutrophil chemotactic activity (NCA), platelet-activating factor (PAF), and basophil kallikreins
Name the major spontaneously generated vasoactive mediator.	Arachidonic acid, leading to formation of leukotrienes, prostaglandins, thromboxane, and prostacyclin
What are the pathologic effects of these mediators?	Increased vascular permeability, vasodilatation, smooth muscle contraction, vasoconstriction
What clinical signs and symptoms of anaphylaxis are caused by increased vascular permeability?	Urticaria, angioedema, laryngeal edema, nasal congestion, gastrointestinal swelling
What clinical signs and symptoms of anaphylactic shock are mediated by vasodilation?	Flushing, headache, reduced peripheral vascular resistance, hypotension, syncope
How does increased vasoconstriction present during anaphylactic shock?	Pulmonary hypertension and edema, decreased cardiac filling pressure, myocardial ischemia, dysrhythmia
What is an anaphylactoid reaction? Name the most common cause.	Similar clinical signs and symptoms as anaphylaxis, but not IgE mediated. Most common causal agent is radiographic contrast media.
What are the clinical signs and symptoms of upper airway obstruction?	Stridor, hypersalivation, hoarseness, angioedema
What are the clinical signs and symptoms of lower airway obstruction?	Coughing, wheezing, rhonchi, decreased air flow

How do you differentiate exercise-induced asthma from exercise-induced anaphylaxis?	In addition to wheezing, the latter manifests pruritus.
How does circulatory collapse present in anaphylactic shock?	Hypotension and tachycardia
How is the diagnosis of anaphylactic shock made?	By recognizing any combination of the above constellation of symptoms and discerning the precipitating antigen
What is the differential diagnosis for signs and symptoms of anaphylactic shock?	Asthma; vasovagal syncope; angioedema; foreign-body aspiration; septic or spinal shock; epiglottitis
What is the initial management of anaphylactic shock?	Stabilize **A**irway, **B**reathing, **C**irculation (ABCs)
What are the steps in airway management?	100% oxygen, jaw thrust, suction, nasopharyngeal or oropharyngeal airway, epinephrine, oral endotracheal intubation
What is the management after the initial ABCs?	2 large-bore IV lines; fluid resuscitation; cardiac and blood pressure monitors; epinephrine; other pharmacologic aids
What pharmacologic aids are used to counteract anaphylactic shock?	Isotonic IV fluids, epinephrine, diphenhydramine, albuterol, methylprednisolone sodium succinate (Solu-Medrol), aminophylline, glucagon, dopamine, cimetidine
What routes of epinephrine are used and why?	Subcutaneous (SC): mild signs and symptoms; normotensive Intramuscular (IM): if generalized urticaria IV: patients in shock (systolic blood pressure <80 mm Hg), respiratory failure, or upper airway obstruction Sublingual or endotracheal: when IV line cannot be established

What is the dosage for epinephrine?	SC or IM: 0.3–0.5 mL of 1:1000 solution; pediatric—0.01 mL/kg IV or sublingual injection: 0.3–0.5 mL of 1:10,000 solution Endotracheal tube: 0.5–1.0 mL of 1:10,000 solution Intraosseous (pediatric): 0.01 mL/kg of 1:10,000 solution

CARDIOGENIC SHOCK

What is cardiogenic shock?	Hypoperfusion of tissues with failure to meet metabolic demand, and systolic blood pressure <90 mm Hg, caused by inadequate myocardial contractility or by mechanical impairment of the heart
What is the incidence of cardiogenic shock after an acute myocardial infarction (MI)?	5–7%
What are some independent predictors of risk for developing cardiogenic shock after acute MI?	Advanced age, female, large or anterior wall MI, previous MI, history of congestive heart failure, multivessel coronary artery disease, proximal occlusion of left anterior descending artery, and diabetes mellitus
What is the predominant cause of cardiogenic shock?	Left ventricular (LV) infarction
What mechanical impairments can lead to cardiogenic shock?	Pericardial tamponade, massive pulmonary embolism (PE), acute mitral valve insufficiency, aortic dissection, ventricular septal wall rupture
In addition to an acute MI, what other causes of decreased myocardial contractility can lead to cardiogenic shock?	Myocardial contusion, toxins or drugs, cardiomyopathy, dysrhythmias, heart block

What blood pressure parameters are more sensitive measures of shock than systolic blood pressure?

Mean arterial pressure: decrease >30 mm Hg; pulse pressure <20 mm Hg

What are the clinical signs and symptoms of cardiogenic shock?

Cool, clammy skin; oliguria; anxiety; confusion, tachycardia, increased vascular resistance

What are the clinical signs and symptoms of pulmonary edema?

Tachypnea, rales, wheezing, frothy sputum

What pathologic process is suggested by jugular venous distention, hypotension, but NO pulmonary edema?

Acute RV failure from either tamponade, infarction, or PE

How can you differentiate mitral regurgitation due to chordae tendineae rupture versus papillary muscle dysfunction?

Chordae tendineae rupture produces a soft holosystolic murmur at the apex, radiating to the axilla. Papillary muscle dysfunction murmur starts with first heart sound, but ends before second heart sound.

What is suggested by an absence of ECG changes with clinical signs and symptoms of shock?

Aortic dissection, PE, pericardial tamponade, acute valvular insufficiency, hemorrhage, or sepsis

What lab studies are ordered to assess cardiogenic shock?

Arterial blood gas; serum bicarbonate or lactate; creatinine kinase (CK); creatine kinase, myocardial bound (CK-MB); and troponin

What are the initial steps for stabilization of cardiogenic shock?

Oxygen, IV access, cardiac monitor, continuous pulse oximetry

What is the first drug given in the setting of an acute MI?

Aspirin, 325 mg orally

What is the first-line treatment for RV infarction with hypotension?	Rapid IV infusion of 1 L 0.9 normal saline, followed by dobutamine if no response
What drug increases myocardial contractility and augments coronary blood flow, but does not induce reflex tachycardia?	Dobutamine
What is the dosage for dobutamine?	2.0–20 μg/kg per minute
What drug is used in the setting of profound hypotension?	Dopamine
If shock persists after giving drugs, what do you use?	Intra-aortic balloon pump (IABP)
What is the reperfusion modality of choice for cardiogenic shock?	Percutaneous transcoronary angioplasty with IABP

HEMORRHAGIC SHOCK

What is hemorrhagic shock?	Tissue hypoxemia and hypoperfusion caused by rapid blood loss of sufficient quantity to overcome the body's compensatory mechanisms
What are the four major sources of acute hemorrhage?	Trauma, gastrointestinal tract, reproductive tract, vascular
What are the classic signs of acute hemorrhage?	Tachycardia, tachypnea, narrow pulse pressure, cool and clammy skin, oliguria, low central venous pressure (CVP), altered mental status, hypotension
What percent blood loss is necessary to produce tachypnea, tachycardia, and orthostatic hypotension?	20–40%

Describe the progression of skin changes noted during hemorrhage.

1. Cool and clammy
2. Capillary refill delayed
3. Mottled
4. Pallor

In a patient with obvious trauma, what is the differential diagnosis of shock?

Hemorrhage, cardiac tamponade, tension pneumothorax, spinal cord injury

How does the endocrine system respond to the acute drop in blood pressure from acute hemorrhage?

Increased renin secretion, leading to increased angiotensin II; increased antidiuretic hormone and aldosterone secretion

What are the end results of endocrine compensation?

Vasoconstriction; sodium and water retention

Name the resuscitation fluid of choice and dosing parameters for initial management of hemorrhagic shock.

0.9 normal saline or Ringer lactate; rapid infusion of 20–40 mL/kg

What percent of normal saline or Ringer lactate remains intravascular? What are the therapeutic implications?

<30%. Total volume replacement should be 3 times blood volume lost.

What natural colloids are available for fluid resuscitation?

Purified protein factor; fresh frozen plasma; albumin

What significant disadvantage is shared by all colloids and crystalloids (except blood)?

Inability to restore oxygen-carrying capacity

Name the advantage(s) and disadvantage(s) of using 3% normal saline.

Advantage—provides prompt, sustained shift of fluid to intravascular space
Disadvantages—confusion, seizures, central pontine myelinolysis

When is transfusion of red blood cells considered?

Continued impaired perfusion after infusion of 30 mL/kg of normal saline or Ringer lactate

What are the indications for using type-specific rather than cross-matched blood?

Profound hypotension on presentation, persistent shock after crystalloid infusion, and rapid ongoing hemorrhagic loss

Define massive transfusion.

Transfusion of 1 blood volume (70–80 mL/kg in adult) in 24 hours

Name the potential complications of massive transfusion.

Bleeding diathesis, electrolyte abnormalities, hypothermia, congestive heart failure, adult respiratory distress syndrome, hemolytic reaction, transfusion-transmitted disease

Name the most common cause of hemolytic reaction.

ABO incompatibility

What complications of resuscitation contribute to cardiac arrhythmias?

Hypocalcemia, hypomagnesemia, hypokalemia/hyperkalemia, acidosis, and hypothermia

What are the risks for the following transfusion-transmitted diseases?

    Hepatitis B virus (HBV)   1/63,000

    Hepatitis C virus (HBC)   1/103,000

    Human immunodeficiency virus (HIV)   1/493,000

    Human T-cell lymphotrophic virus (HTLV)   1/641,000

What physiologic indices are used to assess severity of shock?

Heart rate; blood pressure; capillary refill; urine output; CVP

Which indicators more reliably reflect the presence of hypoperfusion despite normal vital signs?

Mixed venous oxygen saturation and serum lactate concentration

HYPOVOLEMIC SHOCK

What is hypovolemic shock?	A critical reduction of intravascular volume causing circulatory insufficiency or collapse, leading to an imbalance of tissue oxygen demand and supply
What are the major causes of hypovolemia?	Hemorrhage; gastrointestinal losses (vomiting, diarrhea); urinary losses (diabetes insipidus, mellitus); third spacing (ascites, pulmonary edema, sepsis)
What symptoms are associated with volume depletion?	Bleeding; vomiting; diarrhea; excessive urination; insensitive loss secondary to fever; orthostatic light-headedness
Supine tachycardia occurs at what percent volume loss?	10–15%
Supine hypotension occurs at what percent volume loss?	25%
List the basic methods of hemodynamic monitoring for shock.	ECG; pulse oximeter; CVP; end-tidal carbon dioxide; arterial blood pressure; pulse; pulse pressure; respiratory rate
What is the differential diagnosis of hypovolemic shock?	Hemorrhage, sepsis, anaphylaxis, cardiac tamponade, tension pneumothorax, spinal cord injury, endocrine derangement
What are the main priorities in stabilizing a patient in hypovolemic shock?	The ABCs: **A**irway establishment **B**reathing—control work of **C**irculation—restore and optimize
After the ABCs, what are the next priorities?	Prevent inappropriate oxygen consumption; assess adequacy of oxygen delivery and tissue extraction.
What methods are used to control oxygen consumption?	Analgesia; muscle relaxation; warm covers; anxiolytics; paralytic agents if appropriate

What parameters can be monitored in the emergency department to assess tissue oxygen extraction?	Serial lactic acid and central venous oxygen saturation
What are some negative side effects of endotracheal intubation for the patient in shock?	Reduced preload and cardiac output from positive-pressure ventilation; exacerbation of hypotension secondary to vasodilatation and venodilation from sedatives
In restoring circulation, why is the preferred route of venous access two large-bore (16-gauge preferred) peripheral IV lines?	Peripheral IVs instill fluids faster because of their short length and larger diameter.
Name the resuscitation fluid of choice and dosing parameters for the initial management of hypovolemic shock.	0.9 normal saline or Ringer lactate; rapid infusion of 20–40 mL/kg
When giving a fluid challenge, what is the optimal body position?	Supine, with legs elevated
Why should the body not be placed in Trendelenburg position?	May worsen gas exchange and increase risk of aspiration.
When is vasopressor therapy instituted?	If inadequate response to volume resuscitation If patient has a contraindication to volume restoration To prevent lethal consequences of prolonged hypotension

SEPTIC SHOCK

What is sepsis?	Systemic response to infection, exemplified by at least two of the following: 1. Temperature >38°C or <36°C 2. Heart rate >90 beats/min

3. Respiratory rate >20 breaths per minute or $PaCO_2$ <32 mm Hg
4. White blood count >12,000/μL, <4,000/μL or >10% bands

What is septic shock?

Sepsis-induced hypotension, refractory to fluid resuscitation, with perfusion abnormalities as evidenced by lactic acidosis, oliguria, mental status changes

What are the three major organ sources of sepsis?

Abdomen, lungs, urinary tract

What other three organ systems should be focused on?

Central nervous system (CNS), skin, soft tissue

What are two theoretical causes of myocardial depression seen in early septic shock?

1. Decreased coronary perfusion
2. Circulating myocardial depressant substances: nitric oxide, tumor necrosis factor-α, and interleukin-1β

What lung pathology is most closely associated with sepsis?

ARDS

What are the renal manifestations of sepsis?

Oliguria, azotemia, active urinary sediment

What are the most frequent hematologic derangements seen in sepsis?

Neutropenia or neutrophilia, thrombocytopenia, and disseminated intravascular coagulation

How does an arterial blood gas change during the course of septic shock?

Early shock—respiratory alkalosis, with relative or absolute hypoxemia
Worsening shock—lactic acidosis increases, metabolic acidosis develops and worsens

What are the dermatologic manifestations of sepsis?

Acrocyanosis, necrosis, microemboli, and vasculitis

What dermatologic or soft tissue lesions may result in sepsis?	Cellulitis, erysipelas, fasciitis
What is the differential diagnosis of septic shock?	Cardiogenic, hypovolemic, anaphylactic, and neurogenic shock; pulmonary embolism; tamponade; thyroid storm; adrenal insufficiency
Which CNS infection is most closely associated with shock? What are the responsible agents?	Bacterial meningitis; *Streptococcus pneumoniae* or *Neisseria meningitides*
Is meningismus always present in meningitis?	No. Shock and a petechial rash may be the only presenting features.
Name the most common pulmonary pathology leading to septic shock, and the responsible agents in order of frequency.	Acute bacterial pneumonia. Most frequent causes: *S. pneumoniae*, *Haemophilus influenzae*, *Staphylococcus aureus*, miscellaneous gram-negative bacilli, and *Legionella pneumophila*
What diagnoses are primary considerations for septic shock within the biliary tree?	Suppurative cholangitis; empyema of gallbladder
Women of childbearing age are at particular risk for developing septic shock from what disease processes?	Septic abortion; postpartum endometritis or myometritis; toxic shock syndrome
What is the priority in the management of septic shock?	Airway assessment and management
Name the resuscitation fluid of choice and dosing parameters for initial management of septic shock.	0.9 normal saline or Ringer lactate Rapid infusion of 20 mL/kg for children 500 mL every 5–10 minutes for adults

When do you begin inotropic support?

If no response in hemodynamic status after 3–4 L of fluid; or signs of fluid overload as evidenced by pulmonary edema or elevated CVP

What inotropic agents are used, and what is the dosage?

Dopamine is begun at a rate of 5–20 µg/kg per minute. If no response at 20 µg/kg per minute, add norepinephrine at 0.5–1 µg/min (0.1 µg/kg per minute in pediatric patients), increasing by 1 µg to 2 µg/min every 3–5 minutes, until a systolic blood pressure of 80–100 mm Hg is attained.

What guides your decision to begin, and your choice of, empiric antibiotic therapy?

Begin antibiotics on all septic shock patients. Empiric coverage for gram-negative and gram-positive bacteria is based on source of infection.

CARDIAC ARREST

Cardiac arrest patients present with one of two arrhythmias. Name these rhythms.

Either ventricular fibrillation/pulseless ventricular tachycardia (VF/VT) or non-VF rhythms. Non-VF rhythms include asystole and pulseless electrical activity (PEA).

What is the common treatment for both VF/VT and non-VF cardiac arrest victims?

The initial treatment for cardiac arrest is similar regardless of the underlying rhythm: cardiopulmonary resuscitation, tracheal intubation, vasoconstrictors, and antiarrhythmics. Patients presenting with VF/VT also require defibrillation.

When treating non-VT/VF rhythms (e.g., asystole, PEA), it is crucial to look for potentially reversible causes for the arrest. Name the five Hs and the five Ts one must consider in these patients.

The five Hs: hypovolemia, hypoxia, hydrogen ion (acidosis), hypothermia/hyperthermia, and hypokalemia/hyperkalemia
The five Ts: toxins/tablets (drug overdose), tamponade, tension pneumothorax, thrombosis coronary (acute MI), and thrombosis pulmonary (pulmonary embolism)

What is the vasopressor of choice to be used initially in all cases of cardiac arrest, whether VF/VT or non-VF?

Epinephrine 1 mg IV every 3–5 minutes

When a patient presents with VF/VT cardiac arrest, what is the alternative vasopressor according to the 2000 advanced cardiac life support (ACLS) guidelines?

Vasopressin 40 units IV as a one-time dose. Vasopressin is a class II recommendation (may be helpful, probably not harmful) in the 2000 ACLS international guidelines. It is a potent vasoconstrictor with effects similar to epinephrine; repeat doses are not recommended because of its longer half-life of 10–20 minutes compared to epinephrine's 3- to 5-minute half-life. Epinephrine doses at 1 mg IV every 3–5 minutes may be resumed if no response 5 minutes after administration of vasopressin.

When VF/VT are refractory to vasoconstrictors, according to the ACLS guidelines, which medications should be considered?

Administer alternative antiarrhythmics if no response occurs to antiarrhythmics with defibrillation. Recommended antiarrhythmics: amiodarone 300 mg IV (may be repeated once at dose of 150 mg), or lidocaine 1.0–1.5 mg/kg (repeat dose in 3–5 minutes).

Amiodarone has multiple recommended uses in the 2000 ACLS international guidelines. In which clinical situations is this agent indicated?

VF/pulseless VT, with a dose of 300 mg IV, followed by repeat dose of 150 mg. Also recommended in most of the tachycardia algorithms (e.g., medical cardioversion of atrial fibrillation/flutter or Wolff-Parkinson-White syndrome with rapid ventricular response if duration of onset of <48 hours). Other indications: narrow-complex supraventricular tachycardia unresponsive to vagal maneuvers or adenosine; stable VT if baseline QT interval is not prolonged (may indicate torsades).

What is torsades de pointes?

VT subtype with a gradual alteration in amplitude and direction of electrical activity

Which medications are contraindicated in torsades de pointes?

Medications or toxins that effectively prolong repolarization can precipitate it, as well as hypokalemia. Therefore, avoid any antiarrhythmic that further prolongs repolarization of the heart (QT interval): quinidine, disopyramide, procainamide, phenothiazine, and tricyclic antidepressants.

What is the treatment of choice for torsades de pointes?

The first-line treatment is magnesium sulfate 1–2 g IV over 60–90 minutes, followed by 1–2 g IV per hour. If unsuccessful, give IV isoproterenol at 2–10 μg per minute. Most effective treatment: ventricular pacemaker to overdrive the heart at a rate of 90–120 beats/min.

What is an accelerated idioventricular rhythm (AIVR)?

An arrhythmia that may present following reperfusion therapy. It is characterized by a wide QRS and a regular rate, usually 40–90 beats/min.

AIVR should be treated with which pharmacologic agent?

AIVR requires no treatment. The patient is likely dependent on the rhythm for perfusion; eliminating this with antiarrhythmics could lead to asystole.

What interventions can improve neurologic outcome following adequate resuscitation?

Respiratory and cardiac support is essential. Maintain normal ventilatory rates because hyperventilation can decrease cerebral blood flow, leading to ischemia. Treat hyperthermia and tolerate mild hypothermia because hyperthermia causes an increase in overall oxygen demand.

BURNS

What are the six major types of burns?

Scalds, contact, fire, radiation, chemical, electrical

How are burns classified?

By depth of injury:
    First-degree (superficial)—involves only the epithelium

Second-degree (partial thickness)—extends into, but not beyond, the dermis

Third-degree (full thickness)—total destruction of epidermis, dermis, and dermal appendages (e.g., hair follicles, sweat glands)

Fourth-degree—involves underlying connective tissue, muscle, tendons, bone

How are burns distinguished clinically?

First-degree: intact, erythematous, hypersensitive skin without blister formation (e.g., prolonged sun exposure)

Second-degree: reddened, weepy, blistered, and exquisitely sensitive to touch (e.g., scald injuries, flash burns)

Third-degree: dry, pale, leather-like appearance. Upon closer exam, thrombosed vessels are visible and skin is insensate (e.g., prolonged contact with flames, scalding liquid, or corrosive chemicals).

Describe the three concentric areas of a full-thickness burn that can be identified within 24 hours of injury.

1. **Central zone of coagulation:** area of necrotic cells that were most intimately in contact with the insulting substance. Skin appears white or charred; its blood supply has been destroyed.

2. **Intermediate zone of stasis:** pink or red. May blanch with compression, giving observer the impression that blood supply is intact; however, within 3 days, blood flow ceases and tissue becomes white and leathery as the superficial dermis necroses.

3. **Outer zone of hyperemia:** red, has intact circulation, and heals within 1 week.

How long do burns take to heal? Will they leave a scar?

First-degree burns heal completely without scarring in 3–5 days.

Second-degree burns involving less than half the thickness of dermis heal completely in 1–2 weeks without scarring. Deep second-degree burns involving more than half the dermis heal in 2–4 weeks, but likely produce pigment changes and scarring. Skin grafting may be performed to improve functional and cosmetic outcome; graft sites heal in 2 weeks.

Third-degree burns of >2–3 cm require skin grafting to heal; healing time varies based on patient and graft method.

What is the rule of nines?

A quick assessment tool in which each body part represents 9%, or a multiple of 9%, of total body surface area (TBSA). In an adult, the head is 9%, each arm is 9%, the front and back of the torso are each 18%, and each leg is 18%. The genitalia account for 1%. The rule does not apply to children, whose heads and torsos are proportionally larger.

Define and describe the Parkland formula.

0.4 cc/kg/%TBSA burned × weight (kg). A tool for estimating how much fluid (usually Ringer lactate) beyond normal maintenance a burn patient needs in the first 24 hours after injury to avoid burn shock. Does not apply to patients with first-degree burns. Administer half the total amount over the first 8 hours and half over the last 16 hours.

What is burn shock?

Hypovolemic shock caused by increased fluid losses, secondary to increased capillary permeability induced by profound tissue destruction, and increased evaporative losses due to loss of epithelial boundaries

How can you prevent burn shock?

Adequately hydrate burn patients using the Parkland formula as an initial guide. Ultimately adjust rate of fluid administration to ensure urine output of at least 0.5 mL/kg per hour in adults, and 1 mL/kg per hour in children of <1 year.

What are the indications for intubation of a burn patient?

Airway injury may lead to obstruction in 12–24 hours secondary to airway edema. Immediately intubate patients with stridor, voice changes, or respiratory insufficiency despite delivery of 100% oxygen. Strongly consider early intubation of patients with neck or facial burns, carbonaceous sputum, or singed nasal hairs.

What are the criteria for immediate transfer to a burn center?

Major burn injuries as defined by the American Burn Association require transport to specialized burn centers for definitive care:

> Adults with >20% TBSA partial-thickness burns
>
> Burns involving >10% TBSA in patients <10 years and >55 years old
>
> Anyone with full-thickness burns covering >10% TBSA
>
> Significant burns involving face, hands, feet, perineum, or major joints
>
> Significant chemical burns
>
> High-voltage electrical injuries
>
> Burns complicated by inhalation injury or major trauma
>
> Burns sustained in patients with underlying debilitating illnesses

POISONING

Define poisoning.

Exposure to a chemical substance that impairs the normal functioning of an organism, leading to clinical symptoms

At what age is poisoning most common?

<5 years

When should a diagnosis of poisoning be considered?

In a patient with a known or suspected exposure to a toxin, or in a person with sudden onset of mental status changes, respiratory aberrations, abnormal behavior, shock, autonomic dysfunction, vomiting or diarrhea, dysrhythmia, or metabolic derangements not otherwise explained

How does cholinergic syndrome present, and what drugs cause this?	It arises from stimulation of muscarinic and nicotinic receptors. Remember the mnemonic **SLUDGE**: **S**alivation, **L**acrimation, **U**rination, **D**efecation, **G**astrointestinal cramps, and **E**mesis. Pupils are constricted. Drugs causing it include organophosphates, physostigmine, and nicotine.
How does anticholinergic syndrome present, and what drugs cause this?	"Mad as a hatter, hot as a hare, dry as a bone, red as a beet." Tachycardia, hypertension, and dilated pupils are also seen. Drugs to consider are atropine, scopolamine, cyclic antidepressants, jimsonweed, antihistamines, and *Amanita muscaria* poisoning.
How does sympathomimetic syndrome present, and what drugs cause this?	Increased heart rate and blood pressure, and elevated temperature. The patient is diaphoretic and often agitated, with dilated pupils and dry mouth. Drugs include amphetamines, cocaine, phencyclidine, pseudoephedrine, caffeine, methylphenidate, and theophylline.
How does sympatholytic syndrome present, and what drugs cause this?	It is the opposite of sympathomimetic syndrome. Affected patients have bradycardia, hypotension, and hypothermia, with dry skin, constricted pupils, and absent bowel sounds. May be signs of CNS depression. Think of opioids, alcohol, heroin, barbiturates, benzodiazepines, and clonidine.
How do urine and serum toxicology screens differ?	Other than the differing substrate, urine screens are designed primarily for drugs of abuse, whereas serum tests are for over-the-counter products and alcohol.
When should emesis not be induced?	Think of the five **C**s: **C**oma, **C**onvulsions, **C**austics, **C**yclic antidepressants, and hydro**C**arbons

What are the limitations of gastric lavage?

Ingestion must be recent (within 1–2 hours)

Patient must be able to protect the airway (i.e., no depression of sensorium or potential of seizure)

Patient's age and the size of tube that can therefore be used also limit the ability to extract larger pills.

When should activated charcoal not be used?

If endoscopy is a possibility

Drugs for which there is an oral antidote

Hydrocarbons

Those that do not adsorb to it (heavy metals, lithium, iron, acids, alkalis, alcohols, and cyanide)

OTHER EMERGENCY MEDICINE TOPICS

ALTERED MENTAL STATUS

What three broad categories cause acute altered mental status?

Metabolic/toxic causes (65%), focal structural lesions (33%), and psychiatric causes (2%). A decreased level of consciousness can be caused only by global encephalopathy or focal pressure or damage to the reticular activating system in the medulla and midbrain.

What is the most common nontoxicologic cause of altered mental status in the emergency department?

Hypoglycemia

In what order is orientation usually lost?

1. Orientation to time
2. Orientation to place
3. Orientation to person

What are three nonstructural causes of global disorientation?

Toxic ingestions, metabolic encephalopathy, infections

What features of the history and physical exam help differentiate organic from psychiatric disease?

Organic disease—speech often slowed with poor articulation; delirium; hallucinations predominantly visual
Psychiatric disease—speech usually normal with good articulation; hallucinations usually auditory

What distinguishes delirium from dementia?

Delirium—cognitive impairment that is acute in onset with waxing and waning of symptoms; inability to concentrate is the hallmark characteristic.
Dementia—also marked by cognitive impairment, but onset is much slower with less fluctuation of symptoms.

How common is delirium among elderly patients presenting to the emergency department?

10–25% of elderly patients admitted to the hospital meet criteria for delirium; another 30% develop delirium while hospitalized.

What is the differential diagnosis of altered mental status?

Remember the mnemonic AEIOU TIPS:
    A—alcohol
    E—endocrine, electrolytes, encephalopathy
    I—insulin
    O—opiates, oxygen
    U—uremia
    T—trauma, toxins
    I—infection
    P—psychiatric
    S—seizure, stroke, space-occupying lesion, salicylates (overdose)

When should intubation be considered in a patient with altered mental status?

GCS <9, uncontrolled hyperthermia from toxic causes to allow paralysis; agitation uncontrollable with pharmaceuticals to facilitate diagnostic tests and prevent self-injury; need for gastric lavage; elevated intracranial pressure for hyperventilation

What four empiric therapies can be tried initially?

Remember the mnemonic TONG:
    T—thiamine, 100 mg IV (in adults)
    O—oxygen

N—naloxone, 1–2 mg IV if >5 years, 0.1 mg/kg if 0–5 years

G—glucose, 1 ampule D50 (50 mL 50%) IV in adult, 2–4 mL/kg of D10 IV in infants, and 1–2 mL/kg of D25 IV in children

What are the elements of a good mental status exam?

Appearance, general level of consciousness, orientation, speech, memory, attention and concentration, intelligence, mood, affect, perceptions, judgment and insight, suicidal or homicidal thoughts

What lab studies are helpful to determine cause of altered mental status?

Finger-stick blood sugar, complete blood cell count, Chem 7 panel, calcium, arterial blood gases, carboxyhemoglobin, serum osmolality, blood alcohol, serum and urine drug screens, liver function studies, thyroid, cortisol, urinalysis, CSF

What is the imaging study of choice in the emergent evaluation of altered mental status?

Noncontrast CT of head; identifies intracranial hemorrhage, focal infection, tumor, hydrocephalus, and noninfectious inflammatory disorders.

What is the Glasgow Coma Scale?

Widely used method of categorizing patients with altered mental status. Although initially designed for evaluating traumatic brain-injured patients, it is commonly used to evaluate any patient with altered mental status. Maximum score is 15; minimum score is 3.

What is the difference between decorticate and decerebrate posturing?

Decorticate posturing: flexion of upper extremities and extension of lower extremities, caused by lesions to the cerebrum with the brain stem intact.

Decerebrate posturing: extension of both upper and lower extremities caused by lesions to the midbrain and pons; usually carries a grave prognosis.

How does pupil size help your diagnosis?	Small or pinpoint pupils could indicate narcotic overdose, cholinergic crisis, or pontine infarct. Dilated pupils may indicate sympathomimetic overdose (e.g., amphetamines); could also result from anticholinergic toxicity or structural pressure on brain stem or cranial nerves (specifically cranial nerve III).
How does pupil reactivity help your diagnosis?	Pupil reactivity is usually preserved in comas caused by metabolic causes. If pupils are unreactive, it is usually from an intracranial structural cause or direct eye injury or toxin. Fixed and dilated pupils could indicate loss of brain stem function or increased intracranial pressure.

SYNCOPE

Define syncope.	A brief lapse of consciousness caused by transient cerebral hypoxia
Name common causes for the following types of syncope.	
Situational	Micturition, defecation, coughing, or swallowing
Orthostatic hypotension	Dehydration and hypovolemia
Vasovagal	Fear, excitement, fatigue, and stress
Metabolic	Drug toxicity, hypoglycemia (not technically syncope), and hypoxia
Neurologic	Seizures (not technically syncope) and cerebral vascular accidents
Psychiatric	Conversion and anxiety disorders
Decreased cardiac output	Myocardial infarction, pulmonary embolism, hypertrophic cardiomyopathy, valvular stenosis, aortic dissection, and pericardial tamponade
Bradyarrhythmias	Sick sinus syndrome, atrioventricular node disease, conduction system disease, and pacemaker malfunction
Tachyarrhythmias	Supraventricular or ventricular tachycardia

How do the following types of syncope present?

Cardiac
Sudden onset, often with rapid recovery; may accompany chest pain

Vasovagal
Precipitating stressful event followed by nausea, diaphoresis, and syncope

Orthostatic
Prolonged sitting or lying down, precipitating syncope on standing

What physical exam data are especially helpful?
Vital signs with orthostatics and complete neurologic, cardiac, and pulmonary exam

What simple physical exam maneuvers help make the diagnosis?
Valsalva maneuver and carotid sinus massage (reveals carotid sinus hypersensitivity)

What routine tests should be included in the workup?
ECG, complete blood cell count (anemia), and glucose (hypoglycemia)

What additional test should be ordered if the patient has local neurologic findings?
Head CT scan

What additional lab test is important in young women?
Pregnancy test

What further testing is available if initial workup is negative?
Echocardiography, ambulatory cardiac monitoring (Holter), electrophysiologic studies, tilt-table testing, and neurologic or psychiatric testing

How is syncope diagnosed?
History, presentation, supportive lab and radiographic studies

Which conditions are life threatening and require hospitalization for further workup and treatment?
Ischemic heart disease, valvular disease, abnormal ECG, severe anemia, severe hypovolemia (hypotension), suspected cerebral vascular accident (or transient ischemic attack), suspected new onset seizure

**How are the following
non-life-threatening causes
of syncope treated?**

Situational	Behavior modification (e.g., urinate sitting down), stool softeners, and cough suppressants as needed
Orthostatic	Rehydration
Vasovagal	Avoid situations that precipitate syncope.
Diabetic hypoglycemia	Modify therapy.
Neurologic	Neuro consult
Psychiatric	Outpatient therapy

5

Gastroenterology

UPPER GI BLEEDING

AORTOENTERIC FISTULA

Define aortoenteric fistula.	Forms after 2% of abdominal aortic grafts; usually between upper portion of graft and distal duodenum
What is the main risk factor?	Abdominal aortic aneurysm repair in previous 4 years
How does it typically present?	With a "sentinel"—nonexsanguinating initial bleed, melena, hematemesis, or chronic intermittent bleeding; then massive life-threatening hemorrhage
How is it diagnosed?	Angiography or abdominal computed tomography (CT) scan
What is the treatment strategy?	Stabilize with fluids, blood transfusions; then surgery

ANGIODYSPLASIA (ARTERIOVENOUS MALFORMATIONS, VASCULAR ECTASIAS)

Define angiodysplasia.	Abnormal arteriovenous communication
Why does it occur?	Possibly from chronic colonic muscular contractions obstructing venous mucosal drainage
What are the risk factors?	Age >60 years, chronic renal failure, valvular heart disease (especially aortic stenosis), hereditary hemorrhagic telangiectasia, scleroderma
What is the most common anatomic location?	Colon (cecum and ascending colon)

Where else are they found in patients with chronic liver failure?	Stomach and duodenum
How does angiodysplasia commonly present?	Recurrent self-limited hematochezia, melena, or hematemesis; not hemodynamically significant
How is the diagnosis made?	Endoscopically
How is active bleeding treated?	Endoscopic coagulation
What medical therapy decreases recurrent bleeds?	Combined estrogen and progesterone

ESOPHAGEAL CANCER

Name the two most common cancers of the esophagus.	Squamous cell carcinoma (most common) and adenocarcinoma
Incidence of which type is rising in the United States?	Adenocarcinoma (esophageal; gastric cardia), at a rate of 4–10% annually
What are the risk factors associated with squamous cell carcinoma?	Tobacco and alcohol (main risk factors); history of achalasia, head and neck squamous cell cancer, tylosis, lye ingestion, ionizing radiation, Plummer-Vinson syndrome
Describe the premalignant condition associated with adenocarcinoma.	Barrett esophagus, with intestinal metaplasia of esophageal squamous mucosa
Does the incidence of squamous and adenocarcinoma differ by gender and ethnicity?	Both types more common in males; squamous cell more common in African Americans; adenocarcinoma more common in Caucasians
How does esophageal cancer present?	Typically, dysphagia, odynophagia, anorexia, weight loss; also cough, hoarseness, bone pain, nausea, vomiting, hematemesis

What is the diagnostic approach?	Initially, barium esophagram and endoscopy with biopsy
What additional tests are performed for cancer staging?	CT scan of chest and abdomen, endoscopic ultrasound (US) scan, bone scan
What staging system is used for esophageal cancer?	TNM (Tumor, Node, Metastasis)
What is the treatment strategy for early cancer without nodal involvement?	Surgical resection
What is the treatment strategy for locally advanced disease?	Neoadjuvant chemotherapy and radiation therapy followed by surgical resection
How are patients with widespread disease managed?	Palliative treatment: expandable metal stents; laser or bipolar electrocoagulation
With therapy, what is the 5-year survival?	Early-stage cancer: 30–45% Advanced cancer: 5–7%
Is there a role for surveillance in patients with Barrett esophagus?	Yes; endoscopy with biopsy every 2 years to detect high-grade dysplasia

ESOPHAGITIS AND ESOPHAGEAL ULCERS

Name the four most common causes of esophagitis and esophageal ulcers.	Gastroesophageal reflux, radiation, pill-induced chemical injury, infections
What is the role of endoscopy in diagnosing esophagitis?	Most sensitive and specific method, with mucosal biopsy/brush cytology
What causes gastroesophageal reflux disease (GERD)?	An imbalance between the aggressive forces in refluxate and the esophageal defenses (i.e., antireflux barriers, luminal clearance mechanisms, tissue resistance)

What are the common symptoms of GERD?

Heartburn, regurgitation, water brash; worse on bending or lying down
Severe disease: bleeding and dysphagia

What are the extraesophageal manifestations of GERD?

Laryngitis, asthma, chronic cough, hoarseness, aspiration pneumonia
Less common: damage to dental enamel; gingivitis

Which diagnostic tests are helpful in GERD?

Single best test: therapeutic trial of proton pump inhibitors
Standard for confirming pathologic reflux: ambulatory 24-hour intraesophageal pH monitoring

What is the treatment strategy for GERD?

Early endoscopy for dysphagia, odynophagia, weight loss, or gastrointestinal (GI) bleeding; otherwise, empiric therapy

What is the medical management of GERD?

Lifestyle modification, proton pump inhibitors for 8–12 weeks
Prokinetic agents if nonresponsive to therapy
Maintenance therapy needed in some patients

When is surgery warranted in patients with GERD?

If medical therapy fails

What surgical procedure is used most commonly?

Nissen fundoplication

What are the possible complications of GERD?

Peptic strictures; Barrett esophagus (increases risk of adenocarcinoma)

How does esophagitis present if caused by radiation, pill injury, or infection?

Dysphagia, odynophagia, or both
Rarely, bleeding, tracheobronchial fistulae

Who is at risk for esophageal infections?

Immunocompromised individuals

What kinds of esophageal infections occur in immunocompromised persons?	Fungal, viral, bacterial, and mycobacterial
How is esophagitis secondary to infections treated?	Fluconazole for *Candida* infection, acyclovir for herpes simplex; 2 weeks each Ganciclovir or foscarnet for cytomegalovirus, 4 weeks
What are idiopathic esophageal ulcers?	Large, deep ulcers with no specific cause
What patients typically get idiopathic esophageal ulcers?	Up to 40% of those with human immunodeficiency virus (HIV)
How are idiopathic ulcers treated?	Prednisone and thalidomide

ESOPHAGEAL VARICES

What causes esophageal varices to develop?	With portal hypertension, extrahepatic collateral venous channels between portal and systemic circulation dilate and form varices
What is the common anatomic location of varices?	Anywhere in the GI tract
In what locations are varices more likely to bleed?	Distal esophagus; proximal stomach
What is the role of primary prophylaxis in variceal bleeding?	β-Blockers decrease incidence of first bleed in moderate to large varices; if patient intolerant to β-blockers, give long-acting nitrates
Name two contraindications to β-blocker use.	Bronchospasm, cardiac arrhythmias

What are the risk factors for variceal bleeding?

Hepatic venous pressure gradient >12 mm Hg
Large varices
Red color (indicates thin overlying mucosa)
Severe liver disease (Child score)

How common is variceal bleeding? How does it present?

30–50% bleed at some time, presenting with hematemesis of bright red blood or coffee-ground emesis, with or without melena or hematochezia

What is the diagnostic test of choice?

Upper endoscopy

What is the initial therapy?

Fluid resuscitation, then octreotide infusion (first-line agent) to reduce portal pressure, or vasopressin (use with nitroglycerin in patients with coronary artery disease)

What is the typical dose of octreotide?

50-μg bolus, then a drip at 25–50 μg/h

What is the endoscopic management of acute variceal bleeding?

Sclerosant injection or band ligation

If *massive* bleeding continues, what therapy should be considered next?

Temporary placement of Sengstaken-Blakemore tube

When is transjugular intrahepatic portosystemic shunt indicated in management of variceal bleeding?

Uncontrollable acute or significant recurrent bleeding despite endoscopy and medication, with or without placement of Sengstaken-Blakemore tube

What is the prognosis?

The most serious complication of portal hypertension; 40–70% mortality within 6 weeks of acute bleed

GASTRIC CANCER

What are the risk factors for gastric cancer?	Family history, heredity (Asian Americans, Hispanics, and African Americans), gastric polyps, Billroth II surgery, and possibly chronic *Helicobacter pylori* gastritis
What is the most common histologic type of gastric cancer?	Adenocarcinoma (90–95%)
Name two other less common types of gastric cancer.	Leiomyosarcoma (common cause of massive upper GI bleed) and lymphoma
How does the patient with advanced disease present?	Weight loss, abdominal pain (often constant), dyspepsia, early satiety, anorexia, hematemesis, melena
What are the associated lab findings?	Iron deficiency anemia (chronic blood loss), abnormal liver function tests (if metastasis), positive guaiac (50%) and carcinoembryonic antigen (CEA) tests
How is gastric cancer diagnosed?	Upper GI series or endoscopy with biopsy
What additional radiographic studies are performed?	Abdominal and chest CT, for staging
What is the therapy?	Surgery for localized disease; chemotherapy and radiation as adjunctive or palliative therapy
What is the overall survival rate at 5 years?	15%

HEMORRHAGIC GASTRITIS

What is hemorrhagic gastritis?	Inflammatory hemorrhagic mucosal erosion in the stomach, caused by chemical agents or physiologic stress eroding viable tissue

What are the more common risk factors?

Aspirin, nonsteroidal anti-inflammatory drugs [NSAIDs (inhibit prostaglandin synthesis)], alcohol

What are the less common risk factors?

Ischemia, bile acid reflux, physiologic stress, organ system failure, portal hypertension, radiation, trauma [endoscopy, nasogastric (NG) tubes]

What are the signs and symptoms?

Often asymptomatic; may present with dyspepsia

Mild—epigastric pain, anorexia, nausea, vomiting

Severe (rare)—hematemesis, coffee-ground emesis, bloody aspirate in NG tube, melena

What will the physical exam reveal if blood loss is significant?

Pallor, diaphoresis, tachycardia, hypotension, dizziness

What lab tests are helpful?

Hematocrit (anemia), occult blood in stool (guaiac test)

What is the most sensitive diagnostic test? Why?

Endoscopy (upper GI series can miss mild to moderate changes)

What else should be done during endoscopy?

Antral biopsy for *H. pylori*

What distinguishes the erosions of gastritis from those of peptic ulcer disease?

Erosions in gastritis <5 mm in diameter and do not extend through muscularis mucosa

What is the initial therapy in massive GI bleeds?

Stabilize with fluids and packed red blood cells

Continued bleeding—intravenous (IV) vasopressin or endoscopic control

Possibly surgery

What is the treatment for hemorrhagic gastritis?

Antisecretory therapy [histamine (H_2) receptor antagonists or proton pump inhibitor]

Treat for *H. pylori* if present
Sucralfate, especially when NSAID or
   stress induced
Discontinue alcohol and chronic
   NSAID use

What prophylactic treatment is recommended for patients in the intensive care unit?

H_2 receptor antagonists or sucralfate

HEMATOBILIA

Define hematobilia.

Upper GI bleeding from the common bile duct that exits the ampulla (rare)

What are the risk factors?

Gallstones; cancer in the common bile duct

How does hematobilia present?

Jaundice or biliary colic and active GI bleeding

How is it diagnosed?

Endoscopy (reveals blood from ampulla)
Endoscopic retrograde cholangiopancreatography (ERCP; visualizes lesion)

What is the treatment if gallstones are found?

Endoscopic removal of gallstones; then laparoscopic cholecystectomy

What is the treatment if cancer is found?

Surgical consult to determine resectability (most are not); palliative care

MALLORY-WEISS TEARS

What is a Mallory-Weiss tear?

Linear, nonpenetrating mucosal laceration (up to 3 × 20 mm) at the gastroesophageal junction; accounts for 5–15% of upper GI bleeding

What is the cause?

Sudden rise of intra-abdominal pressure (e.g., vomiting, retching, coughing)

What are the risk factors for developing a Mallory-Weiss tear?	Most common—alcohol binges Retching or vomiting Hiatal hernia
Describe the typical patient with a Mallory-Weiss tear.	Male; mean age 40 years
How does it present?	Typically, repeated violent retching, vomiting, or coughing followed by hematemesis; up to 50% have hematemesis on first emesis.
How is the diagnosis made?	Endoscopy
What are the treatment options?	Most stop bleeding spontaneously. If actively bleeding, endoscopically inject 1:10,000 epinephrine, or cauterize.
When is surgery warranted?	Uncontrollable bleeding

PEPTIC ULCER DISEASE

Define peptic ulcer disease.	Lesion in gastric or duodenal mucosa; arises when normal mucosal defenses are weakened by aggressive luminal factors (e.g., acid or pepsin)
Name some common risk factors.	Previous ulcer, chronic NSAID or aspirin use, alcohol, cigarette smoking, physiologic stress (e.g., shock, sepsis), gastrinoma
How do duodenal ulcers present?	Gnawing or burning epigastric pain, relieved by food, recurring 1–3 hours later; nocturnal awakenings
How do gastric ulcers present?	Gnawing or burning epigastric pain, not relieved by food
Which ulcer type is more common?	Duodenal

What findings indicate active bleeding?

Melena or hematemesis, orthostatic symptoms, anemia

What is _H. pylori_?

A noninvasive, gram-negative, urease-producing bacillus

What is the significance of _H. pylori_?

Colonizes antral mucosa in 100% of duodenal and 70–80% of gastric ulcers Associated with higher risk of ulcer recurrence if untreated

Who is at increased risk of _H. pylori_ infection?

Patients 40–50 years old; poorer patients

What may be found on physical exam?

Abdominal tenderness; weight loss; melena or hematemesis in active bleeding; if perforated, sudden severe pain radiating to the back with peritoneal signs

What lab tests should be performed?

Complete blood cell (CBC) count (anemia), pancreatic enzymes, free air x-ray series (if perforation suspected); gastrin level (if gastrinoma suspected)

How is the diagnosis made?

Upper endoscopy to visualize ulcer Antral biopsy, culture for _H. pylori_ Upper GI series if endoscopy fails

What else must be done for all gastric ulcers?

Biopsy to rule out gastric cancer (5% of cases); follow-up biopsies until complete healing is documented

What is the initial therapy in unstable patients?

Fluid resuscitation; packed red blood cells

What is required if the patient is unstable and actively bleeding?

Emergent endoscopy to band or sclerose bleeding vessels; if this fails, emergent surgical gastrectomy

What is the medical treatment?

H_2-receptor antagonists (e.g., cimetidine, ranitidine) and treat for _H. pylori_ if present [(1) amoxicillin, metronidazole, and bismuth, or (2) omeprazole and amoxicillin] for 4–6 weeks; then discontinue and observe for recurrence

What drug can be substituted for amoxicillin if allergic to penicillin?	Tetracycline or clarithromycin
What drug is added if the patient must continue NSAID use and has a high risk of bleeding?	Misoprostol
When is Misoprostol contraindicated? Why?	Women at risk for pregnancy or pregnant; drug causes uterine contractions (abortion risk)
What antiulcer medication is often used in pregnant women? Why?	Sucralfate; coats the ulcer and is not absorbed.
What additional treatment is recommended for all patients?	Stop smoking, drinking, chronic aspirin and NSAID use

LOWER GI BLEEDING

AMOEBIC COLITIS

What is amoebic colitis?	Infectious colitis caused by *Entamoeba histolytica*, an intestinal protozoan
What are the risk factors?	Recent travel (Asia, South Africa, Mexico); male homosexuality; residing in areas with poor sanitation
How does it present?	Abdominal pain and tenderness, rectal pain, diarrhea, bloody stools, possibly systemic toxicity
How is it diagnosed?	Stool studies for ova and parasites Amoebic serologic tests Rectosigmoidoscopy with biopsy
What is the treatment?	High-dose metronidazole (Flagyl)

ANGIODYSPLASIA (ARTERIOVENOUS MALFORMATIONS, VASCULAR ECTASIAS)

(See review of Angiodysplasia, pages 113–114, under Upper GI Bleeding.)

What diagnostic studies are recommended?	Endoscopy, for simultaneous diagnosis and treatment; if endoscopy fails, angiogram
What local agent is used during endoscopy to control bleeding?	Vasoconstrictors (e.g., vasopressin)
What therapy is recommended for massive lower GI bleeding?	Endoscopic fulguration with angiographic control
What medical therapy may decrease recurrent bleeds?	Combined estrogen and progesterone

COLORECTAL CANCER

What is colorectal cancer?	Second most common cancer in United States; usually arises from adenomatous villous polyps (villous polyps are more often malignant than tubular polyps)
What are the risk factors?	Family history of colon cancer, previous adenomatous polyps, long-standing ulcerative colitis, other adenocarcinomas (e.g., breast, ovarian)
What are the colon cancer screening recommendations for patients with no risk factors?	Digital rectal exam, age 40; guaiac test or sigmoidoscopy, age 50, and then every 3–5 years
How does colon cancer present?	Recent change in bowel habits, narrow-caliber stools, abdominal pain, rectal bleeding, weight loss
How is the diagnosis made?	Colonoscopy with biopsy

What lab test results support the diagnosis?	Low mean cell volume (MCV), guaiac-positive stool
After the diagnosis, what other radiographic studies are often performed?	Chest x-ray, bone scan (if patient complains of bone pain), abdominal CT scan (if liver function test results abnormal)
What is the treatment?	Endoscopically resect polyps Surgically resect cancer (if rectal, consider preoperative radiation therapy) Adjuvant therapy [5-fluorouracil (5-FU) and leucovorin] in locally advanced and metastatic disease Routine endoscopic surveillance
What lab test is used to monitor disease activity?	CEA level

DIVERTICULOSIS

What is diverticulosis?	Pouchlike herniation of the colon's muscular layer
What are the risk factors?	Age >60 years
What are the symptoms?	Painless rectal bleeding (large volume, bright red to maroon blood); chronic constipation; postprandial crampy pain in left lower quadrant; dark red stool; dizziness (if hemodynamically unstable)
What is the common anatomic location of bleeding?	Sigmoid colon
Where is the bleeding source, usually?	On a diverticular arteriole; often brisk
What basic physical exam studies should be done?	Vital signs for orthostatics; stool guaiac test

What signifies a positive orthostatic test?	Supine to upright position causes pulse to increase >20 beats/min or systolic blood pressure to decrease >10 beats/min
What laboratory tests should be ordered?	CBC count, type and cross match
What diagnostic studies should be ordered? Why?	Proctosigmoidoscopy or colonoscopy: Identify bleeding as left sided Check for other lesions
Can proctosigmoidoscopy or colonoscopy usually reveal the source of bleeding?	No; bleeding obscures the visual field
What is the therapy?	If hemodynamically stable—supportive; bleeding subsides spontaneously in up to 90% of cases If unstable—angiographic control with intra-arterial vasopressin Recurrent bleeding despite therapy requires surgery
What is the prognosis?	80% of patients have only one episode

HEMORRHOIDS

What is a hemorrhoid?	Swelling due to dilatation of a blood vessel at anus, caused most likely by increased vascular pressure
What are the risk factors?	Straining at stool, constipation, prolonged sitting, congestive heart failure, portal hypertension, pregnancy, obesity, low-fiber diet
How does the patient present?	History of chronic constipation, hemorrhoids, painless bright red rectal bleeding (visible on toilet paper, stool, or in toilet bowl), anal pruritus

What might the rectal exam reveal?	Bluish tense lumps of skin; may be painful (external hemorrhoids are painful; internal ones are not)
What diagnostic study is ordered?	Proctosigmoidoscopy
What is the treatment strategy?	If asymptomatic—no therapy needed If symptomatic—sitz baths, stool softeners, high-fiber diet, increased fluid intake, topical ointments, oral analgesics if needed
What is the treatment in severe cases?	Banding, ligation, and cauterization

INFECTIOUS COLITIS

What are the risk factors for infectious colitis?	Recent travel; contact with infected persons
How does it present?	Abrupt onset of fever, abdominal pain, GI bleeding; toxic appearance
How is it diagnosed?	Stool culture, proctosigmoidoscopy or colonoscopy
What organisms commonly cause infectious bloody diarrhea?	*Shigella* and *Campylobacter* species, and enterohemorrhagic *Escherichia coli*
What is the treatment?	Antibiotics (start ciprofloxacin while awaiting culture)

INFLAMMATORY BOWEL DISEASE

What is inflammatory bowel disease?	Chronic, episodic inflammatory disease of the intestine
What is the main risk factor?	Family history
What are the two common types of inflammatory bowel disease?	Ulcerative colitis and Crohn's disease

What are the characteristic symptoms of ulcerative colitis?

Bloody diarrhea (classic), tenesmus, severe abdominal pain, fever, chills, weight loss, anemia

What are the classic symptoms of Crohn's disease?

Nonbloody diarrhea, severe abdominal pain, anorexia, weight loss, fever, vomiting

What extraintestinal clues suggest inflammatory bowel disease?

Aphthous oral ulcers, corneal ulcers, uveitis, arthritis, erythema nodosum

What diagnostic study is ordered?

Proctosigmoidoscopy or colonoscopy with biopsy; barium x-ray if Crohn's disease suspected

What is the typical radiographic appearance of Crohn's disease?

Skip lesions, cobblestoning, aphthous ulcers

What other test must be ordered in ulcerative colitis? Why?

Stool cultures, to rule out infectious diarrhea

What is the characteristic distribution in Crohn's disease?

Asymmetric disease in any region of GI tract from mouth to anus, but usually not the rectum; terminal ileum in 70% of cases

What is the characteristic distribution in ulcerative colitis?

Starts in rectum; spreads proximally in symmetric, continuous way

Describe two serious complications of ulcerative colitis.

Toxic megacolon (increased risk of septicemia, perforation, death)
Increased risk of colon cancer in long-standing cases

Name four serious complications of Crohn's disease.

Abscess, fistulas, electrolyte imbalance, perforation

What medications are used to decrease abdominal pain and diarrhea?

Anticholinergics, antidiarrheal drugs (Lomotil or loperamide)

What medications are used to treat mild or moderately active disease and to maintain remission?	Sulfasalazine (decreases chronic inflammation); mesalamine (if intolerant to sulfasalazine)
What drug can be added for acute exacerbations?	Oral and topical glucocorticoids
When is surgery warranted in ulcerative colitis?	Life-threatening conditions (severe ongoing hemorrhage, toxic megacolon, cancer)
When might surgery be considered in Crohn's disease?	After medical therapy has failed in treating obstruction, serious complications, or severe ongoing hemorrhage
What is the curative treatment for ulcerative colitis?	Total proctocolectomy and ileostomy
How is toxic megacolon treated?	Nothing by mouth (NPO); IV antibiotics (ampicillin and gentamicin), hydration, steroids Consider total colectomy if medical therapy fails after 48 hours

ISCHEMIC BOWEL DISEASE

What is ischemic bowel disease?	Decreased blood supply to small intestine, colon, or both
What are the risk factors?	Older age, atherosclerotic disease, peripheral vascular disease, hypercoagulable states
How does the patient present?	Low-grade fever, bloody diarrhea or hematochezia, left lower quadrant tenderness
What diagnostic study is ordered? Why?	Flexible sigmoidoscopy or barium enema; shows colitic changes
What risk is associated with sigmoidoscopy?	Perforation

What is the therapy for ischemic bowel disease?	Correct underlying causes; no specific therapy

RADIATION ENTERITIS

What are the risk factors for radiation enteritis?	Radiation exposure; history of cancer (prostate, cervical, uterine) or abdominal lymphoma
How long after radiation therapy can enteritis occur?	Weeks to years
How does radiation enteritis present?	Bleeding, diarrhea, abdominal pain
How is it diagnosed?	Proctosigmoidoscopy or colonoscopy
What is the treatment?	Sulfasalazine, topical steroids Mesalamine (if intolerant to sulfasalazine)

DIARRHEA

ACUTE NONINFLAMMATORY DIARRHEA

What is the definition of acute diarrhea?	Stool >150 mL/day, for <3 weeks
What toxin-producing bacteria can cause it?	Enterotoxigenic *E. coli* (ETEC), *Staphylococcus aureus*, *Bacillus cereus*, *Clostridium perfringens*, and *Vibrio cholerae*
What other organisms can cause it?	Viruses (Norwalk and *Rotavirus*) and protozoans (*Giardia*)
How does noninflammatory diarrhea present?	Watery, nonbloody diarrhea with cramps, bloating, nausea, vomiting; no fever or leukocytosis
What organism is associated with recent travel (especially to Mexico)?	ETEC

What organism is associated with food poisoning?	*S. aureus*
What two organisms characteristically are associated with vomiting?	*S. aureus*; viruses
Which organism can be sexually transmitted?	*Giardia* species
Which organism is associated with seafood ingestion?	*Vibrio cholerae*
What lab tests should be performed in a patient with severe diarrhea who appears dehydrated?	Serum electrolyte levels
How is the diagnosis made?	Stool exam negative for leukocytes and blood
What is the treatment?	Oral rehydration and antidiarrheal agents (loperamide)

INFECTIOUS INFLAMMATORY DIARRHEA

What cytotoxin-producing bacteria cause infectious inflammatory diarrhea?	Enterohemorrhagic *E. coli* 0157:H7 (EHEC), *Vibrio parahaemolyticus*, *Clostridium difficile*
What mucosal invasive bacteria can cause it?	*Shigella* and *Salmonella* species, *Campylobacter jejuni*, and enteroinvasive *E. coli* (EIEC)
What other organisms can cause it?	Viruses (cytomegalovirus) and protozoans (*E. histolytica*)
How does inflammatory diarrhea present?	Fever and bloody diarrhea
What organism is associated with a dysentery-like illness days after food ingestion?	*Shigella* species

Which organism is associated with dairy products or eggs?

Salmonella species

Which organism is often associated with food poisoning?

Campylobacter species

Which organism is associated with recent travel (especially to Asia, India, and South and Central America)?

E. histolytica

Which organism is associated with antibiotic use and pseudomembranous colitis in hospitals?

C. difficile

Which organism is associated with contaminated meat products and hemolytic-uremic syndrome?

EHEC 0157:H7

Which organism is common in immunocompromised and HIV-infected patients?

Cytomegalovirus

How is infectious diarrhea diagnosed?

Positive test for fecal leukocytes

How are infections with *Shigella*, *Salmonella*, *Campylobacter*, and EHEC 0157:H7 diagnosed?

Stool culture

How is *E. histolytica* diagnosed?

Wet-mount exam of stool for amebiasis

How is *C. difficile* diagnosed?

C. difficile toxin in stool or demonstration of pseudomembranes on sigmoidoscopy

How is *Giardia* diagnosed?	Stool parasite exam; if negative, duodenal aspirate exam
What is the treatment for *Giardia*?	Rehydration; empiric antibiotic treatment with ciprofloxacin, trimethoprim-sulfamethoxazole, or erythromycin while awaiting culture results
What is the first-line treatment for *C. difficile*?	Metronidazole
What is the second-line treatment for *C. difficile*?	Vancomycin
What is the treatment for infections with *Salmonella*, *Shigella*, and *Campylobacter* species?	Ciprofloxacin
What is the treatment for cytomegalovirus?	Ganciclovir
What is the treatment for *E. histolytica*?	Metronidazole

HEPATIC INFLAMMATION

ALCOHOLIC LIVER DISEASE

What quantity of alcohol significantly increases risk for alcoholic liver disease?	120 g alcohol (8 oz 100-proof whiskey, 30 oz wine, eight 12-oz beers) daily for >10 years
What sex is at greater risk? Why?	Women, in part due to decreased levels of gastric mucosal alcohol dehydrogenase
How can alcoholic liver disease present?	Fatty liver, hepatitis, or cirrhosis (irreversible disease)
How does fatty liver commonly present?	Usually asymptomatic; may be mild liver enzyme abnormalities and hepatomegaly

How does alcoholic hepatitis present early in the disease?	Usually asymptomatic; abnormal liver enzyme tests
What signs and symptoms may appear as alcoholic hepatitis progresses?	Fever, jaundice, abdominal pain, anorexia, nausea, vomiting, weight loss
What must be ruled out if the patient presents with fever, right upper quadrant pain, and jaundice?	Acute cholecystitis or cholangitis
What tests should be ordered to rule this out?	Hepatobiliary ultrasound; if negative, hepatoiminodiacetic acid (HIDA) scan
How does alcoholic cirrhosis commonly present?	Weakness, fatigue, weight loss, jaundice, hepatomegaly, ascites, palmar erythema, spider angiomata, varices, testicular atrophy
What abnormal lab test results suggest alcoholic hepatitis?	Elevated aspartate aminotransferase [AST ($<$500 μ/L)]; AST:alanine aminotransferase (ALT) ratio ($>$2:1); mean cell volume (MCV); white blood cell (WBC) count; and bilirubin
How is the diagnosis made?	History, presentation, liver enzyme tests; liver biopsy confirms it
What does liver biopsy show?	Fat, polymorphonuclear neutrophils (PMN), and Mallory hyaline
What is the therapy?	Discontinue all alcoholic beverages Give vitamin and nutritional support
Define severe alcoholic hepatitis.	4.6 times prothrombin time (PT) (Δ sec) plus bilirubin $>$32
What medical therapy should be considered in encephalopathic patients with severe disease?	Short course of prednisone

When is transplant recommended?	End-stage cirrhotic liver disease after at least 6 months abstinence from alcohol

α_1-ANTITRYPSIN DEFICIENCY

What is α_1-antitrypsin?	Plasma protein produced in the liver that inhibits proteolytic enzymes (e.g., trypsin)
Name three liver diseases that patients with α_1-antitrypsin deficiency are at risk of developing.	Hepatitis, cirrhosis, hepatocellular carcinoma
Name two other organs that can be affected.	Lungs, pancreas
Do all patients with liver disease have the associated pulmonary emphysema?	No
What tests strongly suggest the diagnosis?	Positive ZZ genotype test and low levels of α_1-antitrypsin (low levels alone not diagnostic; may be heterozygous)
How is the diagnosis confirmed?	Liver biopsy
What is the treatment?	Supportive Consider liver transplant in end-stage liver disease
What additional advantage does transplant offer?	Curative—corrects underlying metabolic defect

AUTOIMMUNE HEPATITIS

Who is at risk for autoimmune hepatitis?	Women predominantly, but both sexes at any age
Name three possible disease presentations.	Asymptomatic, acute, chronic (one-third each)

How do symptomatic patients usually present?	Insidious onset (25% abrupt) of malaise, anorexia, amenorrhea, possibly progressive jaundice
What other extrahepatic autoimmune findings may be found?	Rash, arthritis, thyroiditis, hemolytic anemia, glomerulonephritis
Name four associated lab findings that help make the diagnosis.	Any or all of the following may be positive: anti–smooth muscle antibody, antinuclear antibody, hypergammaglobulinemia (IgG), and anti–liver-kidney microsomal antibody
What diagnostic procedure supports the diagnosis?	Liver biopsy
What is the first-line treatment?	Oral prednisone with or without azathioprine; gradually taper dose of prednisone as serum aminotransferase levels decrease
Why is azathioprine useful?	To facilitate tapering steroid To decrease glucocorticoid-related side effects of prednisone
What maintenance therapy may be needed to prevent relapses?	Low-dose prednisone or azathioprine, or both

DRUG-INDUCED HEPATITIS

Name some dose-dependent hepatotoxins.	Most common—acetaminophen Less common—alcohol, carbon tetrachloride, phosphorus
Name common idiosyncratic (not dose-dependent, difficult to predict patients at risk) hepatotoxins.	Isoniazid, phenytoin, methyldopa, halothane, valproic acid, nitrofurantoin, ketoconazole, diclofenac
How might drug-induced hepatitis present?	Fever, rash, arthralgias, fatigue. May be asymptomatic. Jaundice may evolve.

How does acetaminophen toxicity present	
0–24 hours after ingestion?	Nausea, abdominal pain, lethargy
24–48 hours after ingestion?	Extremely elevated AST, ALT (often >10,000), bilirubin, and PT
3–4 days after ingestion?	Progressive hepatic encephalopathy (confusion, lethargy, coma)
What is a common associated lab finding?	Elevated lactate dehydrogenase (LDH)
Who is at increased risk of fulminant hepatic failure?	Patients who drink alcohol daily and also take acetaminophen in therapeutic doses
What is the treatment for acetaminophen toxicity?	Gastric lavage, activated charcoal, and N-acetylcysteine (Mucomyst). Most effective if given early after ingestion.
What other treatment is available?	Discontinue medication. Consider liver transplant if patient develops fulminant hepatic failure and has no response to N-acetylcysteine.

HEMOCHROMATOSIS

Define hemochromatosis.	Inherited autosomal recessive disorder of iron metabolism; results in excess iron deposits throughout body
Describe the historical presentation.	Hepatomegaly, tanned (bronze) skin, diabetes, cardiomyopathy, arthritis, hypogonadism
How do most patients currently present?	Asymptomatic
Why is it more common in young and middle-aged men?	Women are protected (due to menstruation) until menopause.
What lab test results suggest the diagnosis?	Fasting serum transferrin saturation >45%; positive C282Y (Hfe) gene mutation

What is the therapy?	Phlebotomy at regular intervals removes excess iron Genetic counseling
What is the medical treatment for patients who cannot tolerate phlebotomy?	Deferoxamine (iron-chelating agent)
What are patients at risk for despite adequate therapy?	Hepatocellular carcinoma, but only if cirrhosis has evolved

HEPATITIS A

What causes hepatitis A?	Hepatitis A virus (HAV)
How is it usually transmitted?	Fecal-oral route from contaminated food or water
What are the risk factors?	Recent travel to endemic areas, children in day care, eating raw shellfish
What is the incubation period?	2–6 weeks
How does it present?	Often asymptomatic; may be prodrome of nausea, anorexia, malaise, then dark urine, jaundice (more likely in adults), abdominal pain
What lab tests should be performed?	HAV IgM and IgG serum antibody, AST, ALT, alkaline phosphatase, bilirubin
What is indicated by a positive result in	
HAV IgM serum antibody test?	Diagnostic for acute hepatitis A
HAV IgG serum antibody test?	Previous exposure; immunity to recurring infection

Does HAV pre-exposure prophylaxis exist?	Yes, hepatitis A vaccine should be given to
	  Anyone traveling to endemic areas
	  Anyone with underlying liver disease

What is the treatment?	Supportive for patient with hepatitis A HAV immune globulin for close personal contacts
Are there any long-term sequelae?	No—it is an acute infection. Very rarely causes fulminant/fatal hepatitis or variant (relapsing hepatitis or prolonged cholestasis).
Is there any risk of developing chronic hepatitis, cirrhosis, or hepatoma?	No (unlike hepatitis B and C)

HEPATITIS B

What causes hepatitis B?	Hepatitis B virus (HBV), a DNA virus
How is it usually transmitted?	Contaminated blood; sexual contact; vertical transmission
What are two potential long-term complications of hepatitis B in chronic carriers?	Liver cirrhosis, hepatoma
What is the incubation period?	1–6 months
What are the risk factors?	Injection drug users; men who have sex with men; Native Asians; health care workers; tattoos; vertical transmission in pregnancy
How does it present?	Often asymptomatic (80%); may be typical hepatitis prodrome
What lab tests should be performed?	Hepatitis B surface antigen (HBsAg), AST, ALT, alkaline phosphatase, bilirubin, PT
How is the diagnosis of acute hepatitis B made?	Positive HBsAg, hepatitis B core antibody from IgM class (IgM anti-HBcAb)

Which lab result indicates immunity?

Positive anti-HBs and negative anti-HBc

What lab result indicates previous hepatitis B vaccination?

Positive hepatitis B surface antibody (anti-HBs)

What lab result indicates high infectivity risk from active replication of virus?

Positive hepatitis Be antigen (HBeAg)

What lab result indicates a lower rate of virus replication and lower risk of infectivity?

Positive hepatitis Be antibody (anti-HBe)

Who should receive the hepatitis B vaccine?

Patients at risk of exposure to HBV, as well as organ recipients before transplant

What treatment is available for patients recently exposed to HBV?

Hepatitis B immunoglobulin (HBIG)

What is the medical treatment for acute hepatitis B?

Mainly supportive

What lab tests should be monitored to assess recovery?

AST, ALT, hepatic synthetic function (bilirubin, albumin, PT)

What is the medical treatment for chronic (>6 months) hepatitis B?

Interferon alfa (IFN-α) subcutaneous injections (5 million units daily) for 4 months, or oral lamivudine 100 mg/day

What are the three goals of therapy?

Loss of HBeAg
Development of anti-HBe
Improvement in liver histology

What are the side effects of IFN-α?

Bone marrow suppression, malaise, depression, flulike illness, hair loss

HEPATITIS C

What causes hepatitis C?	Hepatitis C virus (HCV), an RNA virus
How is it usually transmitted?	Contaminated blood transfusions, needles, intranasal cocaine
Who is at risk?	Injection drug users, transfusion recipients (pre-1992), health care workers
What is the incubation period?	1–3 months
How does it present?	Most asymptomatic; may be typical hepatitis prodrome
What lab tests should be performed?	Hepatitis C serum antibody, polymerase chain reaction (PCR) for HCV RNA, AST, ALT, alkaline phosphatase, bilirubin
Which test indicates exposure to the virus?	Hepatitis C antibody (anti-HCV)
What test indicates ongoing viral infection?	PCR for HCV RNA
Does the hepatitis C antibody protect against future infections?	No
What is the treatment for chronic hepatitis C (>6 months)?	Combination therapy: pegylated (long-acting) IFN-α with oral ribavirin for 6–12 months
What are the side effects of	
IFN-α?	Bone marrow suppression, malaise, depression, flulike illness, hair loss
Oral ribavirin?	Hemolytic anemia and fetal malformation

What lab tests should be done while taking interferon?	CBC, platelet count, AST, ALT, quantitative HCV RNA, thyroid function tests (TSH)
What is the therapy for patients with chronic hepatitis C and decompensated cirrhosis?	Consider liver transplant, if no contraindications
Name the relative contraindications to liver transplantation.	Alcohol use in past 6 months, malignancy, HIV infection, or serious comorbid diseases
What long-term risks are associated with hepatitis C?	Cirrhosis and hepatoma
Can patients at risk receive hepatitis C vaccine?	Hepatitis C vaccine has not been developed yet.

HEPATITIS D

Define hepatitis D (previously delta hepatitis).	Occurs only in patients with acute or chronic HBV infection
Who is at risk?	Injection drug users, hepatitis B patients
How does it present?	Severe exacerbation in patient with chronic hepatitis B, or fulminant hepatitis B
How is it diagnosed?	Hepatitis D antibody (IgM for acute, IgG for chronic)
What is the treatment?	Supportive, no specific therapy available Interferon or lamivudine may be helpful in chronic infection
What prophylactic therapy is available?	Immunization with hepatitis B vaccine protects against hepatitis D.

HEPATITIS E

What is hepatitis E?	Self-limited form transmitted by fecal-oral route from contaminated food or water (similar to HAV) usually as an epidemic
What is the main risk factor?	Recent travel to endemic areas
In whom is it associated with a high mortality?	Pregnant women
Are patients at risk of developing cirrhosis or hepatoma?	No; self-limited (no carrier state)
What is the incubation period?	2–6 weeks
How does it present?	Often asymptomatic; may be typical hepatitis prodrome
What lab tests should be performed?	Hepatitis E serum antibody test, AST, ALT, alkaline phosphatase, bilirubin
How is the diagnosis made?	Positive hepatitis E antibody test
What is the treatment?	Supportive; no specific treatment available

ISCHEMIC HEPATITIS

What are the causes of ischemic hepatitis?	Low-flow states [shock (often undocumented), congestive heart failure, myocardial infarction, arrhythmia]
How is it diagnosed?	History of low-flow state (transient hypotension) preceding rapid rise of aminotransferases (usually >1000)
What is the therapy?	Supportive; correct underlying low-flow state

WILSON'S DISEASE

Define Wilson's disease.	Autosomal recessive disorder of copper metabolism; the liver accumulates copper, which is released and taken up by other organs (e.g., brain, cornea, kidney)
Why does copper accumulate in the liver?	It is unable to excrete sufficient copper into bile.
How does Wilson's disease commonly present	
In adolescents?	As liver disease
In young adults?	As neuropsychiatric disease
Patients can present with what four types of liver disease?	Acute hepatitis, chronic hepatitis, cirrhotic liver disease, fulminant hepatic failure (rare)
What ocular findings may be seen on slitlamp exam?	Golden-brown deposits in the cornea (Kayser-Fleischer rings)
What are two possible psychiatric findings?	Depression, psychosis
What neurologic findings may be seen on physical exam?	Parkinsonian tremor, rigidity, choreoid movements (common by age 40)
What lab tests should be performed?	Serum copper level, serum ceruloplasmin level, 24-hour urinary copper levels
What lab test results strongly suggest the diagnosis?	Elevated 24-hour urinary copper levels, low serum ceruloplasmin, Kayser-Fleischer rings
How is the diagnosis confirmed?	Increased copper weight on liver biopsy
What is the medical treatment?	Lifelong copper-chelating agents (D-penicillamine)
When is a liver transplant necessary?	In fulminant hepatic failure or cirrhotic liver despite chelation therapy

What additional advantage does transplant offer?	Curative—corrects underlying metabolic defect

CHOLESTATIC DISEASE

CHRONIC PANCREATITIS

Define chronic pancreatitis.	Inflammation of pancreas from scarring or stricture of distal common bile duct
What cause has the highest mortality?	Cancer at the head of the pancreas
What are common risk factors?	Chronic alcoholism, history of gallstone disease
How do patients present?	Severe chronic abdominal pain (often radiates to back), jaundice, diabetes, weight loss, steatorrhea
What diagnostic studies are helpful? Why?	US scan (rule out gallstones or dilated biliary tree), CT scan (visualize pancreas), ERCP (visualize pancreatic duct)
What is the medical treatment?	Alcohol abstinence, analgesics, oral pancreatic enzyme supplements (steatorrhea and malnutrition), insulin (diabetes)
What intervention should be considered if pain or jaundice persists?	Endoscopic placement of common bile duct stent
When should surgery be considered?	Intractable pain

BILIARY COLIC

What are the risk factors for gallstone formation?	Obesity, Crohn's disease, diabetes mellitus, cirrhosis, pregnancy
How does biliary colic present?	Intermittent right upper quadrant or midepigastric pain, radiating to back or tip of scapula

What causes biliary colic?	Intermittent obstruction by a stone in the cystic duct, without inflammation
How is biliary colic diagnosed?	History, presentation, US scan
How is biliary colic treated?	Laparoscopic cholecystectomy
When is ursodeoxycholic acid useful?	Patients with high surgical risk; those refusing surgery

CHOLECYSTITIS

What causes cholecystitis?	A stone becomes impacted in the cystic duct; inflammation develops behind it (unlike biliary colic, where it only intermittently obstructs it)
What can trigger it?	A large or fatty meal
How does cholecystitis present?	Constant severe right upper quadrant pain (may radiate to right infrascapular area), nausea, vomiting, fever, leukocytosis
What is a key sign on physical exam?	Murphy sign (pain elicited by placing the hand under rib cage on inspiration)
How is acute cholecystitis diagnosed?	History, presentation, US or HIDA scan (more sensitive), elevated WBC count
How is chronic cholecystitis diagnosed?	Recurrent episodes of biliary colic with chronic scarring of gallbladder
What additional diagnostic finding is required in chronic cholecystitis?	Pathology report of gallbladder scarring (thick and fibrous)
What is the treatment for acute and chronic cholecystitis?	NPO; IV fluids, analgesics, antibiotics When stable—laparoscopic cholecystectomy

CHOLANGITIS

How does cholangitis present?	Sudden onset of right upper quadrant pain, fever with rigors, jaundice (Charcot triad); nausea, vomiting
What lab findings suggest the diagnosis?	Bilirubinuria, high conjugated bilirubin and alkaline phosphatase
How is cholangitis diagnosed?	History, presentation, ERCP (US and HIDA scans less reliable)
What is the treatment for cholangitis?	After stabilizing patient, endoscopically (via ERCP) remove common bile duct stone if present; then laparoscopic cholecystectomy

GILBERT SYNDROME

What is Gilbert syndrome?	Decreased uptake and conjugation of bilirubin
How does it present?	Mild elevation of total bilirubin (mostly indirect); asymptomatic
How high does the total bilirubin level rise?	Usually to about 2–3 mg% (total bilirubin value) range
What can trigger an increase?	Infection, exercise, stress, fasting
How is Gilbert syndrome diagnosed?	Asymptomatic patient; mild elevation of indirect bilirubin; no evidence of underlying liver disease
What is the treatment?	None required

HEPATOCELLULAR CARCINOMA (HEPATOMA)

What is the most common cause of primary hepatocellular carcinoma (HCC)?	Cirrhosis

Which cancers commonly metastasize to the liver (not HCC)?	Colon, breast, and lung cancer (stomach, kidney, pancreas less common)
What are the risk factors for primary liver cancer (HCC)?	Chronic hepatitis B or C, alcoholic cirrhosis, α_1-antitrypsin deficiency, hemochromatosis
How might it present early in the disease?	Weight loss, anemia, increased alkaline phosphatase, increased α-fetoprotein
How does it present in more advanced cases?	Jaundice, right upper quadrant pain, hepatomegaly, ascites
Name two other cancers that present with similar advanced symptoms.	Gallbladder, bile duct cancers (cholangiocarcinoma)
What disease is associated with an increased risk of bile duct cancers?	Primary sclerosing cholangitis (which is associated with inflammatory bowel disease)
What are the associated lab test results?	Elevated alkaline phosphatase; slight increase in ALT or bilirubin
What imaging studies are used to help make the diagnosis of cholangiocarcinoma?	US and CT scans, but often not visualized in early stages
What tests are used to monitor cirrhotic patients at risk of hepatoma (HCC)?	US or CT scan, α-fetoprotein at least yearly
What is the treatment?	Surgery for small solitary hepatoma; no effective therapy because often underlying cirrhosis. Chemoembolization or radiofrequency ablation may be tried.

PRIMARY BILIARY CIRRHOSIS

What is primary biliary cirrhosis?	Slowly progressive autoimmune disease characterized by destruction of intrahepatic ducts and cholestasis

Who is at increased risk?	Women >40 years old
What is the classic presenting symptom?	Generalized pruritus
What else may occur as the disease progresses?	Hepatomegaly, fatigue
What features may be seen in more advanced disease?	Jaundice, dark urine, pale stools, portal hypertension
What other diseases may be present?	Autoimmune diseases—scleroderma, Sjögren syndrome, pernicious anemia, thyroid disorders, rheumatoid arthritis, vitiligo, sicca syndrome, CREST syndrome (calcinosis, Raynaud phenomenon, esophageal motility disorders, sclerodactyly, and telangiectasia)
What lab test results suggest the diagnosis?	Increased alkaline phosphatase and bilirubin
What test results confirm the diagnosis?	Positive antimitochondrial antibody, elevated serum IgM levels
What medication may delay progression of early-stage disease?	Ursodeoxycholic acid
What medication is used to treat pruritus?	Cholestyramine
When is liver transplant warranted?	End-stage liver disease

PRIMARY SCLEROSING CHOLANGITIS (PSC)

What is PSC?	Chronic cholestatic disease of unknown cause, characterized by diffuse inflammation, fibrosis, and eventual destruction of extrahepatic and intrahepatic bile ducts

Who typically gets PSC?	Young men, often (50% of cases) with inflammatory bowel disease (IBD)
How does PSC present?	Jaundice or elevated cholestatic liver function tests (especially alkaline phosphatase), pruritus, fever, right upper quadrant pain
What should be suspected if patient also has fever and right upper quadrant pain?	Superimposed cholangitis
How is the diagnosis confirmed?	ERCP
What is the treatment?	ERCP for balloon dilatation of local strictures; liver transplant for end-stage liver disease
Does a colectomy in IBD patients protect against PSC?	No
What are PSC patients at increased risk of developing?	Cholangiocarcinoma

COMPLICATIONS OF PORTAL HYPERTENSION

ASCITES

What is ascites?	Excess fluid in the peritoneum
What are the causes?	Portal hypertension, hypoalbuminemia, increased renal sodium reabsorption
How does it present?	Gradual abdominal distention
What features are commonly found on physical exam?	Shifting dullness, fluid wave
How is it diagnosed?	Abdominal US scan

What is the initial therapy?	Restrict dietary salt
If initial therapy fails, what is the next step?	Diuretics (spironolactone with or without furosemide); monitor serum potassium
What is the treatment for tense ascites with respiratory compromise, if nonresponsive to diuretic therapy?	Large-volume paracentesis with IV albumin

HEPATIC COAGULOPATHY

What is hepatic coagulopathy?	Occurs in severe hepatic disease when synthesis of coagulation factors is impaired
Which clotting factors are decreased?	All, except VIII
Which clotting factors are affected first?	Vitamin K–dependent factors (II, VII, IX, X)
How does the patient present?	Easy bleeding, bruising, prolonged PT
How is it diagnosed?	Increased PT not corrected by vitamin K administration
How is it treated?	Vitamin K (PT should not be affected)
Should transfusions with fresh frozen plasma be considered?	Rarely; consider in face of active bleeding or invasive procedures

HEPATIC ENCEPHALOPATHY

Define hepatic encephalopathy.	Altered mental status, due to inability to clear multiple toxins, in patients with end-stage liver disease
Name two toxins that may be responsible.	Ammonia, endogenous benzodiazepines

What can cause an exacerbation?	Alcohol use, dehydration, diuretics, infection, sedatives, GI bleeding, portosystemic shunt surgery, hypokalemia, alkalosis
How do mild cases present?	Inability to concentrate, irregular sleep patterns
How do more advanced stages present?	Lethargy, obtundation, coma
What laboratory result suggests the diagnosis?	Increased ammonia level
What is the treatment?	Correct underlying cause, restrict protein, give lactulose or neomycin (decreases ammonia-producing bacteria)

HEPATORENAL SYNDROME

What is hepatorenal syndrome?	Worsening renal function of unknown cause
Who is at risk?	Patients with end-stage liver failure
What can trigger syndrome onset?	Hypotensive event, excessive diuresis
How does hepatorenal syndrome present?	Azotemia, oliguria, hyponatremia, low urinary sodium, hypotension
How is it diagnosed?	Exclude other causes of renal failure in patient with end-stage liver failure
Is there effective therapy?	Occasionally reversible if underlying liver disease can be reversed (e.g., alcoholic hepatitis); otherwise, no effective therapy other than liver transplant

SPONTANEOUS BACTERIAL PERITONITIS (SBP)

What causes SBP?	Translocation of enteric bacteria across gut wall or mesenteric lymphatics into peritoneal cavity

Name two bacteria that can cause it.	*E. coli, Streptococcus pneumoniae*
What are the risk factors?	Low-protein ascites in patients with cirrhosis
How does it present?	Often asymptomatic; may be fever, mild abdominal discomfort, mild leukocytosis, hepatic encephalopathy, decline in clinical status
What is the most important diagnostic test?	Abdominal paracentesis
What strongly suggests the diagnosis?	Ascitic fluid PMN count >250/mL
What confirms the diagnosis?	Positive ascitic fluid culture (best obtained after inoculation of blood culture bottles)
What is the treatment?	Start third-generation cephalosporin (cefotaxime) if PMN count is >250/mL; usually 4-day IV therapy required. Thereafter, long-term oral antibiotics (norfloxacin or ciprofloxacin) may prevent recurrent SBP.

VARICEAL BLEEDING

(See Esophageal Varices, page 117.)

OTHER

ACUTE PANCREATITIS

What is acute pancreatitis?	Sudden nonbacterial inflammation of pancreas; occurs when escaped pancreatic enzymes digest the pancreas and surrounding tissue
Name the two most common causes.	Gallstones, alcoholism

What other causes have been implicated?	Hyperlipidemia, drugs (e.g., diuretics, steroids), infections, cardiac bypass surgery, tumors, peptic ulcers
What is the differential diagnosis?	Peptic ulcer disease, gastritis, esophagitis, cholecystitis
How do mild cases present?	Acute epigastric pain radiating to back, nausea, vomiting
What additional symptoms may present in severe cases?	Tachycardia, hypotension, shock, pleural effusion
What two findings on physical exam are unique to acute pancreatitis?	Cullen sign (periumbilical discoloration); Grey Turner sign (bluish discoloration in flank area)
What are the associated lab values?	Increased amylase and lipase
What three radiographic tests are often performed?	Abdominal x-ray, US and CT scans
Why is the US scan useful?	Inexpensive, and gives useful information about bile duct and gallbladder
What are the abdominal x-ray findings?	Sentinel loop (dilated bowel loop near pancreas); colon cut-off sign (right colon distended by gas that stops near pancreas)
Why is a CT scan of the abdomen useful?	Detects extent of pancreatic inflammation, development of sequelae of pancreatitis
How is the diagnosis made?	Presentation, lab values (increased amylase and lipase)
What is the initial treatment of acute pancreatitis?	NPO; nasogastric suction (if vomiting), IV fluids, Foley catheter, antibiotics (if fever), analgesics (narcotics), H_2 blockers

If medical therapy fails, what is the next step?	Surgical consult
What prognostic criteria are used to assess mortality risk?	Ranson's criteria
Define Ranson's criteria within	
24 hours of admission.	Age >55 years, blood glucose >200 mg/dL, serum LDH >350 IU/L, serum AST >250, WBC count >16,000/mL
48 hours of admission	Hematocrit drops >10%, blood urea nitrogen rises >5 mg/dL, serum calcium is <8 mg/dL, arterial oxygen partial pressure is <60 mm Hg, base deficit is >4 mEq/L, fluid sequestration is >6 L
How many of Ranson's criteria are needed to indicate poor outcome and increased risk of mortality?	Three or more

PANCREATIC CANCER

What is the most common histologic type of pancreatic cancer?	Adenocarcinoma (often of ductal origin)
What is the most common location for pancreatic cancer?	Head of the pancreas (80%)
What is a risk factor?	Smoking
How does pancreatic cancer present?	Painless or painful jaundice, icterus, new-onset diabetes, pancreatitis, abdominal pain radiating to back, weight loss
What signs on physical exam suggest metastasis?	Supraclavicular node (Virchow node), periumbilical node (Sister Mary Joseph node), Courvoisier gallbladder (distended gallbladder due to common bile duct obstruction), metastasis to the rectal shelf (Blumer shelf)

What are the associated lab values?	Hyperglycemia; increased bilirubin, alkaline phosphatase, AST, ALT if bile duct obstruction; elevated PT due to malabsorption of vitamin K–dependent factors (II, VII, IX, X)
What tumor markers may be elevated?	CA 19-9, CEA
How is it diagnosed?	US and CT scans (to locate obstruction, determine extent of disease), ERCP with brushings (biopsy confirms diagnosis)
What are the prognostic factors?	Lymph node status (most important), tumor size, local extension, peritoneal invasion
What are the most common metastatic sites?	Liver, lung
What additional test is ordered to determine if metastasis has occurred?	Laparoscopy (inspect liver, peritoneum)
What is the treatment for localized disease?	Surgical resection
What is the medical therapy for metastatic disease?	5-FU
What additional palliative therapies are available?	Biliary bypass (jaundice), celiac blocks (back pain)

ESOPHAGEAL DYSMOTILITY

What differentiates mechanical dysphagia from motility disorder?	Mechanical dysphagia progresses from solid food to liquids; motility disorder exhibits dysphagia for solids and liquids at the same time.
What are two common symptoms of esophageal motility disorders?	Dysphagia, chest pain

What is the test of choice for diagnosing esophageal dysmotility?

Esophageal manometry

What is the typical complaint in diffuse esophageal spasms?

Chest pain

In diffuse esophageal spasms, what findings are expected on esophageal manometry?

Simultaneous contractions and normal peristalsis

What is the treatment of diffuse esophageal spasms?

No effective treatment; calcium channel blockers and nitrates could be tried

In achalasia, what findings are expected on esophageal manometry?

No peristalsis in body of esophagus; incomplete relaxation of lower esophageal sphincter

What treatments are available for achalasia?

Pneumatic dilatation (first-line treatment) or surgical myotomy

What causes functional esophageal dysmotility?

Lowered sensory threshold, abnormal perception of pain

What is the treatment of functional esophageal dysmotility?

No effective treatment; patients may benefit from tricyclic antidepressant.

What establishes the diagnosis of functional esophageal dysmotility?

Absence of both typical dysmotility findings and pain reproducibility during balloon distention

6

Hematology and Oncology

MALIGNANT NEOPLASMS

ACUTE LEUKEMIA

Define acute leukemia.

A malignant neoplasm of the blood cell precursors characterized by diffuse replacement of bone marrow with proliferating leukocyte precursors, resulting in abnormal numbers and forms of immature white cells in circulation

What are the risk factors?

Down syndrome, radiation, and benzene exposure

Name the two forms of acute leukemia.

Acute lymphoblastic leukemia (ALL) and acute myelogenous leukemia (AML)

Which form is more common:
    In children?
    In adults?

ALL
AML

How does the patient with acute leukemia present?

Acutely ill with symptoms of severe anemia (fatigue, pallor, dyspnea), thrombocytopenia (purpura, bleeding, petechiae), and leukopenia (fever, infection, sepsis). Splenomegaly, hepatomegaly, lymphadenopathy, and bone tenderness also may be present.

What dreaded complication may present in patients with AML subtypes M3 or M5?

Disseminated intravascular coagulation (DIC)

Describe the workup.

Complete blood cell (CBC) count, peripheral blood smear, bone marrow aspiration and biopsy

What additional lab tests should be ordered if the patient is febrile?	Pan cultures (blood, urine) and chest x-ray
How is the diagnosis of acute leukemia made?	History, physical exam, and demonstration of blasts in the peripheral blood smear or in bone marrow aspiration (presence of myeloblasts of >30% in the bone marrow)
What is the treatment for fever with a low neutrophil count?	Broad-spectrum antibiotics
What is the treatment for active bleeding or a platelet count of <20,000/μL?	Platelet transfusion
What is the treatment if peripheral blast count is >100,000/dL? Why?	Leukapheresis, to decrease risk of leukostasis
What is the treatment for the underlying acute leukemia?	Chemotherapy and bone marrow transplant

CHRONIC MYELOGENOUS LEUKEMIA

Define chronic myelogenous leukemia (CML).	A malignant myeloproliferative disease of the hematopoietic stem cell that almost always progresses to an acute leukemia usually within 4–5 years
What chromosomal abnormality is associated with CML?	The Philadelphia chromosome (9:22 chromosomal translocation)
What is the median age at diagnosis?	45 years
Name the three phases of CML.	Chronic, accelerated, and blast phase

How do patients present in the chronic phase?

Often asymptomatic with a high white blood cell (WBC) count, but may present with signs and symptoms of anemia (pallor, fatigue, dyspnea on exertion), weight loss, low-grade fevers, night sweats, and mild upper left quadrant discomfort (associated splenomegaly)

How do patients present as they progress from the accelerated phase into the blast phase?

Increased chronic phase symptoms with lymphadenopathy, bone pain, marked anemia, thrombocytopenia (easy bruising), and predominance of blasts

What are blast phase patients at risk for?

Infection and bleeding due to bone marrow failure

What are the associated lab findings?

Leukocytosis with a decreased leukocyte alkaline phosphatase, Philadelphia chromosome

What additional lab results may be found?

Normochromic-normocytic anemia (mild), thrombocytosis, increased lactate dehydrogenase (LDH)

How is the diagnosis made?

Bone marrow biopsy for cytologic and chromosomal analysis (Philadelphia chromosome)

How are chronic phase patients treated?

Chemotherapy with hydroxyurea (decreases leukocytosis and thrombocytosis) and interferon alfa (decreases number of cells carrying Philadelphia chromosome); or combination of interferon and cytosine arabinoside; or STI571, a drug that is a tyrosine kinase inhibitor

What treatment may prevent disease progression?

Bone marrow transplant

What is the treatment for accelerated and blast phases?	Most treatments fail, but the following are available: intensive chemotherapy with STI571, a drug recently approved by the federal Food and Drug Administration for blast crisis; leukapheresis; bone marrow transplant.
As CML progresses, what two types of leukemia are patients at risk for?	AML (70%) and ALL (30%)
What is the median survival after diagnosis?	3–4 years
What do most patients die from if treatment fails?	Infections or bleeding

CHRONIC LYMPHOCYTIC LEUKEMIA

Define chronic lymphocytic leukemia (CLL).	The most common leukemia in adults; characterized by monoclonal expansion of immunoincompetent B lymphocytes (rarely T lymphocytes) into the peripheral blood, bone marrow, spleen, and lymph nodes
What is the median age at presentation?	65 years
How does it present in the early stages?	Often asymptomatic, with an elevated WBC count
How does it present in more advanced stages?	Symptoms of anemia (fatigue, pallor, dyspnea on exertion), thrombocytopenia (easy bruising and gingival bleeding), fever, night sweats, weight loss, splenomegaly, and lymphadenopathy
What are CLL patients at increased risk for?	Infections due to decreased levels of immunoglobulins from neutropenia
What are the associated lab findings?	Normochromic-normocytic anemia and elevated WBC count

How is the diagnosis made?	Lymphocyte count greater than 5000/μL with cell marker studies on peripheral smear demonstrating monoclonality of the cell line
What are the indications for treatment of CLL?	Neutropenia, recurrent infection, anemia, thrombocytopenia, constitutional symptoms, massive splenomegaly, and massive lymphadenopathy causing discomfort
What is the treatment for early stage CLL?	Observation Intravenous (IV) immunoglobulins if hypogammaglobulinemia is present (to decrease risk of infection), and if patient develops frequent infections
What is the treatment for advanced stage CLL?	Chemotherapy (fludarabine single agent, or combination of chlorambucil and prednisone)
What is the median survival after diagnosis?	6 years

HODGKIN LYMPHOMA

Define Hodgkin lymphoma.	Malignancy of the lymphatic system secondary to monoclonal proliferation of Reed-Sternberg cells, which are B cells
How does it present?	With isolated painless swelling of a lymph node in the neck, axilla, or groin, which then spreads to adjacent groups of lymph nodes; hepatosplenomegaly may be found.
What finding suggests advanced disease?	B symptoms (fever, chills, night sweats, weight loss)
How is the diagnosis made?	Painless lymphadenopathy and lymph node biopsy. Presence of Reed-Sternberg cells confirms the diagnosis.

What additional tests are required for disease staging?	Computed tomography (CT) scan, gallium scan, or positron emission tomography (PET) scan, bilateral bone marrow aspiration and biopsy
Define the four stages.	Stage I—1 lymph node region involved Stage II—2 lymph node regions, above the diaphragm Stage III—lymph node regions, both sides of diaphragm Stage IV—disseminated disease, bone marrow or liver involvement
Distinguish stages A and B.	Stage A—absence of constitutional symptoms Stage B—presence of B symptoms (fever, chills, night sweats, weight loss)
What is the treatment for stages I and IIA?	Radiation
What is the treatment for stage IIB?	Radiation and chemotherapy
What is the treatment for stages III and IV?	Chemotherapy

NON-HODGKIN LYMPHOMA

Define non-Hodgkin lymphoma (NHL).	Clonal malignant expansion of B or T cells
Which lymphocytes are most commonly affected?	B cells
What might put someone at risk?	Viral infection or immunocompromise [(e.g., iatrogenic or acquired immunodeficiency syndrome (AIDS)]
How does NHL present?	Painless lymphadenopathy in the neck, inguinal, or axillary regions; hepatosplenomegaly may be present.
Can NHL originate in extranodal sites [e.g., skin, gastrointestinal (GI) tract]?	Yes, but lymph nodes are more common.

What finding suggests advanced disease?	B symptoms (fever, chills, night sweats, and weight loss)
How is the diagnosis made?	Tissue biopsy
Name the three histologic types of NHL.	Low-grade (indolent), intermediate-grade, and high-grade lymphoma
What additional studies are required for staging?	CT scan, bilateral bone marrow aspiration and biopsy
What is the treatment for low-grade lymphoma?	Chemotherapy (chlorambucil or cyclophosphamide) and prednisone
What is the treatment for intermediate- and high-grade lymphomas?	Combination chemotherapy with CHOP (cyclophosphamide, doxorubicin, vincristine, and prednisone)
When is radiation warranted?	Localized disease
When should stem cell or autologous bone marrow transplant be considered?	In the patient who relapses following initial treatment with chemotherapy
What types of NHL have the highest remission and cure rates?	Intermediate- and high-grade lymphomas

ANEMIAS

IRON DEFICIENCY ANEMIA

What are four causes of iron deficiency anemia?	Chronic blood loss (GI bleed most common, menstruation, genitourinary, hookworm) Decreased iron absorption (postgastrectomy, celiac disease) Increased iron demand (pregnancy) Decreased dietary intake (vegetarian diet)
Describe the presentation of mild iron deficiency anemia.	Usually asymptomatic with a low hemoglobin (Hb) found on routine blood work

How does moderate anemia present?	Fatigue and decreased exercise tolerance
What additional symptoms present with severe anemia (Hb <7 g/dL)?	Dyspnea, headache, angina, lightheadedness, dizziness, or syncope
What signs of iron deficiency anemia may be evident on physical exam?	Glossitis, koilonychia ("spoon nail"), and angular stomatitis
What must be included in the workup of all patients?	Stool guaiac exam; if positive, GI workup
What are the associated lab values?	Hypochromic microcytic anemia [low mean cellular volume (MCV)] with low serum iron, low ferritin, low iron saturation, and high total iron-binding capacity (TIBC)
What three tests would confirm the diagnosis?	Bone marrow biopsy, decreased or absent iron stores, low ferritin level
What is the treatment?	Correct underlying cause. Administer oral iron replacement therapy with ferrous sulfate or ferrous gluconate.
What method of iron replacement is used in patients unable to take oral iron or absorb it adequately?	Parenteral iron replacement
What are the side effects of therapy with	
Oral iron replacement?	Dark stools and constipation
Parenteral iron replacement?	Allergic reaction
What lab tests indicate response to therapy?	Increased hemoglobin (1–2 months) and reticulocyte count (5–10 days)
What must be ruled out if the patient does not respond to therapy?	Continued blood loss, poor absorption, or a multifactorial anemia

MEGALOBLASTIC ANEMIA

What can cause megaloblastic anemia?	Deficiency of vitamin B_{12} or folic acid
Which deficiency are patients at greater risk of developing due to lower body reserves?	Folate deficiency
What are the risk factors for folate deficiency?	Decreased intake (alcoholics), increased demand (pregnancy, hemolytic anemia), malabsorption, and drugs (e.g., ethanol, methotrexate, azathioprine, trimethoprim, phenytoin, sulfasalazine)
How long would it take to develop a vitamin B_{12} deficiency?	Years
What can cause a vitamin B_{12} deficiency?	Pernicious anemia, gastrectomy, pancreatic insufficiency, ileal disease or resection, intestinal bacterial overgrowth, and parasites
How does mild megaloblastic anemia present?	Usually asymptomatic with a low hemoglobin on routine lab tests
How does moderate anemia present?	Fatigue and decreased exercise tolerance
What additional symptoms present with severe anemia (Hb <7 g/dL)?	Dyspnea, headache, angina, lightheadedness, dizziness, or syncope
What additional signs and symptoms are seen only in vitamin B_{12} deficiency?	Neurologic manifestations of decreased vibratory and positional sense, ataxia, paresthesias, confusion, and dementia
What finding on peripheral smear supports the diagnosis?	Presence of hypersegmented neutrophils, giant bands

How is the diagnosis made?	Increased MCV with a low folate or vitamin B_{12} level, and typical bone marrow findings (megaloblastic changes)
What test is ordered to determine the cause of the vitamin B_{12} deficiency?	Schilling test, anti–parietal cell antibody and anti–intrinsic factor antibody in the blood
What is the therapy for folate deficiency?	Oral or IV folic acid
What is the therapy for vitamin B_{12} deficiency?	Intramuscular (IM) vitamin B_{12}

APLASTIC ANEMIA

What is aplastic anemia?	A rare acquired disorder of pancytopenia (anemia, leukopenia, and thrombocytopenia) resulting from failure of the bone marrow stem cells
What replaces the normal hemopoietic cells?	Fat
What are the causes of aplastic anemia?	Idiopathic, viral illness [hepatitis, Epstein-Barr virus, and cytomegalovirus (CMV)], drugs (e.g., acetazolamide, chloramphenicol, and penicillamine), or radiation
What are the two most common causes?	Idiopathic (about 50%) Drugs (second most common)
How does it present?	One or all of the following: fatigue and dyspnea (anemia), bleeding (thrombocytopenia), and fever (leukopenia)
What are the associated lab findings?	Pancytopenia with a normal MCV and reduced number of cells of all lines on peripheral blood smear
How is it diagnosed?	Bone marrow biopsy

What is the treatment?	Discontinue offending drugs. Keep red blood cell transfusions to a minimum to avoid iron overload. Transfuse platelets when counts are <10,000. Bone marrow transplant.
What is the therapy for patients unable to receive a bone marrow transplant?	Immunosuppressive therapy with cyclosporine, glucocorticoids, and antithymocyte globulin
What are the indications for empiric broad-spectrum antibiotics?	Fever and neutropenia

SIDEROBLASTIC ANEMIA

What is sideroblastic anemia?	It is a heterogenous group of disorders characterized by failure to incorporate iron into the heme molecule, resulting in deposition of a "ring" of granules around the red blood cell (RBC) nucleus (called ringed sideroblasts, found in bone marrow), increased level of tissue iron, and hypochromic anemia. May be acquired or hereditary (X-linked or autosomal).
What can cause **Primary sideroblastic anemia?**	Myelodysplastic syndrome
Secondary sideroblastic anemia?	Acquired: drugs (e.g., isoniazid, chloramphenicol), chronic alcoholism, lead poisoning, malignancy, chronic inflammation, infection, pyrazinamide, cycloserine, and other pyridoxine antagonists
How does it present?	Possibly with anemia symptoms (e.g., fatigue, dyspnea) depending on degree of anemia. Hereditary disorder usually presents during first few months or years of life.
What are the associated lab findings?	MCV normal, slightly increased or decreased; normal to high-normal serum iron and ferritin saturation (distinguishes it from iron deficiency anemia)

How is it diagnosed?	Bone marrow aspirate shows ringed sideroblasts.

What is the treatment?	Supportive: transfusions as necessary Pyridoxine and erythropoietin may be helpful in myelodysplastic syndrome. Otherwise, treat underlying causes or discontinue drugs that cause the disorder. Pyridoxine, bone marrow transplant for hereditary disorder

What are patients with sideroblastic anemia at risk of developing despite therapy?	Iron overload Rarely, acute leukemia if secondary to myelodysplastic syndrome

THALASSEMIA

What is thalassemia?	An inherited hemolytic anemia characterized by short-lived microcytic hypochromic RBCs

What are the risk factors?	Mediterranean, African, Middle Eastern, Indian, or Asian descent

What causes it?	A genetic mutation in one of the globin genes results in failure to produce one of the globin chains.

How many adult hemoglobin genes are there?	Four α-globin and two β-globin genes

What does the adult hemoglobin molecule consist of?	Two α-globin and two β-globin polypeptide chains

Why do the defective adult hemoglobin molecules hemolyze?	Failure to produce adequate quantities of one globin chain creates a surplus of the other. The additional globin chains precipitate, forming Heinz bodies in the RBCs, and destabilize the membrane, causing hemolysis.

Name the three α-thalassemia syndromes.	α-Thalassemia trait Hemoglobin H disease Hydrops fetalis
Name the three β-thalassemia syndromes.	β-Thalassemia minor (heterozygous) β-Thalassemia intermediate β-Thalassemia major (homozygous, known as Cooley anemia)
Name the most common adult thalassemia.	β-Thalassemia minor (β-chain mutation)
What are the associated lab results?	Microcytic hypochromic (low MCV) RBCs with or without mild anemia, basophilic stippling, target cells on peripheral smear, and normal iron studies
With what other disease is β-thalassemia minor most often confused, and why? What should be avoided in such patients?	Iron deficiency anemia, because of the microcytosis. Do not inadvertently give iron supplementation to these patients.
What additional studies should be done? Why?	Serum iron and ferritin levels, to rule out iron deficiency
How is the diagnosis of β-thalassemia minor made?	Hemoglobin electrophoresis with increased levels of fetal hemoglobin and hemoglobin A_2
What is the treatment for β-thalassemia minor?	Supportive; no specific treatment required

SICKLE CELL DISEASE

What causes sickle cell disease?	A single amino acid substitution on the β-chain of globin in the hemoglobin molecule
How does this affect the RBC?	It polymerizes ("sickles") in the deoxygenated state.
Who is at risk?	Homozygous S patients (HbSS)

How does it present?

Often with fever, malaise, and a painful vasoocclusive crisis in the back, ribs, and extremities lasting for several days

What can precipitate sickle cell pain crisis?

Dehydration, fever, infection, and pregnancy

What is the acute chest syndrome?

An acute vasoocclusive crisis characterized by chest pain, dyspnea, hypoxia, fever, and pulmonary infiltrates

Name two dreaded complications of a vasoocclusive crisis.

Stroke, respiratory failure

What is a common complication of chronic sickling?

Functional asplenia or autosplenectomy from repeated splenic infarctions

Patients with functional asplenia are susceptible to infection from what organisms?

Encapsulated organisms (e.g., pneumococci and *Haemophilus influenzae*) and salmonellae

What are the associated lab values?

Low hemoglobin (5–10 g/dL) with an increased reticulocyte count; MCV may be slightly increased.

What lab values suggest hemolysis?

Increased unconjugated bilirubin and LDH; low serum haptoglobin

What will the peripheral smear show?

Sickle-shaped RBCs with or without Howell-Jolly bodies (indicates functional asplenia)

What radiographic study should be ordered on all patients with pulmonary symptoms?

Chest x-ray and arterial blood gas levels

How is the diagnosis made?

Hemoglobin electrophoresis reveals >90% hemoglobin S (HgS) molecules; heterozygotes have both HgA and HgS in almost equal amounts.

What is the treatment for sickle cell crisis?	IV hydration Analgesics (narcotics) Folate supplements RBC transfusions as needed Antibiotics if infection suspected
What additional treatment is required for acute chest syndrome?	Oxygen and empiric antibiotics
What is the preventative treatment?	Oral fluids to prevent dehydration and hypoxia Folic acid supplements Vaccinations (pneumococcal, hepatitis B, and influenzae) Yearly ophthalmologic examination

ANEMIA OF CHRONIC DISEASE

What are the risk factors for anemia of chronic disease?	Long-standing inflammatory diseases, malignancy, autoimmune disorders, chronic infection
Why does anemia occur?	Decreased delivery of iron to developing erythroblasts, decreased erythropoietin relative to degree of anemia, and impaired bone marrow response to erythropoietin
What are the associated lab values?	Normochromic normocytic anemia, low serum iron and TIBC, with normal or increased iron stores
How is it diagnosed?	Underlying chronic disease with the associated lab values
What is the treatment?	Correct underlying disease, if possible. Consider erythropoietin therapy.
What are the disease states that may benefit from erythropoietin therapy?	Chronic renal insufficiency Chronic infection Chronic inflammatory disease Anemia after chemotherapy treatment Anemia from myelodysplastic syndrome

What are three side effects of erythropoietin therapy?	Hypertension Iron deficiency Seizures from uncontrolled hypertension (rare)
What additional treatment should be considered in patients taking erythropoietin?	Iron supplements

OTHER

HEMOPHILIA

What is hemophilia?	A group of hereditary bleeding disorders characterized by a deficiency of specific plasma clotting proteins required for blood coagulation
Name the two most common hemophilias and their respective deficiency.	Hemophilia A (factor VIII) Hemophilia B (factor IX)
What is the hereditary pattern?	X-linked; male offspring are often affected whereas females are carriers.
In what two ways can it present?	Painful spontaneous bleeding into the joints (hemarthrosis) Prolonged posttraumatic or postoperative bleeding
What are the associated lab values?	Most often, a prolonged partial thromboplastin time (PTT) with normal prothrombin time (PT), fibrinogen level, and bleeding time
How is it diagnosed?	Decreased factor-specific assay test results for factor VIII (hemophilia A) or factor IX (hemophilia B)
What is the treatment?	Replace deficient factor. Avoid platelet-inhibiting drugs (e.g., NSAIDS).

Name other diseases common in patients who were diagnosed with hemophilia before 1985.	Hepatitis B or C, cirrhosis, portal hypertension, and HIV from contaminated blood transfusions

VON WILLEBRAND DISEASE

What is von Willebrand disease?	An autosomal-dominant coagulation disorder characterized by decreased levels of von Willebrand factor (vWF)
What does vWF do?	Facilitates adherence of platelets to injured vessel walls and stabilizes factor VIII in the plasma.
Who is at risk?	Both males and females
How does it present?	Mucocutaneous bleeding (e.g., menorrhagia, GI bleeding, gingival bleeding, epistaxis, easy bruising) and soft tissue bleeding with hemarthrosis
What are the associated lab values?	Prolonged bleeding time, PTT with a normal PT, low vWF antigen, abnormal ristocetin cofactor activity, and abnormal ristocetin-induced platelet aggregation
How is the diagnosis made?	History, physical exam, and associated lab values
What is the treatment?	vWF concentrate, cryoprecipitate, DDAVP for type I vWF disease

7   Infectious Disease

HEAD AND NECK

ACUTE OTITIS MEDIA

What is acute otitis media (AOM)?	Fluid in the middle ear, accompanied by signs and symptoms of acute illness
Name the three most common bacterial causes of AOM.	*Streptococcus pneumoniae, Haemophilus influenzae, Moraxella catarrhalis*. The bacterial etiology is similar in adults and children.
What other pathogens may cause AOM?	Many agents, including viruses, *Staphylococcus aureus, Streptococcus pyogenes*
What is the main risk factor for AOM?	Viral upper respiratory infection
How does AOM most commonly present?	Pain and a sense of fullness in the ear
What other signs and symptoms may occur?	Hearing loss, vertigo, tinnitus, fever, purulent otorrhea
How is the diagnosis made?	Pneumatic otoscopy, with or without tympanometry
What are the clinical findings on otoscopy?	Tympanic membrane (TM) changes: injection, erythema, loss of luster, loss of translucency, bulging, loss of landmarks
Is erythema diagnostic of AOM?	No. Erythema may be caused by inflammation of mucosa throughout the upper respiratory tract.
What is the treatment for AOM?	Oral antibiotics for 10 days

What are first-line treatment options?	Amoxicillin, or trimethoprim-sulfamethoxazole (TMP-SMZ) for penicillin-allergic persons
What are the typical doses of amoxicillin and TMP-SMZ?	Amoxicillin 250–500 mg by mouth 3 times a day TMP-SMZ 1 tablet by mouth twice a day
Do decongestants and antihistamines have a role in treating AOM?	Clinical trials have not demonstrated additional benefit.
What complications may occur in AOM?	Mastoiditis, meningitis, bacteremia, TM perforation
What is the typical outcome of spontaneous TM perforation in AOM?	Most cases resolve spontaneously.
What are three indications for referral after resolution of AOM?	Hearing loss, failure of TM perforation to resolve, and persistent serous otitis
What is a cholesteatoma?	A whitish mass of squamous epithelial cells that may contain cholesterol crystals. Cholesteatoma is a complication of chronic otitis media, and has the potential to erode bone and promote chronic infection.
Where is cholesteatoma found?	In the middle ear, possibly adhering to the TM
How does cholesteatoma occur?	After chronic or repeated ear infections, squamous epithelium of the auditory canal invades or replaces columnar epithelium of the middle ear.
How is cholesteatoma managed?	Surgical intervention

ACUTE SINUSITIS

What is acute sinusitis?	Inflammation of the mucosal lining of the paranasal sinuses, lasting up to 3 weeks
Which four sinuses can be involved in acute sinusitis?	Maxillary, ethmoid, frontal, sphenoid
What is another name for acute viral sinusitis?	Viral rhinosinusitis (VRS)
What agents commonly cause VRS?	Rhinovirus, coronavirus, influenza, parainfluenza, adenovirus, enterovirus, and respiratory syncytial virus
How does VRS most commonly present?	Nasal drainage and cough
What other two signs and symptoms commonly occur?	Fever and sore throat
Define acute bacterial rhinosinusitis (ABRS).	Sinusitis with bacterial superinfection
What is the major risk factor for developing ABRS?	VRS lasting >7–10 days
Name the two most common bacterial agents in ABRS.	*Streptococcus pneumoniae* and nontypeable *Haemophilus influenzae*
What other pathogens may cause ABRS?	*Moraxella catarrhalis*, other streptococcal species, anaerobic bacteria, and *Staphylococcus aureus*
How does ABRS most commonly present?	Purulent nasal drainage and sinus pressure or tenderness
What other signs and symptoms may occur?	Fever is present in about half of cases. Sinus pain may be worse when bending or supine.

What is the "gold standard" for the diagnosis of ABRS?	Sinus puncture with culture of the aspirated fluid
How is a clinical diagnosis of ABRS made?	ABRS is diagnosed when VRS is present for >10 days (or worsens after 5–7 days) and is accompanied by some of the following symptoms: nasal drainage, nasal congestion, facial pain/pressure (particularly with unilateral predominance), postnasal drainage, fever, cough, fatigue, hyposmia/anosmia, maxillary dental pain, ear pressure/fullness.
What is the treatment for ABRS?	Oral antibiotics for at least 10 days
What three major factors influence antibiotic selection?	Exposure to antibiotics in previous 4–6 weeks Severity of illness Antibiotic allergy
What are four first-line treatment options for mild-to-moderate disease in a β-lactam nonallergic adult with no recent antibiotic exposure?	"High-dose" amoxicillin, amoxicillin-clavulanic acid, cefpodoxime, or cefuroxime axetil
What three first-line antibiotics are recommended for a β-lactam allergic patient with mild-to-moderate disease?	Trimethoprim-sulfamethoxazole (TMP-SMZ), doxycycline, or a macrolide (e.g., clarithromycin, azithromycin)
When should a change in antibiotics be considered?	After 72 hours—if ABRS does not improve, or worsens.
What two complications may occur in ABRS?	Meningitis, brain abscess
What is the role of radiographic imaging in the initial diagnosis of ABRS?	None, because VRS appears identical radiographically.

EXUDATIVE PHARYNGITIS

Define exudative pharyngitis.	Inflammation of the pharynx, presenting with sore throat and tonsillopharyngeal exudate
In addition to the presence of exudates, what exam findings should be assessed in a patient with pharyngitis?	Mucosal erythema or ulceration, cervical adenopathy (anterior and posterior), palatal petechiae, mucosal congestion, and lymphoid hypertrophy
What agents are the most common cause of pharyngitis?	Viruses
Which viruses can cause exudative pharyngitis?	Epstein-Barr (infectious mononucleosis), herpes simplex, and adenovirus
What clinical findings are characteristic of Epstein-Barr virus infection?	Fatigue, malaise, and prominent cervical adenopathy (particularly posterior cervical). Exudate is seen in 50% of cases and palatal petechiae in 25%. Splenomegaly also may occur.
What office-based laboratory test can help establish the diagnosis of infectious mononucleosis due to Epstein-Barr virus?	The "spot" test (Monospot) for heterophile antibodies
What is the most common bacterial cause of pharyngitis?	*Streptococcus pyogenes* (group A β-hemolytic streptococci or GABHS). GABHS accounts for 5–15% of cases of pharyngitis in adults.
Name five other bacterial pathogens that cause pharyngitis.	*Neisseria gonorrhoeae, Corynebacterium diphtheriae, Mycoplasma pneumoniae, Arcanobacterium haemolyticum,* and *Chlamydia pneumoniae.* These organisms are infrequent causes of pharyngitis.
What are two major benefits of treating pharyngitis caused by GABHS?	Prevention of suppurative complications and prevention of rheumatic fever

What are the suppurative complications of GABHS pharyngitis?

Peritonsillar or retropharyngeal abscess, otitis media, mastoiditis, sinusitis, and suppurative cervical lymphadenitis

What clinical findings increase the likelihood that pharyngitis is due to GABHS?

Tonsillar exudates; swollen, tender anterior cervical lymph nodes; history of fever; absence of cough

What office-based laboratory test is available for the diagnosis of GABHS?

Rapid antigen detection tests and throat culture

What is the sensitivity of rapid antigen detection tests?

Approximately 85%; therefore, the diagnosis of GABHS cannot be ruled out with certainty based on a negative test, and throat culture is required if clinical suspicion is high. If the rapid antigen test is positive, no further testing is needed.

What is the treatment of choice for pharyngitis due to GABHS?

Oral penicillin for 10 days

What treatment is recommended for GABHS in patients with penicillin allergy?

Erythromycin

When should antibiotic therapy for the prevention of rheumatic fever be initiated after the onset of symptoms?

Antibiotic therapy can begin up to 9 days after the pharyngitis began.

Should suspected GABHS pharyngitis in adults be treated empirically?

A very controversial issue. Some experts believe that all suspected cases should be confirmed by rapid antigen detection or culture before treatment. Others believe that the presence of three of the four clinical findings associated with infection due to GABHS (outlined above) is sufficient to warrant empiric therapy.

ORAL THRUSH

What organism causes oral thrush?	*Candida albicans*
What are the risk factors?	Dentures, diabetes, chemotherapy or local irradiation, steroids (including inhaled steroids), broad-spectrum antibiotics, and human immunodeficiency virus infection
How does it present?	Painful white patches on an erythematous mucosa
Can the patches be scraped off with a tongue depressor?	Yes, unlike leukoplakia or lichen planus. Scraping leaves a raw, bleeding surface in a patient with thrush.
How is the diagnosis made?	Usually a clinical diagnosis. A wet preparation of a smear with potassium hydroxide confirms hyphae, pseudohyphae, and yeast forms.
What is the treatment?	Nystatin "swish and swallow," clotrimazole (Mycelex) troches, or oral azole antifungals (e.g., fluconazole)

OTHER

INFECTIVE ENDOCARDITIS

What is infective endocarditis?	Infective endocarditis (IE) occurs when organisms colonize vegetations (nonbacterial thrombotic endocarditis) composed of fibrin and platelets, which form in response to trauma to the endothelium or in areas of turbulent blood flow.
What is the pathogenesis of IE?	Transient bacteremia secondary to another infection or resulting from invasive procedures involving mucosa normally colonized with bacteria (e.g., mouth, gastrointestinal tract, genitourinary tract) is the usual source of infection. In infected prosthetic

valves, the colonizing organisms may be introduced during valve replacement surgery.

What are the risk factors?

A previous episode of IE; mitral valve prolapse with mitral regurgitation; degenerative, calcific valvular disease; congenital cardiac disease (patent ductus arteriosus, ventricular septal defect, aortic coarctation, bicuspid aortic valve); rheumatic valvular disease; and prosthetic valves. Injection drug users (IDUs) are at risk for right-sided (tricuspid valve) IE.

Do all patients with IE have a risk factor for this infection?

No. Approximately 25% of patients have no known predisposing abnormality.

How does IE present?

Patients may have an acute or subacute presentation. Common symptoms are fever, chills, weakness, dyspnea, sweats, anorexia, weight loss, malaise, myalgia or arthralgia, headache, and stroke syndromes.

What physical findings are suggestive?

Fever, heart murmur, splenomegaly, cutaneous lesions (petechiae, Osler nodes, Janeway lesions, splinter hemorrhages), retinal lesions (Roth spots), clubbing, and focal neurologic findings if central nervous system embolic events have occurred.

What signs and symptoms suggest right-sided IE in IDUs?

In addition to systemic symptoms, they may have pleuritic chest pain due to septic pulmonary emboli.

How is the diagnosis of IE confirmed?

Blood cultures demonstrating persistent bacteremia. A history of a predisposing cardiac lesion and evidence of systemic embolic phenomenon are also significant. Echocardiography, particularly transesophageal echocardiography (TEE), is useful; however, a negative echocardiogram alone does not rule out IE.

What organisms cause native valve IE in persons who are not IDUs?

Streptococci (mainly viridans streptococci) are the most common cause, followed by staphylococci and enterococci. Less common causes are gram-negative organisms (including the "HACEK" group: *Haemophilus, Actinobacillus, Cardiobacterium, Eikenella, Kingella*) and fungi.

What is the most common cause of IE in IDUs?

Staphylococcus aureus

What is the most common cause of early (<60 days after surgery) prosthetic valve endocarditis (PVE)?

Staphylococcus epidermidis. Late PVE has a similar microbiology to native valve IE.

How is IE treated?

Antibiotics are given based on identification and susceptibilities of the infecting organism. Valve replacement may be needed in severe congestive heart failure, paravalvular abscess, more than one major arterial embolic event, inability to sterilize the blood cultures, or relapse after appropriate therapy.

What prevention is available?

Antibiotic prophylaxis is recommended for patients with cardiac abnormalities associated with an increased risk of IE who undergo procedures associated with a risk of transient bacteremia. Specific guidelines are published by the American Heart Association, and are reviewed in most standard textbooks of internal medicine.

HIV AND AIDS

What cell line does human immunodeficiency virus (HIV) primarily infect?

CD4$^+$ T lymphocytes

What are the two most common risk factors for HIV acquisition in the United States?

Injection drug use; men who have sex with men

What additional risk factors exist?

Heterosexual sex, health care workers (e.g., needlesticks), perinatal transmission from an HIV-infected woman, receipt of blood transfusions or blood products prior to 1985 (e.g., hemophiliacs)

How long after contracting HIV does a patient develop the first symptoms?

Time frame varies from months to years. Median incubation period is 10 years.

How does acute HIV infection present?

Mononucleosis-like syndrome of limited duration consisting of anorexia, fever, malaise, lymphadenopathy, pharyngitis, and rash (in 50% of patients)

When does HIV infection become acquired immunodeficiency syndrome (AIDS)?

In one of two ways:
  CD4 T lymphocyte count of <200 cells/mm^3
  Presence of opportunistic infections, regardless of CD4 cell count

With what opportunistic infections can patients present when their CD4 cell counts are
  <500?

  Oral thrush, Kaposi sarcoma, tuberculosis, herpes zoster reactivation

  <200?
  Pneumocystis carinii pneumonia
  <100?
  Toxoplasmosis
  <50?
  Cryptococcus, cytomegalovirus, and *Mycobacterium avium* complex

What basic lab tests should be performed?

Complete blood cell (CBC) count, CD4 cell count, and viral load determination

What diagnostic test result strongly suggests the diagnosis?

A positive enzyme-linked immunosorbent assay (ELISA)

How is the diagnosis confirmed?

Western blot

Do all patients with HIV infection require antiretroviral therapy?

No. Treatment decisions are based on CD4 cell count and viral load.

Name two common starting therapies.

Two nucleoside analog reverse transcriptase inhibitors, like zidovudine (AZT) and lamivudine (3TC), with a protease inhibitor (Indinavir)

Two nucleosides and a non-nucleoside analog reverse transcriptase inhibitor (e.g., efavirenz)

What indicates an adequate initial response to therapy?

A 50% decrease in viral load. Ideally, the viral load should become undetectable in 3–6 months.

How often should CD4 counts and viral loads be monitored?

4 weeks after starting therapy, then every 3 months

What vaccines should be considered?

Pneumococcal vaccine, influenza vaccine, hepatitis B vaccine (if HBs-Ab and anti-Hb_c are negative), and hepatitis A vaccine (if coinfected with hepatitis C and nonimmune)

What prophylactic treatment is given when CD4 cell counts fall below 200?

Trimethoprim-sulfamethoxazole to prevent *Pneumocystis carinii* pneumonia

What is the recommended treatment for individuals with significant occupational exposure to HIV-contaminated fluids?

4 weeks of therapy with zidovudine (AZT), lamivudine (3TC), and indinavir

What treatment is available to prevent perinatal transmission?

Pregnant women receive combination antiretroviral therapy; infants receive a short course of zidovudine after birth.

8

Neurology

INFECTIOUS DISEASES OF THE CENTRAL NERVOUS SYSTEM (CNS)

BRAIN ABSCESS

What are the risk factors?
Dental procedures, artificial heart valves, recent infection, congenital heart defects, paranasal sinus infections, pneumonia

How does brain abscess present?
Headache, nuchal rigidity, focal neurologic deficits with or without fever and seizures

What other diseases present like this?
Rapidly growing brain tumors, meningitis, encephalitis, subarachnoid hemorrhage

What laboratory studies may be helpful?
Lumbar puncture: pleocytosis, low glucose, elevated protein in meningitis
Blood and throat cultures: positive for causative organisms
Chest x-ray: pneumonia

What are the radiographic findings?
Focal brain swelling during cerebritis; with abscess, discrete round ring-enhancing lesion on computed tomography (CT) scan or magnetic resonance imaging (MRI)

What is the medical treatment?
Intravenous (IV) antibiotics
Intraventricular antibiotics
Steroids to reduce mass effect and edema

What is the surgical treatment?
Ventricular drain to reduce acute intracranial pressure (ICP)
Excision, if abscess expands rapidly or unresponsive to antibiotics
Drainage of infected paranasal sinuses

HERPES SIMPLEX VIRUS ENCEPHALITIS

What are the risk factors?	Usually spontaneous; neonates may be exposed in birth canal of infected mothers.
How does it present?	Headache, fever, nausea, vomiting; progressive lethargy, confusion, seizures, personality changes, increased risk of hallucinations
What are the associated cerebrospinal fluid (CSF) values?	Elevated white blood cell (WBC) levels (lymphocytes, monocytes) Red blood cells [RBCs (hemorrhagic component)] Increased protein with decreased or normal glucose level
What are the diagnostic radiographic tests?	CT scan or MRI (T1, T2, and diffusion-weighted image): low-density, nonenhancing lesions in temporal lobe Serial MRI: rapid change
What is the treatment?	Acyclovir; anticonvulsants for seizures
When should acyclovir be administered?	If infection suspected; discontinue if diagnosis not established
What is the reason for early treatment with acyclovir?	To avoid neuronal loss (can occur rapidly, leading to brain damage)
What is the dosage for acyclovir?	10 mg/kg IV infused over 1 hour, every 8 hours for 10 days
Is steroid therapy indicated?	Only in infants and young children
What is the treatment for elevated ICP?	IV mannitol and furosemide Surgical decompression in rapidly increasing ICP

What is the treatment for related seizures?	Fosphenytoin 150 PE/min or phenytoin 50 mg/min IV to a total dose of 10–20 PE or mg/kg; then according to free phenytoin levels
What is the prognosis?	Good for conscious patients. Poor if comatose—70% mortality; survivors have severe neurologic deficits. Mortality is 30% with early acyclovir therapy.

MENINGITIS

What is meningitis?	Inflammation of the meninges
What causes it?	Usually viral, bacterial, mycobacterial, or fungal infection Noninfectious causes: drugs, autoimmune disease, malignancy
What are the risk factors?	Defects of humoral immunity (e.g., splenectomy) may predispose to infection with encapsulated organisms. Defects in cell-mediated immunity (e.g., HIV, corticosteroids) predispose to fungal (e.g., *Cryptococcus neoformans*) or mycobacterial infection. Elderly and immunosuppressed patients. Other: otitis media, sinusitis, mastoiditis, pneumonia, endocarditis. History of head trauma, particularly basilar skull fracture, predisposes to bacterial meningitis.
How does meningitis present?	Headache, stiff neck, photophobia, mental status change
What physical findings suggest the diagnosis?	Fever, nuchal rigidity, mental status abnormalities Focal neurologic findings in about 33% of patients Rash in about 10% of patients; petechial rash highly suggestive but not diagnostic of *Neisseria meningitidis* meningitis

What entities should be considered in the differential diagnosis?	Encephalitis, brain abscess, subarachnoid hemorrhage, cerebral vasculitis (based on presenting symptoms and signs)
How is the diagnosis of meningitis confirmed?	Emergent lumbar puncture shows elevated WBC levels in CSF (bacterial meningitis is a medical emergency)
How can CSF findings help differentiate bacterial from "aseptic" (usually viral) meningitis?	Bacterial meningitis: polymorphonuclear cells (PMNs) predominate; CSF protein level markedly elevated; CSF glucose level depressed (<40% of serum levels) Aseptic meningitis: lymphocytes predominate; CSF protein level normal or slightly elevated; CSF glucose level usually normal
What other laboratory tests should be done on CSF?	Gram's stain or antigen and bacterial cultures; cryptococcal antigen, CSF VDRL, mycobacterial cultures, fungal cultures, and viral PCRs should be considered.
Which two organisms commonly cause bacterial meningitis in adults?	*Streptococcus pneumoniae* and *Neisseria meningitidis*
What other bacterial pathogens should be considered in the elderly and in immunosuppressed patients?	*Listeria monocytogenes*, and enteric gram-negative organisms (e.g., *Escherichia coli*, *Klebsiella pneumoniae*)
What pathogen is most commonly responsible for aseptic meningitis?	Enteroviruses
What empiric therapy is recommended for bacterial meningitis?	Initially: third-generation cephalosporin, reliably active against penicillin nonsusceptible *S. pneumoniae* (ceftriaxone or cefotaxime) plus vancomycin. Add ampicillin if patient at risk for *L. monocytogenes* infection.

What is the rationale for this therapy?	The increasing prevalence of *S. pneumoniae* isolates that are less susceptible to penicillin and other β-lactam antibiotics
What are potential complications of bacterial meningitis?	Early: shock, coagulopathy (due to disseminated intravascular coagulation), adult respiratory distress syndrome, cerebral edema Late: permanent cognitive/behavioral abnormalities, hearing loss, seizures, hydrocephalus Overall mortality: 25%
What preventive strategies are available for bacterial meningitis in adults?	Antibiotic prophylaxis (usually rifampin) for close contacts of patients with *N. meningitidis* meningitis Vaccinate in outbreaks of meningococcal meningitis due to serotypes covered by currently available vaccine (A, C, Y, and W135); however, lack of vaccine that protects against type B limits this as a preventive. Pneumococcal polysaccharide vaccine for all adults at risk for invasive pneumococcal disease

POLIOMYELITIS

What is poliomyelitis?	A viral infection of the spinal cord
How does poliomyelitis infection occur?	Poliovirus enters through the mouth and multiplies in the pharynx and gastrointestinal (GI) tract. It spreads to local lymphoid tissue; enters the bloodstream; then reaches the CNS.
What effect does the virus have?	Replication in motor neurons of the anterior horn and brain stem destroys cells, producing paralytic manifestations
What is poliovirus?	An enterovirus in the picornavirus family. Three poliovirus serotypes (P1, P2, P3) have minimal heterotypic immunity.

How does poliomyelitis present?

Depends on whether illness is inapparent or paralytic (ratio 200:1). In both, incubation period is 3–5 days. Up to 95% of infections are asymptomatic.

How does nonparalytic poliomyelitis present?

Infected asymptomatic persons shed virus in stool, and can transmit virus. Abortive poliomyelitis occurs in 4%–8% of infections and causes minor nonspecific illness (e.g., upper respiratory, GI), with recovery in <1 week. Nonparalytic aseptic meningitis occurs in 1%–2% of infections.

How common are paralytic symptoms?

Occur in <2% of all polio infections

What are the early findings in paralytic poliomyelitis?

Prodromal symptoms for 1–10 days, followed by loss of superficial reflexes, increased deep tendon reflexes, and severe muscle aches and spasms in limbs or back

How does paralytic poliomyelitis progress?

After 2–3 days, flaccid paralysis with diminished deep tendon reflexes; usually asymmetrical. Paralysis lasts for days to weeks, with return of strength in most cases. Many patients recover fully; if weakness or paralysis lasts >12 months, residua usually permanent.

In paralytic poliomyelitis, does sensory loss or change in cognition occur?

No

How is the diagnosis of poliomyelitis made?

Isolation of poliovirus from stool, pharynx, or CSF. Test patients with acute flaccid paralysis using oligonucleotide mapping or genomic sequencing to determine if virus is wild-type or vaccine. Antibody titers rise early; may be high when patient presents, but fourfold rise suggests acute infection.

Differentiate poliomyelitis from acute inflammatory demyelinating polyneuropathy (AIDP; also called Guillain-Barré syndrome).

Sensory symptoms:
  Present in AIDP
  Not present in polio
Nerve conduction study:
  AIDP—slowed conduction velocities consistent with demyelination
  Poliomyelitis—loss of compound motor action potential amplitude consistent with axonal loss, with little slowing of conduction
Leukocytosis:
  AIDP—usually does not cause it
  Poliomyelitis—CSF usually shows leukocytosis (10–200 cells/mm^3, primarily lymphocytes) and mildly elevated protein from 40 to 50 mg/100 mL

How is poliomyelitis prevented?

Humans are the only known reservoir of poliovirus. Systematic vaccination has eradicated virus in the United States.

Name and describe the two types of vaccine.

Both vaccines are trivalent:
  Inactivated (Salk) poliovirus vaccine (IPV)—formaldehyde-inactivated virus; licensed in 1955
  Oral polio vaccine (OPV)—live attenuated virus; in use since 1963; more widely used than IPV but can cause paralytic polio.

How effective are the vaccines?

Both are >95% effective after three doses

Describe the complications related to vaccination.

One case of vaccine-associated paralytic polio (VAPP) occurs for every 2–3 million doses of OPV administered (8–10 cases/year in United States). Since 1980, VAPP has accounted for 95% of all reported U.S. cases of paralytic poliomyelitis. Starting in 2000, it is recommended by the CDC that IPV be used exclusively.

How is poliomyelitis treated?	Acute disease: supportive, with respiratory support if indicated Residual paralysis: physical therapy, braces
What is the prognosis?	Death results from paralytic polio in 2–5% of cases in children and 15–30% of cases in adults (depending on age). It increases to 25–75% with bulbar involvement.

DEGENERATIVE AND HEREDITARY DISEASES OF THE CNS

AMYOTROPHIC LATERAL SCLEROSIS (ALS) AND MOTOR NEURON DISEASE

What is ALS?	An idiopathic lethal neurodegenerative disease affecting both upper and lower motor neurons; most common adult form of motor neuron disease. Some variants present with purely lower motor neuron degeneration (primary lateral sclerosis); many proceed to upper motor neuron degeneration.
How common is familial ALS? Describe its genetic basis.	Seen in 5–10% of patients. Mutations in SOD1, the gene encoding a superoxide dismutase on chromosome 21, are found in 20% of familial ALS patients; rarely, a mutation is present in NFH, the gene encoding the heavy subunit of neurofilament; other genes may be involved.
What is spinal muscle atrophy (SMA)?	Degeneration of anterior horn cells leads to symmetrical muscle weakness and wasting of voluntary muscles. SMA is second most common lethal autosomal recessive disease in Caucasians, after cystic fibrosis.
At what age does SMA present?	Infancy through adolescence
Describe the genetic basis of SMA.	All types map to 5q13; nearly all patients display disruption of the telomeric copy

of the duplicated SMN1 ("survival motor neuron") gene. Most SMA patients are missing the SMN1 gene.

What are the three types of SMA?

SMA I—infantile onset; Werdnig-Hoffman disease
SMA II—intermediate form
SMA III—juvenile onset; Wohlfart-Kugelberg-Welander disease

What are the risk factors for ALS?

Incidence—0.4–1.76/100,000
Affects both men and women
Age of onset—usually 40–70 years, with a peak in the sixth decade

Describe other variants of ALS and their possible cause.

Variants associated with parkinsonism and dementia occur in some Pacific rim countries, especially Guam; may involve both heredity and environment, but current data do not support robust environmental risk factors for sporadic ALS.

How does ALS present?

Upper and lower motor neuron weakness involving any combination of limbs and bulbar innervated muscles. Eye movements and sphincter muscles are spared until very late in the illness; no sensory involvement.

How is the diagnosis made?

Primarily on clinical pattern. Electromyography and nerve conduction studies can demonstrate early lower motor neuron findings and exclude other nerve lesions as cause.

What is the differential diagnosis?

Idiopathic ALS, familial ALS, other motor neuropathies (especially autoimmune multifocal motor neuropathy and toxic neuropathies due to lead or aluminum), spinal cord diseases including cervical stenosis and poliomyelitis, and motor neuron degeneration in other neurodegenerative diseases

What lab studies are helpful?

Electromyography, nerve conduction studies, MRI of cervical and thoracic spine, CSF exam, HbA_{1c}, serum lead, anti-GM1 titer, hexosaminidase A, arylsulfatase A and long-chain fatty acid levels, and immunofixation electrophoresis

What radiographic studies are often performed?

MRI of cervical and thoracic spine (rule out spinal cord lesions); imaging of brain and lower spine (exclude other causes of upper and lower motor neuron findings)

How is ALS treated?

Riluzole, an antiglutamatergic drug, increases life expectancy by 4–6 months, and may improve quality of life during illness.
Other therapy to maximize independence and maintain nutritional status, including physical therapy, occupational therapy, speech therapy, and percutaneous endoscopic gastrostomy.

Is there a role for ventilatory support of ALS patients?

Must be addressed individually. A study of 92 ALS patients receiving long-term assisted ventilation with tracheostomy found 20 lived 8–17 years with the tracheostomy and 9 became "locked in" (conscious, severely paralyzed, unable to communicate except by eye movements). Relatively few patients choose to pursue this type of prolonged survival.

What is the overall prognosis?

Without tracheostomy and ventilatory support, life expectancy of <2 years after bulbar involvement; if predominantly spinal involvement, 5-year survival is approximately 20%

ALZHEIMER'S DISEASE

What is Alzheimer's disease?

The most common cause of dementia; inherited as an autosomal dominant trait in some families

Describe the neuropathology of Alzheimer's disease.	Neuronal loss in hippocampus, frontal and parietal lobes, and subcortical nuclei including basal nucleus of Meynert, locus ceruleus, and brainstem raphe nuclei; formation of β-amyloid containing neurofibrillary tangles and senile (neuritic) plaques
What are the causes of Alzheimer's disease?	Unknown; may be both genetic and environmental. Multiple mutations have been identified in familial Alzheimer's disease.
What are the four important mutation sites?	Amyloid precursor gene at 21q21 Apolipoprotein E-4 allele on chromosome 19 Gene encoding presenilin-1 on chromosome 14 Gene on chromosome 1 that encodes presenilin-2
Who is at risk for Alzheimer's disease?	10% of people >65 years and 50% >85 years have Alzheimer's disease. Age is more important risk factor than female gender and family history. All Down syndrome patients >35 years have neuropathologic evidence of Alzheimer's disease.
What are the symptoms of Alzheimer's disease?	Dementia, implying loss of multiple cognitive abilities in a person without delirium DSM-IV-R requires memory impairment plus impairment in language, judgment, abstract thinking, praxis, constructional abilities, or visual recognition
List the ten warning signs published by the Alzheimer's Association.	1. Memory loss that affects job skills 2. Difficulty performing familiar tasks 3. Problems with language 4. Disorientation to time and place 5. Poor or decreased judgment 6. Problems with abstract thinking 7. Misplacing things 8. Changes in mood or behavior 9. Changes in personality 10. Loss of initiative

How is the diagnosis made?	Difficult to distinguish clinically from other dementias. Definitive diagnosis requires neuropathologic examination at autopsy. Probable diagnosis (80% accuracy) can be made by exam with supporting laboratory studies.
What are the criteria for probable diagnosis?	Dementia by clinical exam, documented by neuropsychologic screens or tests Deficits in two or more areas of cognition Progressive worsening of memory and cognitive functions No disturbance of consciousness Onset between ages of 40–90 years Absence of systemic or CNS disorders that could account for cognitive deficits
What is the differential diagnosis?	Pick's disease (frontotemporal dementia); vascular dementia; dementia with Lewy bodies; Creutzfeldt-Jakob disease, metabolic disease, paraneoplastic disease
What lab tests should be performed routinely in the demented patient?	Complete blood cell (CBC) count; serum electrolytes, glucose, blood urea nitrogen (BUN)/creatinine; serum B_{12} levels; liver function tests; thyroid function tests Neuroimaging to exclude structural lesions leading to cognitive impairment, frontotemporal dementias, and vascular dementia CSF 14-3-3-protein level, if Creutzfeldt-Jakob disease is suspected and recent stroke or viral encephalitis excluded
What other diagnostic tests are helpful?	Depression screening; EEG to rule out other causes of cognitive dysfunction
What diagnostic tests are needed only if there are specific risk factors?	Test for syphilis; lumbar puncture if suspicion of metastatic cancer, CNS infection, or vasculitis, or if there is reactive serum syphilis serology, hydrocephalus, age <55 years, immunosuppression, or rapidly progressive dementia

What is the treatment strategy?	Early diagnosis important. Cholinesterase inhibitors (donepezil, rivastigmine, or galanthamine) improve quality of life and cognitive functions in mild to moderate cases; vitamin E may slow disease progression; there is weaker evidence that selegiline may be helpful. There is insufficient evidence to support use of other medications.
What is the treatment for agitation, psychosis, or depression?	Agitation or psychosis: antipsychotics, if environmental manipulation fails. Atypical agents may be better tolerated than traditional agents. Depression: tricyclics, MAO-B inhibitors, serotonin reuptake inhibitors
What can be done to assist caregivers of patients with Alzheimer's disease and delay nursing home placement?	Short-term educational programs about the disease can improve caregiver satisfaction. Intensive long-term education and support services should be offered to caregivers.

PARKINSON'S DISEASE

What is Parkinson's disease?	A neurodegenerative disease that is the most common cause of parkinsonism (akinetic-rigid syndrome)
What causes parkinsonism?	Apparently multifactorial, but a specific pathology is associated with Parkinson's disease
What is the pathophysiologic basis of Parkinson's disease?	Loss of dopaminergic neurons in the substantia nigra pars compacta and loss of their inputs to the striatum (globus pallidus and caudate nuclei)
Describe the genetics of Parkinson's disease.	Twin studies show that most Parkinson's disease is not heritable. Epidemiologic studies support a multifactorial model in which genetic factors play a role. Familial forms of Parkinson's disease are rare and atypical, most often presenting at an earlier age.

What are α-synuclein and parkin?

Proteins coded for by genes identified in two familial forms of atypical Parkinson's disease; their normal functions are not established.

Where else is α-synuclein found?

The major protein in Lewy bodies (pathologic inclusions found in typical Parkinson's disease)

What are the pathologic findings in Parkinson's disease?

Loss of pigmented neurons in the substantia nigra pars compacta and appearance of Lewy bodies

What are the causes of parkinsonism?

Neurodegenerative diseases including typical and familial forms of Parkinson's disease; Parkinson's Plus diseases; juvenile-onset Wilson's disease and Huntington's disease; toxins including carbon monoxide, manganese, and MPTP (found in "designer drugs" of abuse); structural lesions in basal ganglia including strokes; head trauma; postencephalitic and drug-induced parkinsonism

What are the risk factors for Parkinson's disease?

Increasing age, especially >60 years; family history, particularly of early-onset parkinsonism; rural living

What are the four cardinal signs of Parkinson's disease?

Resting tremor, cogwheel rigidity, bradykinesia/akinesia, and postural reflex impairment

How is the diagnosis made?

Clinically; considered definite if any three cardinal signs are present or any two are present with asymmetry. Diagnostic tests rule out other causes of akinetic-rigid syndrome. Response to dopaminergic medications often used as diagnostic criterion.

Differentiate parkinsonian tremor from essential tremor.

Parkinsonian tremor—with limb at rest; suppresses when limb maintains a posture or is active; supination-pronation morphology in upper extremity ("pill-rolling"), slow frequency (4–6 Hz)

Essential tremor—when maintaining a
posture or during an action; flexion-
extension morphology, faster
frequency (8–12 Hz)

**Which diagnostic tests are
helpful?**

Brain MRI to rule out structural causes
of parkinsonism. Screen patients <40
years old (or older, with liver disease) for
Wilson's disease with ceruloplasmin level,
24-hour urinary copper, and slitlamp
exam for Kayser-Fleischer rings.

**What is the treatment
strategy in early disease?**

Because Levodopa is associated with
motor complications, use of dopa-
sparing medications is advocated.
Anticholinergics are also sometimes
used when tremor is a major symptom.

**Give three examples of
dopa-sparing medications.**

Selegiline, an MAO-B inhibitor that
enhances dopamine activity
    Amantadine, which has some MAO-B
inhibitor activity and some anticholinergic
activity
    Synthetic dopamine agonists
(bromocriptine, pergolide, pramipexole,
ropinirole)

**What is the therapy for
more advanced cases?**

Levodopa/carbidopa (Sinemet), which
remains the single most effective agent,
often combined with long-acting
synthetic agonists because duration of
action for levodopa declines as disease
progresses, and larger doses lead to
peak-dose dyskinesia. Sustained-action
formulations (e.g., Sinemet CR) and use
of catechol-*o*-methyltransferase (COMT)
inhibitors (entacapone, tolcapone) can
extend levodopa's duration of action.

**What surgical treatment is
used in late Parkinson's
disease?**

Pallidotomy; recently, implanted deep
brain stimulators targeting globus
pallidus or subthalamic nucleus have
been effective. Targets for lesions or
stimulators in the thalamus can suppress
tremor but not other symptoms. Tissue
implantation is purely experimental.

NEOPLASMS

BRAIN TUMOR

What are the origins of tumors classified as brain tumors?

Tumors arising with the CNS or from the meninges, intracranial nerves, blood vessels, embryonic cell rests, pituitary gland, and metastatic tumors

What are the percentages of primary and metastatic tumors?

Primary—80%; metastatic—20%

How does a brain tumor present?

Gradual decline in cognitive and intellectual ability, focal neurologic signs, or seizures

What are the four types of glial tumors?

Glioblastoma, astrocytoma, oligodendrogliomas, and ependymomas (in descending order of frequency)

What are the frequencies for nonglial tumors?

Meningioma (10%), pituitary adenoma (10%), acoustic neuroma (5%), miscellaneous tumors (5%)

Are there factors known to precipitate brain tumors?

Yes—embryonic cell rests, neurofibromatosis, tuberous sclerosis, radiation, and genetic factors (production of oncogenes leading to nuclear proliferation and neoplasia)

What is the most common source of metastatic brain tumors?

Lung cancer; increasingly, lymphoma

What are the associated CT or MRI findings?

Irregular lesions with surrounding edema, or ring-enhancing lesions with or without edema, or solid lesions with or without edema. Ventricles displace to opposite side. Hydrocephalus may be present.

How do primary tumors appear on CT scan?

Gliomas: irregular, poorly differentiated boundaries with surrounding edema
Astrocytoma and oligodendroglioma: calcification

What are the findings in meningioma?	Peripheral location pressing into brain; sharp border; little, if any, edema; ventricles not displaced to opposite side
What CT finding should raise suspicion of metastasis?	Multiple brain lesions
What is the treatment?	Steroids to reduce edema Total excision of meningiomas and acoustic neuromas Excision of gliomas and astrocytomas if possible, or debulking followed by radiation and chemotherapy Anticonvulsants for seizure control

DEMYELINATING DISEASES

MULTIPLE SCLEROSIS

What is multiple sclerosis?	An acquired disease causing plaques of demyelination in CNS
What is the mechanism of demyelination in multiple sclerosis?	Believed to be autoimmune. No specific circulating antibodies have been identified, but increased antibody titers to several viruses, including mumps, HSV, rubella and vaccinia, are seen suggesting immune system dysregulation. Increased intrathecal antibodies (oligoclonal bands) are seen, but no specific antigen has been identified. No significant response to most immunosuppressive therapies, however.
How does it present?	With neurologic symptoms caused by white matter lesions: typically, optic neuritis with visual loss, limb weakness, sensory symptoms (numbness, paresthesias, hypesthesia), cerebellar ataxia, nystagmus, and diplopia (due to cranial nerve VI palsy or internuclear ophthalmoplegia)

Who gets multiple sclerosis?

Women are affected twice as often as men are.

Age of onset: 15–50 years, peaking in the 20s

More common in temperate climates; incidence lower in equatorial regions and approaching the poles; regional risk is established by age 15, and emigration after age 15 does not alter risk.

How is the diagnosis of multiple sclerosis made?

By documenting multiple CNS lesions with clinical history, exam, imaging and electrophysiologic tests

What would you expect from:

Imaging tests?

Demyelinating plaques usually seen as areas of increased signal on T2-weighted MRI; active plaques may enhance.

Electrophysiologic tests?

Evoked potential studies [visual evoked potentials (VEP), brainstem auditory evoked response (BAER), somatosensory evoked potentials (SSEP)] can demonstrate subclinical lesions in CNS pathways.

Examination of CSF?

An adjunct in uncertain cases; shows mild pleocytosis (5–50 lymphocytes) during acute attacks, and increased protein and IgG levels with oligoclonal bands persisting between attacks.

What is the course of multiple sclerosis?

Extremely variable. Most common: acute symptom onset, then relapsing/remitting course—episodic exacerbation of new or recurrent symptoms, and eventual burnout of active disease. Many patients develop a secondary course, however, with steady symptom progression without remissions. Some patients have a chronic progressive pattern and never have remissions.

What is the therapy for multiple sclerosis exacerbation?

High-dose IV methylprednisolone may shorten acute exacerbation of symptoms, but has no long-term effect on the disease course.

What other medications exist for multiple sclerosis?

Two forms of interferon beta [interferon beta-1a (Avonex) and interferon beta-1b (Betaseron)] and glatiramer (Copaxone) are effective in reducing severity and frequency of exacerbation; may also slow the course of secondary progressive multiple sclerosis.

How are they commonly known?

As the **ABC** drugs: **A**vonex, **B**etaseron, **C**opaxone

What is the mechanism of action of:
    Interferon beta-1a and beta-1b?

Believed to interfere with the actions of interferon gamma, which appears to provoke exacerbation

    Glatiramer?

A mixture of random polymers of four amino acids (alanine, glutamic acid, lysine, tyrosine); probably inhibits immune response to myelin basic protein and possibly other myelin antigens; has been shown to at least partially cross-react with myelin basic protein on a cellular and humoral level

Besides the ABC drugs, are any others available to slow the course of secondary progressive multiple sclerosis?

Mitoxantrone (Novantrone), a synthetic antineoplastic anthracenedione; use is limited by cardiotoxicity

What other therapy is there for multiple sclerosis?

Symptomatic therapy: antispasmodics (baclofen, tizanidine, benzodiazepines) for limb spasticity; medications for neurogenic pain; catheterization or drugs for neurogenic bladder; bowel regimens; physical and occupational therapy

GUILLAIN-BARRÉ SYNDROME

What is Guillain-Barré syndrome [acute inflammatory demyelinating polyneuropathy (AIDP)]?

A group of acute acquired monophasic polyneuropathies thought to be autoimmune in nature, of which AIDP is the most common in North America and Europe

What is the pathophysiology of AIDP?

An inflammatory demyelination of peripheral nerves, involving both sensory and motor nerves. Spinal roots are often involved early.

What are the causes of AIDP?

All of the Guillain-Barré syndromes appear to involve a transient autoimmune response triggered by an antecedent illness or injury within 1 month of onset. *Campylobacter jejuni* infection is strongly associated with some forms, including AIDP. AIDP is also associated with upper respiratory infections (49%) and diarrheal illness (10%), but no antecedent is identified in 27%, and with cytomegalovirus, Epstein-Barr virus, and *Mycoplasma pneumoniae* infection.

What are the presenting signs and symptoms of AIDP?

Mainly weakness and sensory loss; also ataxia, autonomic dysfunction (postural hypotension and arrhythmias), back pain. "Ascending" neuropathy is classic description, but any multifocal or asymmetric pattern of onset is possible. Progresses rapidly; maximal weakness by 1 week in 50%, by 1 month in 90%.

Who gets AIDP?

Incidence is 1.2 cases/100,000; no gender preference; affects all ages (major peak at 18–30 years, smaller peak at 45–64 years)

How is the diagnosis made?

Physical exam: weakness and sensory loss with early loss of deep tendon reflexes
Nerve conduction studies: slowed conduction consistent with demyelination, especially in distal latencies and f-waves

CSF exam: elevated protein but <10 WBC/mm^3 (pleocytosis suggests HIV seroconversion or poliomyelitis)

What is the differential diagnosis of AIDP?

Other forms of Guillain-Barré syndrome (acute motor-sensory axonal polyneuropathy, acute motor axonal polyneuropathy), chronic inflammatory demyelinating polyneuropathy, acute intermittent porphyria, central pontine myelinolysis, carcinomatous meningitis, poliomyelitis

What is the treatment strategy?

Hospitalize all patients during acute phase because of danger of rapid progression with respiratory compromise and arrhythmia. Plasmapheresis or IV immunoglobulin can shorten and reduce severity of acute phase, but treatment should not be started >3 weeks after onset unless progression continues. Start treatment as soon as possible in patients who cannot walk unassisted; usual treatment course is 5–10 days.

Is there a role for corticosteroids in therapy?

Steroid therapy is not helpful.

What are the possible complications of AIDP?

Respiratory compromise and arrhythmia are serious complications. During acute phase, closely monitor respiratory parameters (forced vital capacity, negative inspiratory force, pulse oximetry) and move patient to intensive care setting if necessary.

What is the overall prognosis?

Recovery begins within 4 weeks after progression ceases; 85% are ambulatory within 6 months, but >50% have residual deficits, 5% remain severely disabled, 16% are handicapped. Mortality is 5%. Indicators of poor prognosis: compound muscle action potentials (CMAP) with amplitudes <20% of normal with distal stimulation; older age; rapid symptom onset; need for ventilatory support.

DISEASES OF NEUROMUSCULAR JUNCTION AND MUSCLE

MYASTHENIA GRAVIS

What is myasthenia gravis?

An autoimmune disease with antibodies against nicotinic receptors at the neuromuscular junction, which causes increased weakness and fatigue of striated muscles

Why does myasthenia gravis cause rapid muscle fatigue and decrementing response to repetitive stimulation?

The normal presynaptic terminal at the neuromuscular junction has ample acetylcholine (ACh) ready for release when an action potential arrives; however, as firing rates increase (due to repetitive stimulation or sustained muscle activity), ACh mobilization becomes rate-limited and the amount released by successive action potentials decreases. This normal decline has no effect with a normal number of postsynaptic ACh receptors, but when myasthenia gravis reduces receptors, transmission at the neuromuscular junction becomes unreliable and some muscle fibers will fail to respond.

What are the risk factors for myasthenia gravis?

Occurs more frequently in young women (third decade) or older men (fifth to sixth decade); associated with thymoma (15–40%), other autoimmune diseases [(15%) e.g., pernicious anemia, rheumatoid arthritis, systemic lupus erythematosus]; can be precipitated by drugs (e.g., penicillamine)

What are the common signs of myasthenia gravis?

Fluctuating diplopia, dysarthria, dysphagia, extremity weakness, and respiratory difficulty. Symptoms are often diurnal, with rapid fatiguing and improvement after rest. Sensation and reflexes are preserved.

How is the diagnosis made?

ACh receptor antibodies are found in 85–90% of cases and are highly specific except in certain groups (elderly Japanese, elderly patients with high antithyroid antibodies, patients with tardive dyskinesia). Decrementing responses to repetitive stimulation on electromyography (decrement of >10% at 3 Hz stimulation) and increased jitter on single fiber electromyography are also used. Use edrophonium test (Tensilon test) if there is a clear, correctable objective finding (diplopia or short arm abduction time).

What is the differential diagnosis of myasthenia gravis?

Lambert-Eaton syndrome, botulism, and drug-induced myasthenia

What is Lambert-Eaton syndrome?

An autoimmune disease with antibodies against presynaptic voltage-gated calcium channels at the neuromuscular junction.

Why do Lambert-Eaton patients become weak?

Failure of the action potential to release sufficient ACh from presynaptic terminals, a calcium-mediated event.

How is myasthenia gravis differentiated from Lambert-Eaton syndrome?

Repetitive stimulation does not produce decrementing response seen in myasthenia gravis, but with rapid repetitive stimulation or sustained muscle activity, calcium can accumulate in presynaptic terminals, resulting in improved ACh release and an incremented response.

What must be ruled out in myasthenia gravis? How?

Thymoma, by chest CT scan

When is surgical therapy indicated?

In thymoma—in patients <45 years old with more than minimal symptoms; in older patients if residual thymus gland found

What is the treatment strategy for:
    Moderate symptoms?

Maintenance on pyridostigmine, an acetylcholinesterase (AChE) inhibitor that enhances transmission at neuromuscular junction

More severe symptoms? Chronic immunosuppression with prednisolone, often with adjunctive azathioprine. CAUTION: Rapid initiation of steroid therapy can cause transient worsening, requiring hospitalization.

Exacerbations (myasthenic crisis)? Plasmapheresis, IV gamma globulin

What is a myasthenic crisis? Immune system activity resulting in exacerbation of myasthenia gravis. Often caused by mild infection, but resulting weakness may lead to respiratory compromise and dysphagia, with secondary pneumonia. Treat underlying infection; give supportive care and additional immunosuppression (plasmapheresis, IV gamma globulin). Reduce AChE inhibitors, as myasthenic crisis can be difficult to distinguish from cholinergic crisis.

What is a cholinergic crisis? Occurs with excess AChE inhibition; causes weakness with increased secretions, fasciculations, and diarrhea. Respiratory compromise and dysphagia can lead to secondary pneumonia. Test doses of edrophonium can distinguish cholinergic crisis (worsens) from myasthenic crisis (improves). Best approach—reduce AChE inhibitors; give supportive care, additional immunosuppression (plasmapheresis, IV gamma globulin).

What drugs must be avoided or used with caution in myasthenia gravis? Drugs that impair neuromuscular transmission: aminoglycosides, tetracyclines, polymyxins, lithium, magnesium, curare, succinylcholine, quinine, quinidine, procainamide, procaine, lidocaine, morphine, meperidine, phenothiazines, phenytoin, β-blockers, chloroquine

What is the overall prognosis?	Most patients do well, but many develop complications from long-term steroid therapy. In addition, intermittent exacerbations, often precipitated by infections, can cause life-threatening respiratory compromise that may progress to pneumonia.

BOTULISM

What is botulism?	An acute, potentially fatal, toxemia caused by ingestion of botulinum neurotoxin, which blocks release of ACh from presynaptic terminals
What is the most common source for the toxin?	Pickled, bottled, or improperly home-canned foods
How does the toxin enter the body?	Botulinum toxin is released on death and autolysis of *Clostridium botulinum* in contaminated food, and is absorbed from the GI tract into general circulation.
How does the toxin act?	By being taken up into presynaptic terminals and cleaving SNARE proteins involved in acetylcholine release.
Are there other sources of infection?	Yes; sinus infection by inhaled contaminated cocaine; contamination of traumatic wounds by *C. botulinum*
How does botulism present?	First symptoms (12 hours to 10 days after ingestion): diplopia, ptosis, blurred vision, photophobia
What are the classic early eye findings?	Fixed dilated pupils
How does the disease progress?	With descending paralysis of caudal cranial nerves (dysphonia, dysarthria, dysphagia) followed by involvement of respiratory muscles

What is the main complication?	Respiratory failure requiring intubation and ventilatory support (40% of cases)
Is the autonomic system involved?	Yes, resulting in constipation, urinary retention, dry mouth, and dry eyes
What are the laboratory findings?	Normal CSF and abnormal electromyography
How is the diagnosis confirmed?	By electromyography usually. When possible, detection of toxin in suspected food, feces, gastric contents; by anaerobic culture for presence of *C. botulinum*
What is the differential diagnosis?	Guillain-Barré syndrome (or its Miller-Fisher variant), brainstem infarction, myasthenia gravis, tic paralysis, diphtheria, familial periodic paralysis, poliomyelitis
Is there a definitive treatment?	Yes; begin with a skin test before giving equine trivalent antitoxin. About 20% of the population are allergic and may require desensitization.
Are other treatments available?	Cathartics to remove toxin from GI tract; high doses of IV penicillin of questionable value; respiratory support if indicated, including mechanical ventilation
What is the mortality rate?	Varies: type A botulism, 50%–70%; type E, 30%; type B, 20%

MUSCULAR DYSTROPHY

What are the muscular dystrophies?	A group of genetically determined progressive myopathies. Important muscular dystrophies include Duchenne and Becker dystrophies, facioscapulohumeral dystrophy, oculopharyngeal dystrophy, and myotonic dystrophy.

What is the genetic basis of Duchenne dystrophy?

Abnormalities in the dystrophin gene, which is X-linked and located at Xp21, and occur in 1:3300 males. Approximately two thirds of mutations are deletions of one or many exons. Although correlation between extent of deletion and severity of disorder is not clear, Duchenne deletions usually shift the reading frame. Dystrophin is virtually absent, with levels <3% of normal in 95% of males with Duchenne dystrophy.

Describe the progression of Duchenne dystrophy.

Normal early development; symptoms appear in second year of life—difficulty standing and walking, waddling gait with lumbar lordosis, and shortened calf muscles with pseudohypertrophy. Most are wheelchair dependent by age 12, with subsequent progressive kyphosis and contractures. Death usually occurs in third decade from respiratory compromise and infections. ECG abnormalities are seen and average intelligence is reduced, but cardiac arrhythmia is rare and there is no cognitive decline.

What is the genetic basis of Becker dystrophy?

Abnormalities in the dystrophin gene (X-linked, located at Xp21) as with Duchenne but less severe. Patients have abnormal or reduced amounts of dystrophin.

Describe the symptoms of Becker dystrophy.

Similar to Duchenne, but less severe with later onset. Most can walk until at least age 16; average intelligence is not reduced; less tendency to form contractures.

What is the genetic basis of facioscapulohumeral dystrophy?

The gene is located at 4q35; shows an autosomal dominant inheritance pattern with variable penetrance. Affects 1:200,000 people; third most common hereditary disease of muscle after Duchenne and myotonic dystrophy.

Describe the symptoms of facioscapulohumeral dystrophy.

Begins in second decade of life and gradually progress; facial weakness, scapular winging, and proximal muscle weakness in both upper and lower extremities. Heart rarely involved; intellect normal; most patients lead full and productive lives.

What is the genetic basis of oculopharyngeal dystrophy?

Oculopharyngeal dystrophy is probably caused by mutation in the gene encoding poly(A)-binding protein-2 located at 14q11.2-q13. It is autosomal dominant.

Describe the symptoms of oculopharyngeal dystrophy.

Age at presentation >50 years; characterized by dysphagia and progressive ptosis of eyelids. May develop external ophthalmoplegia, facial and sternocleidomastoid weakness, diffuse wasting in limbs. Many patients are of French-Canadian descent.

What is the genetic basis of myotonic dystrophy?

Most common form of muscular dystrophy in adults; prevalence of 1:8500. One form is caused by an expanded CTG repeat in the 3-prime untranslated region of the dystrophia myotonica protein kinase gene located at 19q13; severity varies with number of repeats. A genetically distinct form has been mapped to a region of 3q. It is autosomal dominant.

Describe the symptoms of myotonic dystrophy.

Myotonia, muscular dystrophy, cataracts, hypogonadism, frontal balding, ECG changes. Muscle loss in face and frontal balding causes typical "hatchet face" appearance. Reduction in intelligence with more severe disease; frequently associated neuropathy.

How is the diagnosis of muscular dystrophies made?

First on clinical grounds: most patients have elevated creatine phosphokinase (CPK), which can be quite high in early Duchenne dystrophy but declines as disease progresses. Genetic testing is available for Duchenne, Becker, myotonic, facioscapulohumeral, and oculopharyngeal dystrophies.

What lab tests should be performed?

ECG, to look for changes seen in many muscular dystrophies

What are the treatment options in muscular dystrophy?

Largely supportive:
  Duchenne and Becker dystrophies—physical therapy, bracing, Achilles' tendon release, pulmonary care; prednisone can temporarily slow progression
  Facioscapulohumeral dystrophy—scapular fixation for arm abduction; dysphagia management
  Oculopharyngeal dystrophy—dysphagia management
  Myotonic dystrophy—prolongation of PR interval can progress to heart block, requiring pacemaker placement

MYOPATHY

What is myopathy?

Diseases of muscle. Major categories: inflammatory, endocrine, metabolic, toxic, congenital, muscular dystrophies, periodic paralyses. Inflammatory myopathies (Myositis) and Muscular Dystrophies are covered as separate topics in this chapter.

How does myopathy present?

With progressive weakness, usually involving proximal muscles first. Except for the inflammatory myopathies (myositis), presentation is usually painless. Reflexes are preserved until muscle weakness is severe; sensory examination is intact. Some myopathies also cause acute recurrent weakness, often precipitated by exercise. Many causes of myopathy (endocrinopathies, mitochondrial cytopathies, metabolic enzyme deficiencies, toxin exposures) also have manifestations in the nervous system and other organ systems.

What are the causes of endocrine myopathy?

Cushing disease (50–80% have myopathy, as do 2–21% of patients treated with chronic steroids); Addison disease (25–50% have myopathy that improves with steroid replacement); thyrotoxicity (60% develop myopathy); hypothyroidism, acromegaly, hypopituitarism, hypoparathyroidism

What are the causes of metabolic myopathy?

Abnormalities of muscle energy metabolism involving glycogen or lipid metabolism, or respiratory chain (mitochondria). Glycogenoses are mostly autosomal recessive; include deficiencies of phosphorylase (McArdle's), phosphorylase b kinase, phosphofructokinase, phosphoglycerate kinase, phosphoglycerate mutase, lactate dehydrogenase, acid maltase (Pompe's), and debrancher and brancher enzymes. Disorders of lipid metabolism: primary carnitine deficiency, carnitine palmitoyltransferase deficiency, and long-chain and very-long-chain acetyl-CoA dehydrogenase (fatty acid oxidation) deficiencies. Most mitochondrial disease shows a maternal inheritance pattern (although some mitochondrial enzymes are coded by autosomal genes); usually CNS dysfunction also.

What are the causes of toxic myopathy:
  With neuropathy?

Amiodarone, organophosphates, zidovudine, vincristine

  With cardiomyopathy?
  With both neuropathy and cardiomyopathy?

Emetine (ipecac) and metronidazole
Chloroquine, clofibrate, colchicine, doxorubicin, ethanol, hydroxychloroquine

What are the causes of congenital myopathy?

Central core disease, nemaline rod myopathy, myotubular myopathy, and congenital fiber-type disproportion

What are the causes of periodic paralysis?

Associated with abnormalities of voltage-gated ion channels. Hyperkalemic periodic paralyses are due to sodium channel mutations; hypokalemic periodic paralyses are due to calcium channel mutations.

How is the diagnosis of myopathy made?	On clinical grounds, but specific testing is required to establish cause. Important factors: age at onset; temporal pattern of symptoms (progressive weakness vs. acute, recurrent dysfunction and myoglobinuria); fatigability; factors precipitating weakness (e.g., cold and carbohydrate loading); toxin exposures; family history. Assess for: pattern of muscle weakness and fatigability; associated central and peripheral nervous system signs; myotonia; organomegaly.
What lab tests help to establish the cause?	Venous lactate levels with ischemic exercise testing show decreased rise in glycogenoses, except acid maltase deficiency; resting venous lactate elevated in mitochondrial disease. Elevated CPK and electromyography abnormalities can help to distinguish among the myopathies. Specific genetic tests are available for mitochondrial diseases, channel mutations, and some other metabolic myopathies; muscle biopsy and enzymatic testing can be used to diagnose others.
What is the treatment strategy?	Endocrine myopathies generally improve with treatment of underlying endocrine abnormality. Most toxic myopathies respond to withdrawal of offending agent. Effects of metabolic myopathies and periodic paralyses can be modulated by diet and exercise modifications and, in some cases, use of specific cofactors. Physical and occupational therapy can help in coping with effects of disease.

MYOSITIS

What is myositis?	An inflammation of muscle, generally either infectious, drug induced, or autoimmune
What are the causes of infectious myositis?	Viral: influenza virus A and B, parainfluenza virus, Coxsackie virus, echovirus, adenovirus

Bacterial: *Staphylococcus aureus,
Streptococcus pyogenes*
Parasitic: toxoplasmosis, cysticercosis,
trichinosis

**What are the causes of
drug-induced myositis?**

D-Penicillamine, cimetidine,
ranitidine, procainamide, statins,
and gemfibrozil are associated with
autoimmune myositis and toxic
myositis/myopathy.

**What are the causes of
autoimmune myositis?**

Polymyositis, dermatomyositis, and
inclusion-body myositis. Polymyositis and
dermatomyositis are the most common
inflammatory myopathies, with an
incidence of 0.5–1.0/100,000.

**How does myositis
present?**

With progressive weakness of muscles,
often with myalgia and muscle
tenderness; elevation of CPK and
other muscle enzymes. Infectious, and
sometimes drug-induced, myositis can be
localized; autoimmune myositis is usually
generalized and symmetric. Systemic
manifestations of inflammation are
often present, and dermatomyositis
is associated with a distinctive
erythematous dermatitis.

**How does autoimmune
myositis present?**

With progressive symmetric weakness
of limb girdle and neck flexor muscles,
and sometimes dysphagia. Reflexes are
decreased only when muscles are
markedly weak; no sensory involvement.
Dermatomyositis presents more acutely
than polymyositis, and is more often
associated with systemic symptoms.

**What are the dermatologic
manifestations of
dermatomyositis?**

Erythematous dermatitis over neck,
upper trunk, and extensor surfaces
of posterior interphalangeal,
metacarpophalangeal, elbow, and knee
joints; heliotrope discoloration of upper
eyelids. Other manifestations: nailbed
infarcts, periorbital edema.

How should myositis be evaluated?

History: exposures to causative infections and drugs

Systems review: symptoms of infection or vasculitis

Physical exam: assess pattern of muscle tenderness, weakness; possible compartment syndromes; rashes, arthropathies

What lab tests should be performed?

Serum CPK establishes active muscle breakdown; serum aldolase level. If CPK is high or course is acute, assess for myoglobinuria. A CBC count with differential helps to identify an infectious cause. The erythrocyte sedimentation rate (ESR), positive antinuclear antibody panel, and positive test for syphilis help to identify autoimmune causes. Serum creatinine and electrolytes to exclude vasculitic renal disease. In acute disease, serum antibody titers for relevant viruses should be performed. Electromyography shows "irritative" myopathy; muscle biopsy is often needed for definitive diagnosis of autoimmune myositis.

What are the biopsy findings in autoimmune myositis?

Segmental myonecrosis and regeneration with mononuclear inflammatory exudates. Vasculopathic changes suggest dermatomyositis; CD8+ T cells suggest polymyositis. Rimmed vacuoles and eosinophilic inclusions are seen in inclusion body myositis; granulomas are seen in sarcoidosis and other granulomatous diseases, but are infrequent causes of myositis and often do not cause CPK elevation.

How is myositis treated?

Treatment of infectious or drug-induced myositis is directed at the causative agent. Treatment for polymyositis or dermatomyositis begins with prednisone, 1 mg/kg per day orally; gradually taper once response is obtained. Add immunosuppressive medications when needed: azathioprine (100–250 mg/day orally), methotrexate (weekly, IV or orally, doses increasing up to effectiveness or 50 mg/wk), and cyclosporine (125–200 mg twice daily orally). Plasmapheresis and IV immunoglobulin may be helpful, especially in dermatomyositis. Immunosuppression has not been effective for inclusion body myositis.

What are the complications of immunosuppressive therapy for autoimmune myositis?

Side effects of chronic steroid therapy (i.e., hypertension, diabetes, peptic ulcer disease, weight gain, steroid psychosis). Steroid myopathy is the most difficult situation to detect and manage, and must be considered whenever weakness progresses despite increasing steroid doses.

VASCULAR DISEASES OF THE CNS

ARTERIAL STENOTIC STROKE

What are the risk factors for arterial stenotic stroke?

Atherosclerosis, predisposed by smoking, hypertension, diabetes mellitus, hypothyroidism, hyperuricemia, hypercholesterolemia, or hypertriglyceridemia

How does it present?

Transient ischemic attack (TIA), stroke, amaurosis fugax (often described by the patient as a shade coming down over the ipsilateral eye) indicating possible internal carotid stenosis

What findings may be appreciated on auscultation?

Bruit (murmur) over carotid artery

What diagnostic tests are indicated?

Duplex ultrasound (real time and Doppler) of all four neck vessels or magnetic resonance arteriography; transesophageal echocardiography (TEE)

Why perform ultrasound of all four vessels?

Present status of collateral circulation important to surgeon

Why perform TEE?	High incidence of coronary artery disease and myocardial infarction (MI) in patients with severe carotid stenosis
How do you detect emboli breaking off the carotid plaque?	Transcranial Doppler studies of circle of Willis
What additional studies should be done in younger patients with family history of stroke?	Antithrombin III, anticardiolipin, serum homocysteine, factor V Leiden, protein C, protein S, sickle cell
What is the medical treatment?	Treat for risk factors; give aspirin, aspirin plus dipyridamole, or clopidogrel to decrease platelet aggregation
What surgical treatment is available?	Carotid endarterectomy if stenosis of >50% lumen
Why perform surgery for ulcerated plaques?	To remove source of platelet or thrombotic emboli

CARDIOEMBOLIC STROKE

What is it?	Cerebral infarction and loss of neurologic function due to embolism of a cerebral artery
What is embolism?	The passage of a blood clot through the circulation; in this case, a blood clot enters the cerebral circulation and lodges in a major cerebral artery (e.g., middle cerebral or basilar artery), impeding further blood flow through the artery.
What are the risk factors predisposing to embolism?	Atrial fibrillation, diseased heart valves (rheumatic fever, bacterial endocarditis), recent MI with mural thrombosis, ventricular aneurysm, patent foramen ovale, artificial heart valves, ulcerated atheromatous plaques in ascending aorta or internal carotid artery

How does it present?

With any of the following: acute onset hemiparesis, hemianesthesia, impaired or decreasing level of consciousness (cerebral edema), loss of vision (homonymous hemianopia), loss of language (dysphasia or aphasia), neglect on paralyzed side (anosognosia, autotopagnosia)

What are findings on neurologic examination?

Hemiparesis or hemiplegia with flaccid limbs and depressed reflexes; extensor plantar responses on affected side; gradual development of spasticity and increased reflexes on affected side after 72 hours

What should be ordered if patient has a fever?

Blood cultures (rule out endocarditis), urinalysis with culture and sensitivity, chest x-ray (rule out pneumonia)

What additional tests are helpful?

Noncontrast CT scan of head to determine if ischemic or hemorrhage infarction and anatomic site; ECG; two-dimensional echocardiogram; TEE; four-vessel (carotid and vertebral arteries) duplex ultrasound (Doppler and real time); cardiology consultation (rule out or detect associated heart disease; stroke patients high risk for MI)

What is the treatment?

Supportive: head of bed elevated at least 35 degrees at all times; establish airway; evaluate swallow before initiating oral intake; begin rehabilitation program on day 1

What is the treatment strategy if atrial fibrillation develops?

Assume cardiac embolism, administer anticoagulants

When else is anticoagulation treatment warranted?

If studies reveal source embolism (i.e., valvular disease), patent foramen ovale, mural thrombus, cerebral arteritis, recent MI

When should anticoagulants be prescribed?

In proven embolus; anticoagulants not indicated in nonembolic stroke; begin with intravenous heparin, convert to warfarin (coumadin). Assume embolism in patients with atrial fibrillation.

What tests should be ordered when patient is receiving anticoagulants?

For heparin therapy: activated clotting time or partial thromboplastin time (PTT)
For coumadin therapy: prothrombin time (PT) with international normalized ratio

What additional therapy is indicated for long-term prevention of recurrent stroke or MI?

Treat atrial fibrillation; may need cardioversion or antiarrhythmic drugs. Treat hypertension, diabetes mellitus, hyperlipidemia, hyperuricemia, hypothyroidism, obesity, tobacco abuse, and alcoholism, if present.

When is surgical treatment indicated?

Patent foramen ovale repair; heart valve replacement

What therapy is available for patients who cannot (or refuse to) take anticoagulation?

Aspirin, aspirin plus dipyridamole, clopidogrel, or ticlopidine

Are there additional factors in younger persons with cardioembolic stroke?

Check ESR, antinuclear antibodies, anticardiolipin, antithrombin III, serum homocysteine, factor V Leiden, antiphospholipid, protein C, and protein S; test for syphilis.

What is the prognosis?

10–25% will have a recurrence of stroke within 1 year unless treated
   10% return to work without impairment
   30% have mild residual disability
   50% have severe residual disability and require an assisted-living situation or home care
   10% need permanent care in an extended-care facility

LACUNAR STROKES

What are the risk factors for lacunar strokes?	Hypertension, atherosclerosis, diabetes mellitus, carotid artery stenosis
What pathologic changes are seen with lacunar strokes?	Small vessel vasculopathy due to atherosclerosis, arteriosclerosis, or embolism of terminal penetrating arteries
What is the usual presentation of lacunar strokes?	Clumsy hand with dysarthria, dysphasia, or ataxia
How are lacunar strokes classified?	Pure motor—no sensory impairment Pure sensory—paresthesias and mild sensory loss; clumsy hand with dysarthria Ataxia with mild hemiparesis
What radiographic studies should be ordered?	CT scan shows small, localized lesions, usually subcortical, or located in deeper structures (internal capsule, caudate nucleus putamen, brainstem, cerebellum)
What is the medical treatment?	Control hypertension in high normal-low hypertensive range. Treat diabetes, hypercholesteremia. Stop smoking. Give aspirin or clopidogrel.
What is the surgical treatment?	Carotid endarterectomy in patients with >50% stenosis to eliminate repeated embolism
What is the prognosis for patients with mild symptoms?	Most improve rapidly, but major stroke or MI is a risk

VERTEBRAL BASILAR SYSTEM STROKES

What is the frequency of vertebral basilar strokes?	Figures vary; 18–50% of strokes

How does occlusion of the vertebral artery present?	Asymptomatic, if adequate circulation through remaining artery
How does a vertebral basilar system stroke usually present?	Sudden onset of vertigo, vomiting, ataxia, diplopia, facial weakness, nystagmus, dysarthria, dysphonia, dysphagia
What is the pathology?	Small infarct in medulla or pons
What is the prognosis?	Good recovery over period of months
What is lateral medullary syndrome?	Occlusion of posterior inferior cerebellar artery or terminal portion of a vertebral artery
What are the early symptoms of lateral medullary syndrome?	Sudden onset with intense vertigo, vomiting, diaphoresis, unilateral facial pain
What are the later symptoms of lateral medullary syndrome?	1. Dysarthria, dysphonia, nystagmus due to ipsilateral paralysis of palate, tongue, pharynx 2. Nystagmus and ipsilateral ataxia (infarction of ipsilateral cerebellar peduncle) 3. Contralateral loss of pain and temperature sensation (infarction of lateral spinothalamic tract) 4. Ipsilateral loss of pain and temperature sensation of face (involvement of spinal tract and fifth nerve) 5. Ipsilateral Horner syndrome (involvement of ipsilateral descending sympathetic fibers)
What is the territory of the anterior inferior cerebellar artery?	Anterior surface and inferior surface cerebellum, vermis, and lower pons
Give the symptoms of occlusion of the anterior inferior cerebellar artery.	Vertigo, nausea, vomiting, dysarthria, dysphagia, ipsilateral Horner syndrome, facial numbness, facial weakness, hearing loss, contralateral hemiparesis

What is the most common presentation of basilar artery disease?

Thrombosis of small penetrating vessels entering the pons, resulting in vertigo, ataxia, contralateral hemiparesis, ipsilateral cerebellar signs, and partial Horner syndrome

What happens with thrombosis of the short circumferential arteries arising from the basilar arteries?

Infarction of the ventrolateral pons with vertigo, diplopia, ipsilateral sensory loss over face, ipsilateral cerebellar signs, dysarthria, Horner syndrome, contralateral hemiparesis

What are the distinct findings in infarction of the tegmentum of the pons?

Loss of sensation of face, facial weakness, diplopia, dysarthria, vertigo, internuclear ophthalmoplegia, contralateral hemisensory loss, ipsilateral cerebellar signs, and mild contralateral hemiparesis

Can occlusion of the superior cerebellar artery produce distinct signs?

Yes; ipsilateral or contralateral rubral tremor or myoclonus, contralateral hemiparesis, and loss of pain and temperature sensation

What causes complete occlusion of the basilar artery?

Thrombosis or embolism (saddle embolism in terminal portion of basilar artery)

Describe the signs of basilar artery occlusion.

Rapid onset of coma. Survivors are quadriplegic and may show locked-in syndrome. Occipital lobe involvement produces severe visual impairment or cortical blindness.

What happens to survivors?

Some improve slightly over several months. Most exhibit severe deficits with multiple bilateral cranial nerve involvement, bilateral corticospinal tract involvement, and spastic quadriparesis.

What are the diagnostic procedures for basilar artery occlusion?

All patients with vertebral basilar disease need full evaluation for diseases of heart and blood vessels, abnormalities of blood constituents, and reduced cerebral perfusion.

OTHER STROKES

Define antiphospholipid syndrome.	A heterogenous population of antiphospholipid antibodies directed against phospholipids and their complexes with plasma proteins
What are the effects of antiphospholipid antibodies?	They are associated with thrombotic complications in the venous and arterial systems of affected persons.
What are the major conditions in the syndrome?	Lupus anticoagulant syndrome, anticardiolipin syndrome, and systemic lupus erythematosus
How does the lupus anticoagulant syndrome present?	History of spontaneous abortions, recurrent venous thrombosis (particularly of deep veins), decreased platelet count, positive test for syphilis
Are other entities involved?	Yes: systemic lupus erythematosus, drug-induced lupus, autoimmune diseases, neoplasia, use of phenothiazines, stroke in young persons, rheumatoid arthritis, and Sjögren syndrome
What are the laboratory findings?	Elevated ESR and C-reactive protein, presence of lupus anticoagulant, and anticardiolipin
How does antiphospholipid syndrome present?	Similar to lupus antiphospholipid syndrome
Can the syndrome present as idiopathic conditions?	Yes. Each is a potent cause of stroke in young adults.
What is the treatment?	Immunosuppression for lupus erythematosus, aspirin for mild cases, anticoagulation for thrombosis
What are the causes of stroke in young adults or children?	Sickle cell disease or trait, factor V Leiden, factor VII deficiency, protein C and protein S deficiency, MELAS syndrome

What is MELAS syndrome?	Mitochondrial encephalomyopathy-lactic acidosis- and stroke-like symptoms
Can congenital cardiac anomalies cause stroke?	Yes; congenital heart disease with right-to-left shunt, atrial myxoma, and mitral valve disease
What congenital abnormalities are associated with hemorrhage?	Atrioventricular malformation, congenital aneurysm, Sturge-Weber disease, and spontaneous arterial dissection
Can trauma cause stroke?	Yes; head trauma with subdural hematoma, subarachnoid hemorrhage, or direct trauma to carotid or vertebral arteries
In children, can infection lead to stroke?	Yes; especially serious bacterial or viral infection (e.g., pneumonia, viral encephalitis, bacterial endocarditis); HIV infection can cause thrombotic or hemorrhagic stroke.
Can migraines cause stroke?	Yes; hemiplegic migraine may be followed by permanent hemiparesis.
What other conditions can cause stroke?	MELAS syndrome; history of severe migraine headaches, vasculitis

INTRACRANIAL HEMORRHAGE

What are the main sites of nontraumatic intracranial hemorrhage?	Intracerebral hemorrhage involving thalamus and internal capsule; basal ganglia and external capsule; or a combination of these sites resulting in a large quadrilateral hemorrhage
Name three other locations of nontraumatic intracranial hemorrhage.	Pontine hemorrhage; cerebellar hemorrhage; lobar hemorrhage confined to one lobe of brain
What pathologic changes precede intracranial hemorrhage?	Arteriolosclerosis of penetrating vessels entering the brain, leading to weakness of vessel walls and occasionally aneurysm formation (Charcot-Bouchard aneurysm)

How do intracerebral hemorrhages present?	Sudden onset of headache, nausea, vomiting; focal neurologic deficits then rapid development of stupor and coma
List the three important questions in these cases.	1. Is the patient chronically hypertensive? 2. Has there been head trauma? 3. Is the patient receiving anticoagulants?
What are the three initial procedures in the emergency department?	1. Establish airway. 2. Obtain coagulation profile (PT and PTT). 3. Obtain head CT scan.
What are the CSF findings?	CSF clear, unless there was associated bleeding into subarachnoid space
What is the treatment for intracerebral hemorrhage?	Control hypertension, maintain airway, monitor heart. Stabilize coagulation deficits; lower ICP, if necessary.
What is the main cause of lobar hemorrhage?	Amyloid angiopathy with deposits of amyloid weakening intracerebral vessels
What are the symptoms of lobular hemorrhage?	Headache, focal neurologic deficits; coma less of a problem
What is the treatment for lobular hemorrhage?	Supportive; prognosis often good
What is the main complication?	Recurrence from additional bleeding of weakened vessels
What is the main cause of pontine hemorrhage?	Arteriolosclerosis due to chronic hypertension
What are the symptoms of pontine hemorrhage?	Sudden onset with rapid progression to hemiplegia or quadriplegia; coma offers poor prognosis
What is the cause of cerebellar hemorrhage?	Rupture of arteriosclerotic vessel in cerebellum

How does cerebellar hemorrhage present?	1. Onset of severe headache with rapid progression to coma and death
	2. Abrupt onset of occipital headache, severe vomiting, vertigo, and ataxia. Progressive loss of consciousness, brainstem compression, and death.
	3. Slowly developing occipital headache, vomiting, and vertigo, followed by obtundation leading to coma.
How do you diagnose cerebellar hemorrhage?	CT scan or MRI shows blood in cerebellum
What is the treatment for cerebellar hemorrhage?	Depends on diameter of hematoma: <40 mm—treat conservatively >40 mm—perform surgical evacuation unless patient comatose

SUBARACHNOID HEMORRHAGE

Define subarachnoid hemorrhage.	A syndrome with bleeding into subarachnoid space
What is the most common cause of subarachnoid hemorrhage?	Head trauma
What is the most common cause of nontraumatic (primary) subarachnoid hemorrhage?	Rupture of saccular (berry) aneurysm
What are other frequent causes of subarachnoid hemorrhage?	Bleeding from an arteriovenous malformation; rupture of intracranial hemorrhage into subarachnoid space
Are saccular aneurysms usually single?	Yes, but 15% are multiple
What is the pathology of aneurysm formation?	Degenerative changes in vessel wall leading to weakness and dilatation
What are the predisposing factors?	Atherosclerosis or weakening vessel wall

Is heredity a factor?	Only in a minority of cases
What other factors predispose to aneurysm formation?	Hypertension, smoking, elevated serum lipid levels, alcohol consumption
What are the changes in the vessel wall?	Lack of internal elastic lamina; thin wall of fibrous tissue lined by laminated blood clot
Describe the clinical features of a ruptured aneurysm.	Sudden onset of severe headache lasting a few hours to several days, often with focal neurologic deficits or coma
What is a sentinel headache?	An acute but transient headache that may precede aneurysm rupture by several hours to a few days
Describe other prodromal symptoms of aneurysm rupture.	Pressure on third nerve, producing diplopia, ptosis, and pupillary dilatation; pressure on fifth nerve, producing facial pain
When does a ruptured aneurysm occur?	During physical activity (e.g., work, exercise), but can occur at rest
What are the symptoms of a ruptured aneurysm?	Sudden onset of severe headache with pain spreading to occiput and neck, and nuchal rigidity, often rapidly leading to coma
What percent of patients have rapid loss of consciousness	20%
What are additional symptoms in conscious patients?	Photophobia, nausea, vomiting, lethargy, confusion
Do funduscopic changes occur?	Yes. Subhyoid hemorrhages and papilledema can develop as early as 6 hours after rupture of aneurysm.

What is the main complication in survivors?	Development of arterial vasospasm sufficient to cause cerebral infarction
What is the cause of vasospasm?	Large volume of blood in subarachnoid space
What is the pathogenesis of vasospasm?	Oxyhemoglobin leads to production of endothelin, which results in intense vasospasm.
Are there other complications?	Bleeding into brain or subdural space, acute hydrocephalus, cardiac arrhythmias, inappropriate secretion of antidiuretic hormone, seizures
What is the prognosis with ruptured saccular aneurysm?	Poor; 30% die within 24 hours; 40% die within 7 days; 50% of survivors have second bleed; 60% die within 6 months
What is the treatment for subarachnoid hemorrhage with unruptured aneurysm?	If neurologic examination normal, or mild impairment of consciousness or mild focal neurologic deficits (Hunt and Hess classification grades 1–3), immediate surgical or coil obliteration of aneurysm
What is the treatment for patients with severe neurologic deficits?	Medical management: 3 weeks of strict bed rest, adequate nursing care, pain control; treat hypertension and cerebral edema; prophylaxis for vasospasm with nimodipine 60 mg every 4 hours for 21 days.
How do you treat vasospasm?	Start intraarterial infusion of papaverine, 300 mg in 1 hour, or perform transluminal balloon angioplasty.
What other measures are used?	Avoid infection; Guglielmi coils inserted into aneurysm in surgically inaccessible cases
What is arteriovenous malformation (AVM)?	A congenital non-neoplastic mass of tortuous blood vessels with absent capillary system

Where are cerebral AVMs located?	90% supratentorial, usually in parietal lobe; others can occur elsewhere in brain or spinal cord.
What are the symptoms of an AVM?	Partial or generalized seizures, migraine-like headaches
What is the risk of bleeding from an AVM?	3–4% percent per year
Is there increased risk of bleeding during pregnancy?	No
What is the treatment for cerebral AVM?	Control seizures with anticonvulsants.
Is surgical treatment feasible for cerebral AVM?	Yes, when risk of surgical treatment is less than risk from no treatment.
What methods are used to reduce volume of AVM before surgery?	Embolization of bleeding vessels with plastic beads or detachable coils
What is a mycotic aneurysm?	An aneurysm resulting from repeated infection of vessel wall
What are prgdisposing factors for mycotic aneurysm?	Drug addiction, repeated use of contaminated needles
How is a mycotic aneurysm detected?	Usually after subarachnoid hemorrhage
What is the treatment for mycotic aneurysm?	Antibiotics to control infection, particularly of heart valves
What is the prognosis?	Mortality is high after subarachnoid hemorrhage. Mycotic aneurysm may respond to antibiotic therapy.

EPISODIC DISORDERS

EPILEPSY

What is epilepsy?	A group of conditions characterized by recurrent seizures, which are clinically manifested abnormal electrical discharges in the brain. Epilepsies are classified by type of seizure and cause.
Describe the three types of epilepsies.	Primary—genetic predisposition without structural, metabolic, or pathologic abnormality Symptomatic—seizures consequent to known brain disease Cryptogenic—seizures thought to be symptomatic but underlying brain disease not established
What types of seizures are there?	Partial (focal), generalized, or unclassified.
What types of partial seizures are there?	Partial seizures are simple (no alteration in consciousness) or complex (alteration in consciousness); either type can evolve secondarily to generalized seizures.
What are the types of generalized seizures?	Generalized seizures include absence seizures, tonic-clonic, tonic, clonic, myoclonic and atonic, depending on the presence and type of motor activity.
What are the causes of seizures:	
In infancy (0–2 years)?	Congenital maldevelopment, birth injury, metabolic (hypocalcemia, hypoglycemia), vitamin B_6 deficiency, phenylketonuria
In childhood (2–10 years)?	Birth injury, trauma, infection, cerebral artery or vein thrombosis, onset of idiopathic epilepsy
In adolescence (10–18 years)?	Trauma, onset of idiopathic epilepsy, congenital defects

In early adulthood (18–35 years)?	Trauma, neoplasm, onset of idiopathic epilepsy, alcoholism, drug addiction
In middle age (35–60 years)?	Neoplasm, trauma, vascular disease, alcoholism, drug addiction
In late life (>60 years)?	Vascular or degenerative disease, neoplasm

How is the diagnosis of seizures made?

History (including witness accounts), physical exam, and laboratory testing to establish underlying cause. EEG helpful but often normal interictally (between seizures); abnormal EEG, even with epileptiform discharges, does not always indicate occurrence of clinical seizures. Provocation during EEG (hyperventilation, photic stimulation with strobe light, sleep deprivation) may cause epileptiform activity and overt seizures. In difficult cases, prolonged video and EEG monitoring needed to establish diagnosis and type of seizures.

What is the differential diagnosis of seizure?

Syncope, transient ischemic attack, migraine, metabolic derangements, parasomnias, transient global amnesia, paroxysmal movement disorders, nonepileptic seizures (pseudoseizures)

Which diagnostic tests are helpful?

CBC count; chemistry studies (electrolytes, glucose, calcium, magnesium, uremia, and hepatic encephalopathy); toxicology screen, MRI, EEG in patients with new-onset seizure. Lumbar puncture if possible meningitis. In patients with known seizure disorders or when history not available, obtain antiepileptic drug levels. EEG, video monitoring useful in selected cases.

How are seizures treated?

Seizures of unknown cause or secondary to specific or treatable causes do not require initiating anticonvulsant therapy; but consider risk of seizures in certain patients (e.g., heavy machinery operators, roofers). Treat recurrent seizures with chronic anticonvulsant therapy; base drug selection on seizure type.

What drugs are available for seizure treatment?

Many newer drugs are available for all seizure types. Commonly used drugs for simple or complex partial and generalized tonic-clonic seizures: phenytoin, carbamazepine, and valproic acid. Commonly used drugs for absence, myoclonic, and atonic seizures: valproic acid and ethosuximide.

How are anticonvulsant drug levels used in treating epilepsy?

Recommended therapeutic ranges are a general guide; therapy can be individualized based on previously documented levels at which a given patient either had seizures or developed toxicity.

When is surgery warranted?

If seizures are refractory to medical treatment, and a resectable focus of seizure onset can be identified

What is status epilepticus?

A state of continuing or recurring seizures without complete recovery between attacks, lasting >20 minutes. Can occur with any seizure type; is a true emergency only if there is generalized tonic-clonic status.

How is status epilepticus treated?

Start IV; draw baseline labs (CBC count, chemistry panel, anticonvulsant drug levels, arterial blood gas, toxicology screen, finger stick for glucose). Obtain vital signs. Assess patient quickly for infection, respiratory compromise, head trauma, and focal neurologic signs. With resuscitation equipment at bedside, begin fosphenytoin IV push at 150 mg/min or less, to 20 mg/kg in an adult (15 mg/kg in children). Monitor blood pressure, pulse, ECG, respiration; slow infusion if necessary. If status continues, begin IV lorazepam at 2 mg/min to 0.1 mg/kg; monitor blood pressure and respiration. Refractory status requires intubation and continued IV lorazepam, general anesthesia, or pentobarbital coma.

POSTICTAL STATES

What is a postictal state? — A constellation of symptoms—headache, drowsiness, disorientation, poor recall, delusions—following a partial or generalized seizure

What are the predisposing factors? — Simple or complex partial, or generalized tonic clonic (grand mal) seizure

What causes a postictal state? — Exhaustion of neurons involved in seizure activity

What is the duration of a postictal state? — Several hours; sometimes several days

What can be found in the patient's history? — Epilepsy (i.e., multiple seizures in the past); occasionally occurs after a single recorded seizure

What other symptoms can occur in a postictal state? — Hemiparesis (Todd's paralysis) resolving in a few hours to several days. Some patients have mild difficulty with memory and cognitive functioning for up to 1 week.

What should you be aware of with elderly patients? — Prolonged postictal state accompanying minor subclinical seizures can cause a pseudodementia.

What laboratory tests are helpful? — Electrolytes, BUN, creatinine, liver function test; toxicology screen if drugs of abuse suspected

Why should you monitor anticonvulsant drug levels? — Overdoses can mimic postictal state. Be aware of drug interaction in polypharmacy.

What diagnostic studies should be done?

CT scan, MRI, EEG. Imaging emphatically indicated in recent-onset seizures with postictal state. Assume tumor until ruled out.

What is the treatment?

Appropriate testing; treatment of underlying cause of seizures; anticonvulsant therapy to prevent recurrence

9

Obstetrics and Gynecology

UTERUS

ENDOMETRIOSIS

What is endometriosis?

Ectopic growth of uterine glands and stroma

What is the incidence of endometriosis?

Depends on population studied: estimated at 5%–10% in the general population; higher in infertile women and those with pelvic pain

What are the most common locations?

Pelvic peritoneum, ovary

Name the main risk factors for endometriosis.

Family history, reflecting altered immune system that is ineffective at removing retrograde menstrual debris, or endometrium that is inherently more likely to attach to ectopic tissues. Other risk factors: uterine, cervical, or vaginal obstruction (either congenital or acquired), both of which make retrograde menstruation more likely.

How does endometriosis present?

Dysmenorrhea, dyspareunia, infertility, and other pelvic pain (e.g., constant diffuse pain, lower back pain, dysuria, dyschezia), or acute or chronic intestinal pain syndromes. Dysmenorrhea and dyspareunia usually begin in late second or early third decades, earlier than is seen with adenomyosis.

What are the common physical exam findings?

Fixed, enlarged, tender adnexa, uterosacral nodularity on rectovaginal exam, or a fixed retroverted uterus; no pathognomonic signs or symptoms

What is the differential diagnosis?	Pelvic inflammatory disease, adenomyosis, pelvic adhesions, functional ovarian cysts, leiomyomas, ovarian neoplasms
How is endometriosis diagnosed?	Laparoscopy to inspect pelvis directly; biopsies of suspected lesions to confirm presence of ectopic endometrial glands and stroma. Pelvic sonography may reveal adnexal cysts suspicious for ovarian endometriomas, but is not diagnostic; other imaging modalities rarely helpful. No blood tests are useful for diagnosis.
What medications are used for the treatment of endometriosis?	GnRH analogs, Danazol, progestins, and oral contraceptives produce a hypoestrogenic state, by different mechanisms. GnRH analogs produce profound hypoestrogenic state that causes endometrial implants to resolve. Also, danazol, progestins, and oral contraceptives suppress endometrial growth and ultimately result in endometrial atrophy.
What alternative therapy is available if medical therapy fails or is not indicated?	Surgical excision of endometrial implants and adhesions (either by laparoscopy or laparotomy)
What definitive therapy exists?	Total abdominal hysterectomy and bilateral salpingo-oophorectomy (TAH-BSO) along with lysis of adhesions and excision of endometrial lesions
What medical treatment should be considered after TAH-BSO?	Estrogen replacement therapy, but use caution in initiating therapy too soon after definitive surgery (may stimulate regrowth of hidden foci of endometriosis)

LEIOMYOMA (MYOMA, FIBROID, FIBROMA)

Basic Science

What is a leiomyoma?	Frequent, usually asymptomatic, benign tumor of the uterus. Usually appear as multiple, well-vascularized masses with

pseudocapsules; easily scooped out intact on biopsy. May be calcified or degenerate, causing acute pain. Estrogens regulate growth. Most common reason for hysterectomy.

Risk Factors and Presentation

What causes a leiomyoma?

Unknown. High-dose exogenous estrogens can increase growth; but low-dose oral contraceptives do not. Myomas are more common in obese women. Smokers and thin women may have a lower incidence due to decreased androgen conversion to estrogen.

What are the risk factors?

Black race; obesity; perimenopausal age group; nonsmoking

Do leiomyomas become cancerous?

After menopause, risk of conversion to a sarcoma doubles, but is still extremely low (<1%).

What unusual complications may be seen?

Polycythemia (mainly in menopausal women) secondary to increased erythropoietin production by tumor

With large tumors: carneous degeneration with pain, abruption/abortion, malpresentation, failure of cervix to dilate, preterm contractions, and increased cesarean section rates

Rarely, benign metastasizing uterine leiomyomas may produce multinodular lung lesions or attach to other pelvic organs.

What are the symptoms and signs of leiomyomas?

Major presenting symptoms: abnormal uterine bleeding; pelvic mass; sensations of pressure in pelvis. The uterine mass is usually centrally located, firm, nontender, irregular, and attached to the uterus. Pressure on other organs (e.g., ureters, colon, bladder) can cause symptoms. Pain is rare; occasionally, acute pain from torsion of a pedunculated stalk or degeneration.

Diagnostic Tests/Studies

How is the diagnosis made?

Usually by abdominal and pelvic exam. Imaging studies show discrete calcified, round masses on ultrasound (US); submucous fibroids may appear as distinct areas lacking contrast on hysterosalpingography.

What additional workup may be needed for a large myoma?

Imaging of adjacent structures by intravenous pyelography, or barium enema

Therapy

What is the treatment strategy for leiomyomas?

Usually, none needed; myomas shrink after menopause. Before menopause, gauge progression at 6-month intervals. Treatment rarely needed for asymptomatic myomas of <280 g (weight equivalent to 12-week gestation). Symptomatic fibromas may be treated either medically or surgically, depending on the woman's preference about further childbearing.

What are the indications for hysterectomy?

A rapidly growing myoma; large number of mitoses [>10/10 high-power fields (HPFs)] suggest possible transformation to sarcoma.

What is the medical treatment?

Gonadotropin-releasing hormone (GnRH) agonists to decrease luteinizing hormone (LH) and follicle-stimulating hormone (FSH), with resultant hypoestrogenic menopause-like state; also progestins (e.g., medroxyprogesterone)

What are the side effects of treatment with GnRH agonists?

Menopausal symptoms: hot flushes, vasomotor instability, pelvic tissue atrophy with dysuria and dyspareunia, memory loss, osteoporosis, hyperlipidemia

What are the advantages of medical treatment?

Medical treatment option associated with decreased bleeding, and allows treating the patient until natural menopause

What is the surgical treatment:

If maintaining fertility is a concern?

In women past childbearing age, or not wishing to have children? If abnormal bleeding has occurred? For asymptomatic fibroma?

Myomectomy with anterior incision of the uterus is a conservative approach; laparoscopic and hysteroscopic myomectomy in selected situations. Hysterectomy is the procedure of choice; ovaries and fallopian tubes are usually left intact, unless abnormal. Endometrial biopsy to rule out cancer should precede hysterectomy. American College of Obstetricians and Gynecologists (ACOG) recommends avoiding removal unless the size is greater than that of a 12-week gestation (280 g).

Are there any other treatment options?

Laparoscopic bipolar coagulation of the uterine vessels in symptomatic fibroids to shrink tumors. Relatively new procedure; recommended only for women past childbearing. Vascular embolization also used to shrink symptomatic tumors.

Are there contraindications to hormone replacement in the postmenopausal woman with fibromyomas?

No. If irregular bleeding develops, submucous fibromas can often be removed via hysteroscopy.

What is the pregnancy rate following myomectomy?

Up to 60%. Cesarean section is often needed after extensive myomectomy.

UTERINE CANCER

Basic Science

Which sporadic oncogenes play a role in endometrial cancer?

HER-2/neu, c-*fms*, K-*ras*, c-*myc*

Name two tumor suppressor genes in endometrial cancer.

p53, PTEN

Name two DNA repair genes responsible for microsatellite instability in endometrial cancer.

MSH2, MLH1

Name the histologic types and frequencies of endometrial cancer.

Endometrioid adenocarcinoma, 75%; papillary serous adenocarcinoma, 10%; clear cell, 5%; stromal and smooth muscle malignoma are rare.

Risk Factors and Presentation

What is the strongest risk factor for endometrial cancer?

Unopposed estrogen

What are other risk factors?

Nulliparity, early menarche, late menopause, exogenous estrogen use, diabetes mellitus, obesity, polycystic ovary syndrome

What is the prevalence in asymptomatic women?

Low, because women present even in early stages with abnormal bleeding

Diagnostic Tests/Studies

How is endometrial cancer diagnosed?

Endometrial biopsy

What is the false-negative rate of office endometrial biopsy?

10%; therefore, symptomatic patients with negative office endometrial biopsy must be followed with fractional curettage under anesthesia.

What test is useful to screen for metastasis?

Chest x-ray

What is the significance of the presence of endometrial cells in a pap smear?

If obtained during second half of cycle, or in postmenopausal women, possibility of endometrial disease

What is the significance of normal endometrial cells in a pap smear in a postmenopausal woman?

Approximately 6% of these patients have endometrial carcinoma; approximately 13% have endometrial hyperplasia.

Therapy

When endometrial cancer is diagnosed, what are some prognostic variables?

Age, histologic type, histologic grade, nuclear grade, myometrial invasion, vascular space invasion, tumor size, peritoneal cytology, hormone receptor status, DNA ploidy, therapy (surgery vs. radiation)

What is the therapy for International Federation of Gynecology and Obstetrics (FIGO) stage I?

Total abdominal hysterectomy plus bilateral salpingo-oophorectomy

What additional therapy should be considered if lymph node biopsy is positive?

Localized radiation therapy

What is the treatment if endometrial cancer has metastasized?

Radiation, chemotherapy, and hormone therapy (high-dose progestins and antiestrogens)

OVARY

OVARIAN CANCER

Basic Science

Which genes located on which chromosomes are known to play a role in hereditary ovarian cancer?

Breast/ovarian cancer susceptibility genes BRCA1 and BRCA2; BRCA1 is located on chromosome 17q, BRCA2 on chromosome 13q.

What is the most frequent genetic event described in ovarian cancer to date?

Alteration of the p53 tumor suppressor gene

From which tissues are ovarian cancers derived?

Around 90% originate from cells derived from celomic epithelium

What is the percentage distribution of histologic types of epithelial ovarian cancer?

75%–80% serous carcinomas; 10% mucinous; 10% endometrioid; rest are clear cell, Brenner, and undifferentiated carcinomas

What is peritoneal carcinoma?	A primary malignant transformation of the peritoneum that simulates ovarian cancer clinically

Risk Factors and Presentation

What is the common denominator of reproductive events protecting from ovarian cancer?	Decrease of lifetime ovulatory cycles: late menarche, early menopause, pregnancy, breast-feeding, oral contraceptives
At what FIGO stage is ovarian cancer detected most of the time?	FIGO III (out of FIGO I–IV)

Diagnostic Tests/Studies

Define "multimodal approach" to early ovarian cancer detection.	Combining imaging studies (e.g., transvaginal US) with biochemical markers (e.g., CA125) to improve prediction of true positive cases
What is CA125 most useful for?	Evaluating response to treatment
How does ovarian cancer present in early disease?	Asymptomatic
How does it present in late disease?	Vague gastrointestinal (GI) symptoms, abdominal discomfort, fullness, early satiety, ascites, pain, pelvic mass, weight loss
What imaging studies in the workup are helpful in monitoring therapy?	Chest x-ray and computed tomography (CT) scan of pelvis and abdomen as baseline studies for comparison in recurring disease
What are pelvic washings?	Irrigation of pelvis, aspiration of irrigation fluid, and examination for malignant cells

Therapy

What is the goal of surgical intervention?	Optimal tumor debulking (i.e., reduce tumor to <2 cm), if macroscopically complete removal cannot be accomplished

What is the current standard therapy for FIGO stage III ovarian cancer?	Total abdominal hysterectomy with bilateral salpingo-oophorectomy, and omentectomy followed by combination chemotherapy with intravenous platinum/paclitaxel

CERVIX

CERVICAL CANCER

Epidemiology

What factors are associated with cervical cancer?	Human papilloma virus (HPV) infections, multiple sexual partners, early age of first intercourse (coiarche), short interval between menarche and coiarche, smoking, low socioeconomic status, malnutrition, and immunocompromise (e.g., HIV-positive)
What HPV subtypes are highest risk?	HPV types 16, 18, 31, and 41
How does HPV induce malignancy?	Interaction of HPV E6 and E7 proteins are thought to bind to and inactivate Rb and p53, transforming and immortalizing cells
At what age does it present?	Average age at diagnosis, 52 years; bimodal distribution of cases (peaks at 35–39 years and at 60–64 years)
What are the major histologic types?	Squamous cell and adenocarcinoma (glandular)
What is the most common histologic type?	Squamous cell carcinoma
Where does it originate?	At the squamocolumnar junction or transformation zone of the uterine cervix, where columnar cells are exposed to acidic vaginal pH, transforming into metaplastic squamous cells

Clinical Presentation and Diagnosis

How does cervical cancer present?	Early stage disease may be asymptomatic; postcoital bleeding, intermenstrual bleeding, or menorrhagia; vaginal discharge; constant gnawing lumbosacral or gluteal pain, signaling involved iliac or para-aortic lymph nodes impinging on nerve roots; or urinary and rectal symptoms of hematuria or rectal bleeding
What are the physical findings?	Normal physical exam; visible lesions on cervix, which may be exophytic or ulcerative; or palpable masses
How is it commonly diagnosed?	Abnormal pap smear followed by colposcopic or cone biopsy

Staging and Treatment

How is cervical cancer staged?	Clinically with speculum and bimanual pelvic and rectal exam, cystoscopy, rectosigmoidoscopy, chest x-ray, intravenous pyelogram, and barium enema
Define the following stages of cervical cancer:	
Stage 0	Carcinoma in situ
Stage I	Confined to uterus
Stage II	Invades beyond uterus, but not to pelvic wall or lower third of vagina
Stage III	Extends to pelvic wall, or involves lower third of the vagina, or causes hydronephrosis or nonfunctioning kidney
Stage IV	Invades mucosa of bladder or rectum, or extends beyond true pelvis
What is microinvasive carcinoma?	Measured stromal invasion of <5 mm with horizontal spread of <7 mm (stage IA)
What is the most effective prevention for cervical cancer?	Early diagnosis of preinvasive disease with yearly screening pap smears, colposcopy, and ablation or excision (conization) of dysplasia

What is the treatment for microinvasive disease?	Cone biopsy for those wishing to maintain fertility; hysterectomy, either vaginal or abdominal, for definitive treatment
What is the treatment for stages IB-IIA?	Hysterectomy and lymph node resection
What is the treatment for stages IIB-IV?	Pelvic radiation
When is pelvic exenteration, or en bloc removal of pelvic viscera, appropriate treatment?	Central recurrences for curative purposes only (i.e., with no evidence of lymphatic involvement or distant metastases)

MENSTRUAL DISORDERS

AMENORRHEA

Define amenorrhea.	The absence or cessation of menstrual cycles. Differentiated from oligomenorrhea: amenorrhea is complete absence of menstrual cycles; oligomenorrhea is the condition in which menstrual cycles have an interval of >35 days.
What is primary amenorrhea?	Absence of menses by age 16 in a girl without secondary sexual characteristics (e.g., breast and pubic hair development), or absence of menses by age 18 in a girl with secondary sexual characteristics.
What is secondary amenorrhea?	Cessation of menses (in a woman who previously had menses) for either 6 months or three menstrual intervals if she had oligomenorrhea
How are the causes of primary amenorrhea categorized?	Based on absence or presence of secondary sexual characteristics

If secondary sexual characteristics are absent (suggesting either absent or quiescent ovaries):

What are the causes of primary amenorrhea?

Either congenital ovarian failure or failure of the hypothalamic-pituitary axis to awaken and stimulate the ovaries.

What are some possible diagnoses?

Gonadal dysgenesis (e.g., Turner syndrome, pure gonadal dysgenesis), hypothalamic or pituitary failure (e.g., tumors, medications, eating disorders, excessive athletic exercise, stress), or postablative ovarian failure due to chemotherapy or radiation therapy

If secondary sexual characteristics are present (presuming some ovarian function):

What are the causes of primary amenorrhea?

Hypothalamic or pituitary dysfunction (ovaries not being cyclically stimulated), or genital tract abnormalities interfering with menstruation.

What are some possible diagnoses?

Hypothalamic-pituitary dysfunction (either idiopathic or due to eating disorders, weight gain or loss, excessive athletic exercise, stress); imperforate hymen, transverse vaginal septum, segmental or complete mullerian agenesis

How is primary amenorrhea evaluated?

History and physical exam; then, order lab tests based on presence or absence of secondary sexual characteristics

What tests are done to evaluate primary amenorrhea if secondary sexual characteristics are absent?

Serum FSH to determine whether cause is ovarian or central. Elevated FSH suggests ovarian failure; karyotype is then indicated to look for Y chromosome. If found, then gonadectomy is indicated to prevent malignant degeneration. Normal FSH suggests central problem; perform additional endocrine tests (serum gonadotropins, GnRH stimulation test).

What tests are done to evaluate primary amenorrhea if secondary sexual characteristics are present?

Progestin challenge test. If patient bleeds after progestin administration and withdrawal, an outflow abnormality is excluded; then evaluate hypothalamic-pituitary axis. Failure to bleed, without withdrawal bleeding to estrogen and progestin, suggests a congenital abnormality of genital tract; perform further imaging studies.

What are the causes of secondary amenorrhea?

Pregnancy, hypothalamic-pituitary dysfunction or failure (hyperprolactinemic conditions, pituitary necrosis following shock), ovarian failure (e.g., chemotherapy, radiation, autoimmune, surgery), and acquired genital tract abnormalities [e.g., cervical stenosis, intrauterine adhesions (Asherman syndrome), uterine fibroids]

Why is secondary amenorrhea an important problem?

Two important concepts must be stressed to the patient:

1. Hypoestrogenic amenorrhea can have significant sequelae (bone demineralization, osteoporosis, and atherogenesis) with a resulting increased risk of coronary artery and cerebrovascular disease.
2. When the woman is amenorrheic and euestrogenic, prolonged periods of amenorrhea increase her risk of endometrial proliferative diseases (e.g., hyperplasia, malignancy).

What tests are done to evaluate secondary amenorrhea?

First, pregnancy test. If negative, then progestin challenge test. If the patient bleeds after progestin administration and withdrawal, anovulation is diagnosed; determine why. If the patient does not bleed, then differentiate ovarian failure from genital abnormalities preventing menstruation by the estrogen-progestin challenge test. If the patient bleeds, this signals ovarian failure due either to a primary ovarian problem or a failure of the hypothalamic-pituitary axis. Differentiate by FSH level (elevated in primary ovarian problem). If the patient does not bleed, a genital tract abnormality is diagnosed and additional imaging is needed.

How is primary amenorrhea treated?

Depends on the cause. If gonadal dysgenesis, then hormone replacement therapy (HRT). If central (hypothalamic-pituitary) failure, then treat to restore normal function or replace missing gonadotropins if the goal is to restore ovarian function; alternatively, if ovarian function not required, give hormone replacement alone if the goal is to prevent hypoestrogenic complications and establish menses.

How is secondary amenorrhea treated:
  If fertility is not requested?

If significant conditions affecting general health can be excluded, then begin either cyclic progestin therapy (to prevent endometrial hyperplasia) or estrogen-progestin replacement (to prevent hypoestrogenic problems).

  If fertility is requested?

Induce ovulation, either with clomiphene citrate or exogenous gonadotropin therapy.

Is surgery ever indicated for treatment of secondary amenorrhea?

Yes, when anatomic problems are the cause.

DYSFUNCTIONAL UTERINE BLEEDING

What is dysfunctional uterine bleeding?

Abnormal uterine bleeding, often with anovulation, in the absence of other anatomic lesions. It is therefore a diagnosis of exclusion.

What other factors need to be excluded?

Foremost is pregnancy. Other causes: fibroids, polyps, endometrial cancer, infection, genital trauma, foreign bodies

What causes dysfunctional uterine bleeding?

Dysfunction of the hypothalamic-pituitary-gonadal axis resulting in continuous noncyclic estrogen stimulation of the endometrium. This leads to constant endometrial stimulation and subsequent irregular endometrial shedding.

Name other causes of irregular bleeding.

Any medical substance with estrogenic effects (e.g., ginseng)
20% of teens with dysfunctional uterine bleeding have a coagulation defect.

How does dysfunctional uterine bleeding often present?

Irregular, often heavy uterine bleeding with anovulation

What basic tests can be ordered to determine whether ovulation is occurring?

Pregnancy should always be considered; exclude using a serum β-hCG determination. Exclude hypothyroidism or hyperprolactinemia by determining serum thyroid-stimulating hormone and prolactin. Document anovulation using daily basal body temperature graph and day 23–35 serum progesterone level. Exclude leiomyomata and polyps with US of uterus, sonohysterogram, or both. Exclude infection using endometrial biopsy. Pap smear can exclude cervical dysplasia and cancer.

How is dysfunctional uterine bleeding treated?

Progestational agent (e.g., medroxyprogesterone acetate) orally for minimum of 10 days during luteal phase for several cycles

What is an alternative treatment?

Oral contraceptives, 1 tablet 2–4 times/day for 1 week, then immediately begin a normal regimen (i.e., do not allow endometrium to bleed) for at least 3 months. Bleeding should stop 12–24 hours after starting this regimen, with about 60% reduction in blood flow.

What if bleeding is heavy?

25 mg conjugated estrogen IV every 4 hours for 24 hours. If bleeding not controlled: dilatation and curettage is appropriate for diagnosis and therapy. If bleeding controlled: initiate oral contraceptives, continue for 3 months.

MENOPAUSE

MENOPAUSE AND THE CLIMACTERIC

Define menopause.

Literally, cessation of menses, equivalent to intractable amenorrhea. Usually used in the context of a woman at the end of reproductive life, when irreversible ovarian failure causes her to stop menstruating.

Define the climacteric.

The transitional phase in a woman's life when her normal reproductive (i.e., ovarian) function starts to decline, ending when a new postreproductive steady-state is reached.

Define perimenopause.

The transition years in a woman's life when normal reproductive function starts to decline, ending at menopause. Perimenopause does not include the postmenopausal years of the climacteric.

At what age does menopause usually occur?

In developed countries, menopause typically begins between ages 50 and 52; about 95% of women reach menopause between ages 45 and 55.

What specifically causes the climacteric and menopause?

The climacteric begins when follicles no longer respond to normal FSH stimulation; functional follicles are exhausted, and estrogen production from the ovaries declines. When circulating estrogens fall low enough, as ovulation ceases, that endometrial proliferation stops, menstruation ceases; menopause is said to have occurred.

What are the typical symptoms of the climacteric?

During perimenopause, highly variable changes in menstrual cycles are common, including changes in interval, amount, and associated perimenstrual molimina. As the degree of hypoestrogenism increases, more hypoestrogenic symptoms occur during the perimenopausal years, including hot flushes, genitourinary atrophy (e.g., dyspareunia, pruritus, urinary frequency, atrophic vaginitis and vulvitis, urgency and stress incontinence, pelvic organ prolapse), skin changes, hirsutism, breast reduction, and emotional symptoms. Over 95% of perimenopausal and postmenopausal women have hot flushes.

Aside from hypoestrogenic symptoms, what two other conditions are commonly seen in perimenopausal and postmenopausal women?

Osteoporosis
Cardiovascular lipid changes causing atherosclerotic vascular disease

How are the climacteric and menopause diagnosed?

Because ovarian failure is the hallmark of the climacteric, diagnostic tests are aimed at demonstrating irreversible ovarian quiescence. Serial elevated FSH levels (>45 mIU/mL) with concomitant low estradiol levels confirm ovarian failure. Testing is unnecessary in most patients, however, because onset of hypoestrogenic symptoms and physical findings in a woman >40 years is the hallmark.

What is premature ovarian failure?

Refers to women who have menopause before age 40. Incidence is about 1%.

What are the causes of premature ovarian failure?

Genetic factors (e.g., mosaicism for Turner syndrome), gonadotropin ovarian resistance syndrome (Savage syndrome), autoimmune disorders, smoking, chemotherapy, radiation therapy, hysterectomy, low body weight, rare glycogen or lipid storage diseases

How are patients with premature ovarian failure treated?

Treatment is identical to that for postmenopausal ovarian failure.

Describe the therapeutic goals in treating patients in the climacteric.

Ameliorate symptoms, prevent osteoporosis, and prevent atherosclerotic cardiovascular disease; all met simultaneously with estrogen replacement therapy.

Besides decreased circulating estrogen levels, what are some other risk factors for osteoporosis?

Reduced weight, family history, early menopause (natural or postsurgical), low calcium intake, cigarette smoking, nulliparity, high caffeine or alcohol intake, and Caucasian or Asian race

How is osteoporosis diagnosed?

By using imaging modalities that evaluate bone density at sites at risk (trabecular bone in vertebral bodies, trochanter of femur, distal radius, and calcaneus). Comparison is usually to bone density of women at peak bone mass, age mid-30s. The imaging modality most commonly used is dual-energy x-ray absorptiometry (DEXA), although dual photon absorptiometry (DPA), single photon absorptiometry (SPA), quantitative CT scan, and even plain films can be used.

How does the risk of atherosclerosis change in postmenopausal women?

With prolonged hypoestrogenism, the circulating lipid profile in postmenopausal women shows increased total and low-density lipoprotein cholesterol, and decreased high-density lipoprotein cholesterol. This favors atherogenesis, and is the basis for the increase in atherosclerotic coronary artery and cerebrovascular disease in postmenopausal women not on estrogen replacement therapy (ERT); compared to this group, women on HRT have a lowered risk of angina, myocardial infarction, and stroke.

How and why does hormone treatment differ based on the presence or absence of the uterus?

Estrogens (natural or synthetic) cause endometrial proliferation. In the reproductive years, this proliferation is checked monthly by the endometrial shedding that occurs when progestogens (secreted by the corpus luteum after ovulation) are added to the estrogens stimulating the endometrium, and then withdrawn. Thus, when postmenopausal women are placed on ERT, those with a uterus are also prescribed a progestogen to prevent endometrial proliferation. Large cohort trials have shown that this regimen decreases the risk of endometrial cancer.

Describe the difference between cyclic and continuous hormone replacement with progestogens.

Cyclic: administer for 7–10 days each month; when completed, the patient has a uterine bleeding episode.

Continuous: daily administration does not result in cyclic "menses," but irregular bleeding commonly occurs during early months of therapy.

How are progestogens and estrogens usually administered?

Progestogens: Primarily orally; less frequently by transdermal route; depot formulations are available as contraceptives, but are not usually used as hormone replacement.

Estrogens: Available for oral, transdermal, and intramuscular depot administration (intramuscular used less commonly)

What are the advantages and disadvantages of oral administration of estrogens?

Advantages: ease of use, generally lower cost, and extensive experience

Disadvantages: GI side effects (especially early in treatment) and lower efficacy in some women due to wide variations in blood levels after ingestion

What are the advantages and disadvantages of transdermal administration of estrogens and progestogens?

Transdermal estrogens are relatively new; both 3.5- and 7-day systems are available.

Advantages: continuous peripheral delivery; bypasses GI tract and hepatic circulation; theoretically, more convenient to use, fewer side effects (but this is variable)

Disadvantages: more expensive than oral formulations; local irritation from the patch in some patients. New patch formulations now available, with both estrogens and progestogens for transdermal uptake.

What are some equivalent estrogen replacement doses?

Conjugated estrogens (Premarin) 0.625–1.25 mg daily by mouth, esterified estrogens (Estratab) 0.625–1.25 mg daily by mouth, micronized estradiol (Estrace) 0.5–1.0 mg daily by mouth, and 17β-estradiol transdermal patch (Climara, Vivelle) to deliver 0.05–0.10 mg daily are equivalent in terms of estrogenic effect, side effects, and risks.

What are the doses of oral progestins for hormone replacement regimens?

Medroxyprogesterone (Provera, Cycrin) 2.5–5.0 mg by mouth daily throughout month or 5.0–10.0 mg by mouth daily for 7–10 days; norethindrone acetate (Aygestin, Norlutate) approximately half the medroxyprogesterone dose is equivalent.

What are the common side effects and risks of HRT?

Side effects: water retention with weight gain, nausea, abdominal discomfort, headache, breast fullness, and mastalgia

Risks: exacerbation of gallbladder disease, endometrial hyperplasia, and breast neoplasia. Relationship of increased risk of breast neoplasia to estrogen or estrogen-progestogen therapy is very controversial and unsettled at present.

What adjunctive therapy is recommended in addition to HRT for postmenopausal patients?

Supplementation with approximately 1000 mg of absorbed calcium, to optimize effects of ERT on preventing osteoporosis; weight-bearing exercise to stimulate bone remodeling; drugs (e.g., calcitonin) in selected patients to prevent or treat osteoporosis

What are the alternatives to traditional HRT?	Some suggest natural forms of estrogens (e.g., phytoestrogens from soy products) and vegetable-derived progestogens; however, their efficacy is unproved at present. Other drugs can provide some benefits of HRT in selected patients (e.g., bisphosphonates or selective estrogen receptor modulators in patients who cannot or will not take HRT with estrogen).

BREAST CANCER

EPIDEMIOLOGY

What factors are associated with breast cancer?	Age, history of prior breast cancer, family history, alcohol intake, (possibly) postmenopausal estrogen use; also BRCA1, BRCA2, and the Lynch II syndrome
At what age does breast cancer present?	Uncommon before age 45; incidence increases steadily after age 55.
What are the major histologic types of breast cancer?	Ductal, intraductal, lobular, medullary
What is the most common histologic type?	Ductal; also has the worst prognosis.
Where does it originate?	Ductal epithelium (ductal) or terminal lobules (lobular)

CLINICAL PRESENTATION AND DIAGNOSIS

How does breast cancer present?	Usually with an irregular, painless mass
What are the physical findings?	Most patients present with a painless, irregular, dominant mass. Advanced findings include chest wall fixation, palpable axillary nodes, and skin and nipple involvement.

How is breast cancer commonly discovered?	Mammography is the most sensitive test, but most commonly the patient finds it during self-examination.
How is a diagnosis of breast cancer confirmed?	Mammography NEVER diagnoses breast cancer; tissue diagnosis mandatory. Biopsy (either needle or excisional) is the diagnostic method.

Staging and Treatment

How is breast cancer staged?	The staging is both clinical (i.e., fixation to chest wall) and surgical (involvement of lymph nodes).

Define the following stages:

Stage 0	Either DCIS (ductal) or LCIS (lobular) carcinoma in situ. Both may be associated with invasive cancer in the ipsilateral (ductal) or contralateral (lobular) breast.
Stage I	Tumor of <2 cm, no positive nodes
Stage II	Combination of tumor of <2 cm with positive nodes (IIA), OR a tumor of >2 cm with negative nodes (IIB)
Stage III	Combination of tumor of >2 cm with fixed nodes, OR a tumor of >5 cm with positive nodes, OR chest wall fixation, peau d'orange, or skin nodules
Stage IV	Any primary tumor with distant metastases

What is the treatment for stages I–IIA?	Either modified radical mastectomy or combination of lumpectomy, axillary node dissection, and postoperative radiation
What is the treatment for stages IIB–IV?	Postoperative chemotherapy is offered to patients with high-risk prognostic factors; may be given preoperatively to shrink tumor.

FEMALE INFERTILITY AND PELVIC INFLAMMATORY DISEASE

INFERTILITY

What is the definition of infertility?	Inability to conceive a viable pregnancy during 1 year of regular, unprotected

sexual intercourse. The time period is derived from knowledge of the optimal human monthly probability of conception (fecundity), which is approximately 20%; thus, after 1 year of attempting pregnancy, roughly 85–90% of normal couples will succeed, and failure to conceive after 1 year suggests an abnormality.

What is the difference between primary and secondary infertility?

Primary infertility—inability to ever conceive; secondary infertility—the couple has conceived before but is subsequently infertile

What is the incidence of infertility?

Occurs in approximately 1 in 10 reproductive-age couples

What are the causes of infertility?

4 categories: male, ovulatory (female), mechanical, and immunologic

Describe the causes of male-factor infertility.

Disorders of sperm production leading to low sperm count, low motility, low normal morphology (teratozoospermia), or sperm function abnormalities; these may be caused by varicoceles, sexually transmitted diseases, mumps orchitis, medications, alcohol or recreational drugs, gonadal dysgenesis, pituitary dysfunction or failure, and hypothalamic failure (Kallmann syndrome).

Describe the ovulatory factors in infertility.

Commonly, uncharacterized hypothalamic-pituitary dysfunction. Other possible causes: pituitary (e.g., tumor, infarction); hypothalamic (e.g., anorexia, weight gain or loss, medications); ovarian (e.g., premature ovarian failure); polycystic ovarian syndrome (a neuroendocrine disturbance causing ovulatory dysfunction, infertility, dysfunctional uterine bleeding, and variable insulin resistance)

What are the mechanical factors in infertility?

Cervical stenosis or mucus abnormalities (after infection or surgery), uterine causes (e.g., congenital abnormalities,

Asherman syndrome, uterine fibroids), tubal disease (after other pelvic or abdominal surgery with postoperative adhesions, or infection), pelvic factors (e.g., endometriosis, pelvic adhesions)

What are the immunologic factors in infertility?

Disorders of the immune system that produce a cellular or humoral immune response interfering with sperm migration, sperm-oocyte interaction, fertilization, conceptus transport, implantation, or early embryonic development

What are the basic tests for evaluating an infertile couple?

Semen analysis; ovulatory confirmation; endocrine tests to explain known or suspected ovulatory dysfunction; evaluation of the uterine cavity and tubal patency; postcoital test to evaluate sperm-cervical mucus interaction; laparoscopy to exclude pelvic adhesions or endometriosis

How is ovulation assessed?

Basal body temperature charting, urinary LH surge detection, and/or serial pelvic US to assess follicle growth during periovulatory phase of cycle. Postovulatory endometrial biopsy showing secretory phase endometrium and elevated midluteal phase progesterone levels indicate corpus luteum progesterone secretion, and are evidence that ovulation has occurred.

What is the postcoital test used for, and how is it done?

It assesses sperm–cervical mucus interaction, necessary for sperm capacitation. The woman is examined 2–10 hours after having sexual intercourse in the periovulatory phase of the cycle; the presence of motile sperm in the endocervical specimen constitutes a normal test.

How are the shape of the uterine cavity and tubal patency determined?

Hysterosalpingogram (HSG) and sonohysterogram are used to evaluate the uterine cavity for congenital or acquired abnormalities. HSG is superior to sonohysterogram in providing information about tubal architecture and tubal patency.

How is HSG done?

HSG requires an x-ray facility with fluoroscopy. A balloon-tip catheter is inserted into the uterine cavity and radio-opaque contrast material (dye) is inserted in a retrograde fashion into the upper genital tract, outlining the uterine cavity, and then the fallopian tubes; dye spilling from the fimbriated ends of the tubes confirms tubal patency.

How is a sonohysterogram done?

Similar to HSG, except the contrast agent is normal saline and US is used instead of x-ray fluoroscopy.

Describe how laparoscopy is done.

Either regional (spinal or epidural) or general anesthesia is administered; a needle is inserted through the umbilicus into the peritoneal cavity, and a pneumoperitoneum is induced by filling the space with carbon dioxide gas. The laparoscope is then placed through the umbilicus into the pneumoperitoneum, and the pelvic and abdominal cavities are inspected. Additional puncture sites allow placement of accessory sheaths to introduce instruments for operative laparoscopy.

How is male-factor infertility treated?

Depending on the cause, treatment could include clomiphene or gonadotropin therapy to improve semen parameters; varicocelectomy; intrauterine insemination of the female partner; in vitro fertilization (IVF); IVF with intracytoplasmic sperm injection; or use of donor semen for insemination.

How is ovulatory dysfunction treated?

First, evaluate the patient to determine underlying cause of the ovulatory problem; treat complicating conditions; and then choose an appropriate ovulation induction agent (e.g., clomiphene citrate, urinary or recombinant gonadotropins). Bromocriptine and corticosteroids can be used to induce ovulation in women with hyperprolactinemia and congenital adrenal hyperplasia.

How is clomiphene citrate administered?

Clomiphene is marketed as a 50-mg pill; usual dosage required to induce ovulation is 50–150 mg daily for cycle days 5–9. Ovulation typically occurs 7–10 days after the last pill is taken.

What are the side effects and risks of clomiphene therapy?

Side effects are attributed to antiestrogenic effects (hot flushes, vaginal dryness, insomnia) of the drug while administered, and the hyperestrogenic response (nausea, breast tenderness, water retention) it produces as ovulation is stimulated. Risks: ovarian cyst production; multiple births.

How are cervical factor infertility problems treated?

Ovulation induction, if the problem is poor mucus production secondary to ovulatory dysfunction. When the cervical factor is due to semen or sperm abnormalities, intrauterine insemination, IVF, or donor sperm may be used.

How are uterine problems that cause infertility treated?

Surgical treatment is almost always needed to correct the anatomic defect. Myomectomy is done for uterine fibroids; metroplasty is done for congenital uterine defects.

How are tubal problems and pelvic adhesions that cause infertility treated?

These are now common indications for IVF. Otherwise, tuboplasty by either laparoscopy or laparotomy is needed to repair the tubes and restore tuboovarian relationships. The same surgical approaches are used to treat pelvic adhesions interfering with normal tuboovarian function.

What are the steps needed to complete the IVF procedure?

IVF requires a specialized human embryology laboratory, numerous trained personnel, and 6–7 weeks to complete:

1. Administration of a GnRH analog to downregulate the pituitary gland, blocking the patient's own feedback and subsequent LH surge.
2. After successful pituitary downregulation, administration of exogenous gonadotropins to directly stimulate multiple follicular development; response assessed by daily serum estradiol assay and follicular US.
3. Once optimal follicle number and size are reached, transvaginal oocyte retrieval is initiated.
4. With US guidance, a long needle is advanced through the vagina into the ovarian follicles, which are aspirated.
5. Oocytes are identified and prepared for in vitro insemination using the male partner's sperm; fertilized oocytes develop in the laboratory for several additional days.
6. Early embryos (8–12 cells) are transferred to the uterine cavity using a transcervical catheter.

How is infertility due to endometriosis treated?

Medication and surgery; choice of treatment is highly individualized; for severe cases, surgery to excise or destroy the implants and restore normal anatomic relationships is preferred. IVF is also an option.

PELVIC INFLAMMATORY DISEASE (PID)

What is PID?

Upper genital tract infection and inflammation, resulting from microorganisms colonizing the endocervix and ascending to the endometrium and fallopian tubes; inflammation produces clinical conditions of endometritis, salpingitis, and peritonitis.

What is the cause of PID?

Usually, sexually transmitted microorganisms.

What are the most common infectious agents?

Most common organisms: *Neisseria gonorrhoeae* and *Chlamydia trachomatis*. Later, intestinal flora may be cultured from the endosalpinx and pelvic peritoneum, and anaerobes such as *Bacteroides* and peptostreptococci are commonly found in tuboovarian abscesses. *Actinomyces* is associated with PID complicated by foreign body [e.g., intrauterine device (IUD)].

What is the typical clinical presentation of PID?

Varies, but triad of pelvic pain, cervical motion tenderness, and bilateral adnexal tenderness (with or without rebound tenderness suggesting pelvic peritonitis) is common. Fever and mucopurulent endocervicitis are common. Presentation may include urinary symptoms or abnormal uterine bleeding (menorrhagia, metrorrhagia). Mild cases of PID may go unrecognized, or are asymptomatic.

How is the diagnosis of PID confirmed?

Diagnosis is clinical, supported by triad of signs and symptoms. No absolute, confirmatory or pathognomonic tests, but helpful tests include elevated c-reactive protein or erythrocyte sedimentation rate, leukocytosis, positive cultures for gonorrhea or chlamydia, sonography (tubo-ovarian abscess), endometrial biopsy (endometritis), and laparoscopy to confirm salpingitis (and obtain endosalpingeal and peritoneal Gram stain and cultures).

What is the goal of PID therapy?

Resolve acute infection, prevent progression of infection with increased morbidity and even mortality, and maintain reproductive potential (i.e., prevent loss of ovarian and tubal function). Therapy regimens provide empiric, broad-spectrum coverage of likely pathogens (e.g., *N. gonorrhoeae*, *C. trachomatis*, gram-negative bacteria, anaerobes).

When is hospitalization recommended for treatment of PID?

When clinical presentation is severe, pelvic abscess is suspected or proven, diagnosis is uncertain, outpatient treatment has failed, or compliance with outpatient regimen is questionable. Criteria for discharge: patient afebrile for at least 24 hours; resolution of leukocytosis, rebound tenderness, and pelvic organ tenderness.

Describe the specific treatment regimens commonly used for outpatient therapy of PID.

One common regimen combines ceftriaxone 125 mg IM as a single dose with doxycycline 100 mg by mouth twice a day for 7 days, to treat gonorrhea and chlamydia, respectively. Instead of ceftriaxone, can use ofloxacin, cefixime, or ciprofloxacin; instead of doxycycline, can use azithromycin, ofloxacin, clindamycin, metronidazole, or erythromycin.

Describe several equivalent inpatient treatment regimens for PID.

Typically, triple-antibiotic therapy with clindamycin 900 mg IV every 8 hours, gentamicin 1.5 mg/kg IV every 8 hours, and ampicillin 1 g IV every 6 hours. An alternative is cefoxitin 2 g IV every 6 hours or cefotetan g IV every 12 hours, along with doxycycline 100 IV or by mouth every 12 hours.

When is surgery indicated for treatment of tubo-ovarian abscess in PID patients?

With appropriate inpatient antibiotics, about 75% of patients with tubo-ovarian abscess will respond to medical therapy alone. If antimicrobial therapy fails, surgical exploration with drainage or extirpation of abscess and involved tissues is indicated.

COMPLICATED PREGNANCY

ECTOPIC PREGNANCY

Basic Science

What is ectopic pregnancy?

Pregnancy outside the uterine endometrium

What is heterotopic pregnancy?	Multiple pregnancy with implantation occurring in the uterus along with pregnancy outside the lining of the endometrium (commonest in fallopian tube)

Risk Factors and Presentation

What are the causes of ectopic pregnancy?	PID, previous tubal pregnancy, history of tubal ligation or tubal surgery, and presence of IUD
What are the risk factors?	Besides the above causes, infertility and assisted reproductive techniques
Name the two major risk factors.	Tubal surgery and previous ectopic pregnancy
Which uterine device has highest risk of ectopic pregnancy?	Progesterone-containing IUD
How does ectopic pregnancy present?	Ranges from vaginal spotting to hemorrhagic shock. Patients may be asymptomatic; may be diagnosed due to high suspicion leading to evaluation and subsequent diagnosis.
What are signs and symptoms of ectopic pregnancy?	Delayed menses, spotting, abdominal pain, shoulder tip pain, and hypovolemic shock symptoms. Physical exam: shock findings, abdominal tenderness, guarding, and rebound tenderness. Pelvic exam: uterus soft, enlarged, and tender; adnexal mass may be palpable.
What are the risk factors for heterotopic pregnancy?	In vitro fertilization and controlled super ovulation. Incidence up to 1% in these patients.

Diagnostic Tests/Studies

How is the diagnosis of ectopic pregnancy made?	Inappropriate rise or fall of human chorionic gonadotropin (hCG) is

suggestive. When beta hCG (bhCG) is ≥1500 mIU/mL, absence of intrauterine pregnancy on US is suggestive. Presence of free fluid and adnexal mass on US are suggestive. Occasionally one can see a fetal heart or fetus outside the uterus, which is diagnostic.

What is the differential diagnosis?

Normal intrauterine pregnancy, ruptured ovarian cyst, bleeding corpus luteum, spontaneous abortion, adnexal torsion, and endometriosis

What is your diagnostic approach?

Pregnancy test. If unstable, consider immediate laparoscopy or laparotomy depending on clinical situation. If stable, consider vaginal US; if no intrauterine pregnancy is seen, a bhCG level of >1500 IU/L is consistent with ectopic pregnancy. Depending on clinical situation, institute medical or surgical management at that time. If bhCG is <1500 IU/L and patient remains stable, follow bhCG levels every 48 hours to >1500 IU/L, then proceed as above.

How do you differentiate missed abortion with ectopic pregnancy?

Missed abortion has minimal abdominal pain and some evidence of pregnancy (sac or debris in uterus). Dilatation and curettage can confirm villi in missed abortion.

Which tests are helpful in the diagnosis of ectopic pregnancy?

Pregnancy test, quantitative bhCG, transvaginal US

How do you diagnose heterotopic pregnancy?

Diagnosis is difficult. A fetus or fetal heart outside the uterus or hemoperitoneum with an intrauterine pregnancy raises suspicion of heterotopic pregnancy.

**How common is
heterotopic pregnancy?**

Spontaneous heterotopic pregnancy
is rare (1 in 30,000 pregnancies). In
patients undergoing assisted reproductive
techniques (IVF and controlled super
ovulation), can be as high as 1 in 100
pregnancies.

**How do you differentiate
a ruptured corpus luteum
from ruptured ectopic
pregnancy?**

Differential may be difficult because
both may have hemoperitoneum.
Sonographic findings of intrauterine vs.
extrauterine fetus or fetal heart activity
may be required.

**What is an appropriate
rise in bhCG in a normal
intrauterine pregnancy?**

66% increase in 48 hours; doubling every
3 days

**What are the chances of
inappropriate rise of
bhCG in patients who
have intrauterine
pregnancy?**

12%

**Does progesterone have a
role in differentiating a
viable from a nonviable
pregnancy?**

Progesterone value of 5 ng/mL or less is
suggestive of a nonviable pregnancy.

What is culdocentesis?

Passing a needle (e.g., an 18G
Angiocath) from the posterior vaginal
fornix into the peritoneal cavity to allow
aspiration of cul de sac fluid

**What does it mean if
blood obtained from
culdocentesis clots after
removal?**

The blood sample is an aspirate from a
vein or artery.

**What is the interpretation
of finding free-flowing,
nonclotting blood during
culdocentesis?**

There is blood in the abdominal cavity
that clotted and then lysed after
collecting, suggesting that there was
a source of intraperitoneal bleeding,
suggestive of ruptured ectopic
pregnancy.

Therapy

What is the treatment of stable ectopic pregnancy?

Depends on patient's condition, compliance with follow-up, and wishes for future childbearing; medical management with methotrexate is preferred.

What is the medical management of ectopic pregnancy?

Treat with methotrexate, a folic acid antagonist.

What are the prerequisites of medical management of ectopic pregnancy?

1. Stable, reliable, and compliant patient.
2. US fails to find intrauterine pregnancy, or no villi seen in uterine curetting.
3. Ectopic pregnancy measures <4 cm in greatest diameter.
4. No evidence of rupture (i.e., hemoperitoneum).
5. HCG titers of <10,000 IU/L and no fetal cardiac activity.

What are the contraindications of methotrexate for ectopic pregnancy?

Unstable, noncompliant patient; ruptured ectopic pregnancy; adnexal mass of >4 cm; patient on folic acid; patient with liver disease

When is surgical therapy warranted?

Hemodynamically unstable patient; suspected ruptured ectopic pregnancy; medical therapy contraindicated

When is laparoscopy or laparotomy appropriate?

Depends on patient's condition and operator's skill. If possible, laparoscopy is preferable.

When is linear salpingostomy or partial salpingectomy appropriate?

Salpingostomy is preferred if patient wishes future childbearing and has unruptured ectopic pregnancy. Partial salpingectomy is advisable if childbearing is complete or the tube is ruptured.

What is the treatment of heterotopic pregnancy?

Surgery—partial salpingectomy

What is the risk of recurrence of ectopic pregnancy?	After one ectopic pregnancy: 15%

ABRUPTIO PLACENTAE

Define abruptio placentae.	Premature separation of a normally implanted placenta
What is the incidence?	1/86–1/206
What is the presenting clinical triad?	1. External or occult uterine bleeding 2. Uterine hypotonus/hyperactivity 3. Fetal distress/death
What are the grades of abruptio placentae?	Grade I: slight vaginal bleeding; maternal and fetal status stable Grade II: mild external vaginal bleeding; maternal tachycardia, tetanic uterine contractions, fetal distress Grade III: moderate to severe vaginal bleeding, tetanic and painful uterine contractions, fetal distress, and coagulation abnormalities
What is the primary cause?	Unknown
What are risk factors?	Maternal hypertension, crack/cocaine use, maternal abdominal trauma, multiple gestation, cigarette smoking, and polyhydramnios
How is the diagnosis made?	By history in a patient with risk factors. There are no pathognomonic tests for abruptio placentae. One classic clue to diagnosis: presence of hemodynamic shock out of proportion to blood loss in a patient with third-trimester uterine bleeding; this is caused by concealed retroplacental hemorrhage.

What are the typical objective findings?	Firm, tender uterus with or without vaginal bleeding and fetal heart rate decelerations
Which labs need to be drawn?	Complete blood cell (CBC) count, type and screen, coagulation studies, urine drug screen
How do you rule out a previa as a cause of bleeding?	US
If mother and fetus are stable, what is the intrapartum management of abruptio placentae?	Continuous electronic fetal and uterine monitoring, anticipating spontaneous vaginal delivery
If mother, fetus, or both are not stable, what is the management of labor and delivery?	Immediate cesarean section
What confirms the diagnosis of abruptio placentae?	Gross and pathologic examination of the placenta after delivery

PLACENTA PREVIA

What is placenta previa?	Implantation of the placenta over the cervical os
What is the incidence?	1/200 live births
What are the three types?	1. Total: cervical os completely covered by placenta 2. Partial: cervical os partially occluded by placenta 3. Marginal: encroachment of placenta to the margin or edge of the cervical os
What are potential risk factors?	Maternal age of >35 years, African American race, previous cesarean delivery, multiparity, and previous placenta previa

What is the classic presentation?	Painless third-trimester vaginal bleeding
How is the diagnosis made?	US is the only reliable method.
What labs should be ordered?	CBC count, prothrombin time/partial thromboplastin time, with preparation for transfusion if massive hemorrhage should occur
In what instance can a vaginal exam be performed?	NEVER
What are the options for mode of delivery?	Cesarean section is the only option for safe delivery of mother and fetus.

PREGNANCY-INDUCED HYPERTENSION

What is the classic triad of preeclampsia?	Hypertension, proteinuria, nondependent edema
What is eclampsia?	Seizure activity in a pregnant or postpartum woman with hypertension
How is hypertension defined in pregnancy?	Blood pressure of >140/90, or a 30 mm Hg increase in systolic or 15 mm Hg rise in diastolic pressure from prepregnancy baseline. Elevation must be present on two measurements 6 hours apart.
How many grams of protein in a 24-hour urine are needed to make the diagnosis of preeclampsia?	>0.3 g
How is chronic hypertension distinguished from preeclampsia?	Chronic hypertension is hypertension that occurs before the 20th week of gestation.

What are the criteria for severe preeclampsia?

Blood pressure: ≥160 mm Hg systolic or 110 mm Hg diastolic recorded on two separate measurements 6 hours apart. Proteinuria: >5 g in 24 hours or 3–4+ on qualitative exam. Oliguria: <400 mL in 24 hours. Other criteria: cerebral or visual disturbances, epigastric pain, pulmonary edema or cyanosis, cardiac abnormalities, thrombocytopenia, impaired liver function, intrauterine growth restriction, oligohydramnios, eclampsia, and microangiopathic hemolysis

What are risk factors for preeclampsia?

Multiple gestation, hydatidiform mole, preexisting hypertension, nulliparity, family history, extremes of age, African American race, diabetes, chronic hypertension, previous preeclampsia, antiphospholipid syndromes

What are the classic symptoms of preeclampsia?

Headache, blurred vision, scotomata, edema, nausea and vomiting, malaise, epigastric pain

What lab tests are needed to evaluate a patient with preeclampsia?

Urinalysis for protein, serum transaminases, and platelets

What is the management of mild preeclampsia?

Delivery (if term), hospitalization with bed rest, consider medical antihypertensive treatment if remote from term, IV magnesium sulfate for seizure prophylaxis. Always consider delivery for worsening maternal or fetal status.

What is the management of severe preeclampsia/ eclampsia?

Stabilize mother, IV magnesium sulfate therapy, deliver fetus; antihypertensive medication if needed for blood pressure control

What are the complications of preeclampsia?

Abruption; disseminated intravascular coagulation; hemolysis, elevated liver enzymes, and low platelet count (HELLP) syndrome; eclampsia; increased risk of preterm birth; Couvelaire uterus; renal failure; stroke

PREMATURE LABOR

What is the definition of preterm labor?	Labor that occurs between 20 and 37 weeks gestation.
What are the risk factors associated with preterm delivery?	History of previous preterm birth, premature rupture of membranes, low socioeconomic status, nutritional status, African American race, maternal age of <18 or >35 years at first delivery, preeclampsia, placental abruption, placenta previa, fetal growth restriction, inadequate weight gain, uterine anomalies, cervical procedures, second-trimester abortion, smoking, cocaine use, multiple gestations, congenital anomalies, incompetent cervix, intrauterine infection, systemic infection, diethylstilbestrol exposure, inadequate or excessive amniotic fluid, shortened cervix
What symptoms are associated with preterm labor?	Uterine contractions, menstrual-like cramps, backache, pelvic pressure, increased vaginal discharge, and bloodstained vaginal discharge
How is preterm labor diagnosed?	Documented persistent uterine contractions and evidence of cervical change with intact membranes between 20 and 37 weeks gestation; or cervical dilatation of 2 cm or effacement of 80%.
What should be included in the initial patient assessment?	History and physical including examination of cervix, determination of gestational age, assessment of fetal well-being with external tocography and fetal heart rate tracing, cervical cultures, urinalysis and culture, urinary drug screen, identification of clinical signs of intra-amniotic infection including fever and fundal tenderness, identification of subclinical infection, including amniotic fluid cultures via amniocentesis and urine cultures
What is the management of preterm labor?	Bed rest, hydration, and tocolytic therapy

What pharmacologic agents are currently in use for preterm labor tocolysis?	Magnesium sulfate, prostaglandin inhibitors (indomethacin), calcium channel antagonists (nifedipine), and β-adrenergic agonists (ritodrine and terbutaline)
What are the major neonatal complications of prematurity?	Respiratory distress syndrome, intraventricular hemorrhage, necrotizing enterocolitis, neonatal sepsis, patent ductus arteriosus, bronchopulmonary dysplasia, retinopathy of prematurity, and neonatal death
What are the long-term morbidities associated with preterm birth?	Mental retardation, cerebral palsy, seizure disorders, chronic pulmonary disease, blindness, and deafness
What are the current recommendations for antenatal corticosteroid therapy?	Patients at risk of delivering preterm are candidates for antenatal corticosteroid therapy if >24 weeks and <34 weeks gestation with intact membranes, or <30–32 weeks with premature rupture of membranes.
What are the current recommendations for antenatal antibiotic therapy?	Patients with preterm labor are candidates for intravenous prophylactic therapy for group B β-hemolytic streptococci.

PRENATAL TESTING

Basic Science

What is prenatal testing?	The use of noninvasive and invasive testing to determine the viability of a fetus in utero, detect congenital fetal and placental anomalies, and monitor fetal development.
What percentage of newborns have a detectable genetic defect?	Approximately 1 in 20

Risk Factors and Presentation

Name three clinical parameters used to screen for an abnormal pregnancy.

1. Blood pressure usually decreases in second trimester. An increase of 30 mm Hg diastolic or 15 mm Hg systolic is considered abnormal.
2. Fetal heart rate outside normal range of 120–160 beats/min
3. Fundal height (in centimeters) outside normal range (approximately equal to gestational age between 16 and 36 weeks)

What is the significance of fundal height and how is it confirmed?

Small-for-dates: intrauterine growth retardation, fetal anomaly, oligohydramnios, abnormal fetal lie, or premature fetal descent into pelvis

Large-for-dates: leiomyomata or other pelvic tumor, multiple fetuses, polyhydramnios, or macrosomia

Confirm either small-for-dates or large-for-dates impression by abdominal or transvaginal US.

When do most chromosomal aberrations occur?

During first trimester of pregnancy

Define chorioangioma and name the major types.

Most common primary nontrophoblastic tumor of the placenta; angioma, cellular, degenerate

Name eight major complications of chorioangiomas.

Hydramnios (most frequent), antepartum hemorrhage, premature labor, fetal congestive heart failure, fetal thrombocytopenia, hemolytic anemia, intrauterine growth failure, and fetal death (due to preeclampsia or intrauterine cardiac death)

What are the presenting signs of preeclampsia?

New onset edema of face and/or hands in the presence of proteinuria and hypertension

Diagnostic Tests/Studies

When should prenatal testing begin?

First prenatal visit: 6–8 weeks after first missed menses

What tests should be done at the first prenatal visit?

Complete history, blood pressure check, height, weight, body mass index, breast exam, fundal height, cervical exam. Test for fetal heart tones if beyond first trimester, and fetal position if beyond second trimester

Lab tests: hemoglobin/hematocrit, Rh factor, blood type, antibody screen, Pap smear, urine dipstick for protein, sugar, culture, and urinalysis, and tests for rubella, syphilis, hepatitis B, and human immunodeficiency virus

What are additional important laboratory tests?

1. Maternal serum α-fetoprotein to detect neural tube defects, at week 15–20
2. A 1-hour, 50-g oral glucose intolerance screen: if blood sugar is $\geq$140 mg/dL after 1 hour, proceed to a 3-hour, 100-g test.
3. All Rh-negative women should be retested at 26–28 weeks. If still antibody negative, give Rho(D) immune globulin, 300 mg, at 28 weeks to prevent isoimmunization.
4. Pelvic exam and wet mount (and possibly Gram stain) late in second trimester to detect bacterial vaginosis (with test of cure), to decrease incidence of preterm labor, endometritis, and premature rupture of membranes.
5. Testing for group B β-hemolytic streptococci with antibiotic prophylaxis during labor. Serum total bhCG and unconjugated estriol in women of <35 years. Amniocentesis (after 14 weeks) or chorionic villous sampling (10–12 weeks), with possible karyotyping for genetic screening, in women of >35 years.

What types of genetic conditions can be diagnosed prenatally?	Autosomal dominant: myotonic dystrophy, Marfan syndrome, neurofibromatosis, achondroplasia, and Huntington's disease Autosomal recessive: cystic fibrosis, sickle cell anemia, Tay-Sachs disease, and phenylketonuria X-linked recessive: hemophilias, Duchenne muscular dystrophy X-linked dominant: Alport syndrome, vitamin D-resistant rickets, incontinentia pigmenti
What are the indications for obtaining a fetal karyotype?	Advanced maternal age ($\geq$ 35 years: increased risk of trisomy), previous child with an abnormal karyotype, parental chromosome rearrangements, fetal structural anomaly on US, unexplained intrauterine growth restriction, abnormally low serum maternal α-fetoprotein
How is transvaginal sonography used in the evaluation of fetal placement?	Normal: gestational sac (echogenic ring with hypoechoic center) in uterus confirmed as early as 5–6 weeks. If ectopic: absence of a gestational sac with bhCG levels of 1500–3000 mIU/mL (with subsequent plateau and decrease).
What is the screening test of choice for Down syndrome?	Second-trimester sampling of hCG or (preferably) free bhCG. Second-line tests: α-fetoprotein (AFP) and unconjugated estriol (uE_3). Blood samples for AFP at or after 15 weeks for neural tube defects.
What is the diagnostic test of choice for chorioangiomas?	Ultrasonography (preferred), ultrafast magnetic resonance imaging, color flow mapping, and Doppler velocimetry

Therapy

What interventions are available prenatally to reduce risk of fetal loss or defect?	All women of reproductive age who have the potential to become pregnant should take 0.4 mg (400 μg) of folic acid daily. Women with previous pregnancies affected by neural tube defects should take 4 mg of folic acid daily.

OTHER GYNECOLOGIC ISSUES

CONTRACEPTION

Contraceptive Efficacy

What percentage of pregnancies in the United States are unplanned?

50%

What is the Pearl Index?

The number of contraceptive failures per 100 woman-years of exposures to a contraceptive device

What is a life-table analysis?

The failure rate for a contraceptive device for each month of use

Contraceptive Methods

IUD

How many years is a copper-containing IUD approved for use?

10 years

What is the 10-year cumulative failure rate of a copper-containing IUD?

2.1%

What is the effect of copper on sperm?

Copper reduces sperm motility and capacitation.

What percentage of IUDs will be fully or partially expelled during the first year of use?

5.5%

Complications related to IUD use generally occur at what time?

Uterine perforation, expulsion, and infection usually occur at or close to the time of insertion.

Barrier Methods

What is the failure rate of the male condom?

10–12%. Rates as high as 20% have been reported.

What female barrier methods are currently available?	Diaphragm, cervical cap, female condom, spermicidal agents

Long-acting Contraceptives

What long-acting progestin contraceptives are currently available?	Subdermal implants and intramuscular injection
What is the effect of progestins on cervical mucus?	Thickens cervical mucus, which impedes sperm penetration
What is the effect of progestins on the endometrial lining?	Progestin-exposed endometrium atrophies over time, and does not support implantation.

Oral Contraceptives

What hormones do combination oral contraceptive pills contain?	A synthetic estrogen and progestogen
How much estrogen do current oral contraceptive pills contain?	20–35 mg
How much estrogen did oral contraceptive pills contain in the 1960s?	150 mg
At what point in a pack of oral contraceptive pills does missing pills result in the greatest risk for pregnancy?	The beginning and end of the pill pack
What side effects are reported to occur with oral contraceptive pills?	Headaches, weight changes, mood changes, changes in libido, and GI problems

What is the incidence of venous thromboembolism with estrogen-containing contraceptive pills?	25–30 per 100,000 woman-years
At what age should smokers discontinue oral contraceptive pills?	Age 35 years
What effect do oral contraceptive pills have on benign breast disease?	Oral contraceptives decrease benign breast disease.
What gynecologic malignancies are reduced by oral contraceptive pills?	Epithelial ovarian cancer and endometrial adenocarcinoma
Do oral contraceptives cause increased fibroid growth?	No

Emergency Contraception

What is emergency contraception?	A postcoital method of contraception involving a dose of combination oral contraceptive pills taken within 72 hours of unprotected coitus, followed by a second dose 12 hours later
Emergency contraception with combination birth control pills reduces pregnancy rates by what percentage?	75%

Other Methods

What percentage of U.S. women use permanent sterilization?	25%
What is natural family planning?	Periodic abstinence during the fertile interval in a woman's menstrual cycle

What is the typical failure rate of natural family planning?	18–20%
What is the failure rate of withdrawal or coitus interruptus?	18%

ABORTION

What is the definition of an abortion?	Termination of a pregnancy before viability, usually defined as 20–24 weeks. Definition varies based on legal jurisdiction.
How are abortions categorized?	According to the underlying cause or complicating factor
Define the following types of abortion:	
Threatened abortion	Any uterine bleeding during first half of pregnancy (before attainment of viability)
Inevitable abortion	Uterine bleeding during first half of pregnancy with cervical dilatation
Incomplete abortion	Uterine bleeding during first half of pregnancy with cervical dilatation and partial expulsion of products of conception. Also called a miscarriage. Without removal of remaining products of conception, continued bleeding and other sequelae are possible.
Complete abortion	Same as incomplete abortion, except that all products of conception are expelled and hence uterine bleeding resolves.
Habitual abortion	Three or more incomplete spontaneous abortions. Causes include genetic factors, autoimmune problems, genital system infection (TORCH, cervical, ureaplasma, chlamydia), uterine or cervical abnormalities (uterine septum, fibroids, cervical incompetence), endocrine causes (diabetes mellitus, hypothyroidism, ovulatory dysfunction), and chronic systemic disease.

Induced abortion	A voluntary termination of pregnancy
Septic abortion	An abortive process complicated by intrauterine infection

What is the incidence of spontaneous abortion?

15–20% of all known pregnancies. If sensitive hCG testing is used to detect early subclinical pregnancy, incidence rises to approximately 30%. Approximately 80% occur in first trimester. Threatened abortion is seen in 40–50% of pregnancies, depending on the population studied.

What is a blighted ovum?

A pregnancy in which the embryo has failed to form. Usually diagnosed sonographically beyond 7.5 menstrual weeks as an empty gestational sac without embryonic or fetal pole.

What is the typical clinical presentation of a spontaneous abortion?

Usually crampy midabdominal or midpelvic pain and vaginal bleeding. The pain is variable both in severity and character; may be constant or episodic, mild or intense. Similarly, bleeding may range from minimal spotting or staining to severe hemorrhage.

How is the diagnosis of a spontaneous abortion (either threatened, inevitable, incomplete, or complete) made?

The hallmark is uterine bleeding during the first half of pregnancy. Strictly speaking, pelvic exam is required to confirm that vaginal bleeding identified by the patient is not due to either a vaginal or cervical lesion.

When uterine bleeding is confirmed, how does the clinical evaluation continue?

Bleeding from the external cervical os confirms uterine bleeding, and defines a threatened abortion. If the cervical os is dilated, then an inevitable abortion is diagnosed. Expulsion of some but not all of the products of conception, determined either by inspection or US, confirms diagnosis of incomplete spontaneous abortion. The diagnosis of a complete abortion is most often made retrospectively.

Besides a history and simple physical exam, what additional tests are employed in evaluation of an abortion?

Ultrasonographic exam (transvaginal or transabdominal) to aid in diagnosis or confirmation of abortion. Presence of an irregular or collapsed gestational sac, absent embryo or fetus, or absent fetal cardiac activity support the impression of an abortion. Slowly rising serum hCG levels (slower than a doubling time of 2–3 days) or falling hCG levels

What is the differential diagnosis of uterine bleeding in the first trimester?

Vaginitis, cervical polyps, cervical carcinoma, gestational trophoblastic disease, ectopic pregnancy, trauma, and foreign body

How is a threatened abortion managed?

No effective therapy. The clinician should attempt to confirm viability of pregnancy with serial hCG determinations or ultrasonographic exams. For example, if a gestational sac is seen, the loss rate drops to about 11%, and if the fetus is larger than 5 mm, the loss rate is only 3%. An empty sac of >17 mm diameter, or a sac of >14 mm without a yolk sac, predicts nonviability. Supportive measures with unproven efficacy include bedrest and progesterone therapy.

How is inevitable abortion managed?

Sonographic exam is used to determine viability of pregnancy. If nonviable, curettage is generally recommended to terminate the pregnancy and prevent further (possibly severe) bleeding. Otherwise, the patient is managed expectantly, as in threatened abortion.

How is an incomplete abortion managed?

Decide the need for curettage with the patient:

For curettage: possibility of hemorrhage or infection if tissue remains in the uterus; emotional impact of continued vaginal bleeding with a nonviable pregnancy remaining in utero

Against curettage: some patients will resolve spontaneously; curettage is an invasive procedure with occasional complications of perforation and scarring (Asherman syndrome)

What is important in the management of all abortion patients?

All Rh-negative patients should receive Rho(D) immune globulin (RhoGAM) for any abortive process, even an early threatened abortion. Follow-up to confirm completion of the abortion, inspect the pathology report to confirm intrauterine products of conception (and thereby exclude ectopic pregnancy), and provide supportive care.

10 Pediatrics

NORMAL GROWTH AND DEVELOPMENT

INFANTS

What is the best sleeping position for the newborn? Why?	Supine; reduces risk of sudden infant death syndrome (SIDS)
What is the typical developmental progress of a 2–4-week-old child?	Raises head slightly from prone position, blinks in response to light, focuses and follows with eyes, and responds to sound by quieting or turning toward the noise.
Which infants need supplementation with vitamin D?	Breast-fed infants who are dark skinned or have limited sunlight exposure
What is the typical developmental progress of a 2 month old?	Holds head erect temporarily, can briefly hold a rattle, tracks and follows objects visually, looks at faces and responds to sound, will coo, has a social smile
What motor skills are typical for a 4 month old?	Holds head erect, no head lag when pulling to a sitting position, raises body using arms in prone position, may roll one or both ways, may support weight on legs, reaches for and grabs objects, puts hands together
What social and communication skills are typical of a 4 month old?	Tracks and follows objects visually to 180°, coos reciprocally, blows bubbles, makes "raspberry" sounds, smiles readily, may laugh or squeal, differentiates individuals
When and how should solid foods be introduced?	At 4–6 months of age. Introduce foods one at a time, beginning with rice cereal.

What food should be avoided until after 1 year of age?	Honey and corn syrup, because of their association with botulism
When do infants normally sleep through the night?	Usually between 3 and 4 months of age
What motor skills are typical for a 6 month old?	Holds head high when prone, holds head steady when pulled up to sit, rolls over both ways, sits with support, uses raking grasp to grab objects, transfers objects from one hand to the other
What social skills are typical for a 6 month old?	Takes initiative in vocalizing or babbling at others; imitates sounds; smiles, laughs, and coos to initiate social contact; recognizes parents; shows pleasure and excitement at interactions with parents.
What motor skills are typical for a 9 month old?	Sits well, crawls or creeps on hands, may begin cruising furniture, begins to use pincer grasp, feeds self, bangs objects together
What social skills are typical for a 9 month old?	Enjoys games such as peek-a-boo and pat-a-cake, may react to unfamiliar adults with fear or anxiety
What communication skills are typical for a 9 month old?	Responds to name, understands a few words such as "no" and "bye-bye," imitates vocalizations, babbles using several syllables
What motor skills are typical for a 12 month old?	Sits well, crawls, pulls self up and walks with support, feeds self, has a mature pincer grasp
What social skills are typical for a 12 month old?	Plays games (e.g., peek-a-boo, pat-a-cake), waves bye-bye, looks at books, points to named body parts or animals, follows simple commands, likes to play with adult-type objects (e.g., phone, hairbrush)

What communication skills are typical for a 12 month old?	Uses "mama" and "dada" correctly, has 3–5 additional words
When should the infant be able to drink from a cup and be weaned from the bottle?	Between 9 and 12 months
When is an infant allowed to graduate to a toddler car seat?	Keep infants in a rear-facing infant car seat until age 1 year and a weight of >20 pounds.
When should children be screened for lead poisoning?	At age 1 year; repeat after age 2.
What questions are important for lead toxicity screening?	Does the child spend time in any building built before 1950? Does the child spend time in a house built before 1978 with recent or ongoing renovation? Does the child have a sibling or playmate with lead poisoning?
At what level is a child considered to have lead poisoning?	A level of 10 or greater is considered elevated and needs follow-up.

TODDLERS

What motor skills are typical for a 15 month old?	Feeds self with fingers or spoon, scribbles with crayons, stacks two blocks
What are typical communication skills of a 15 month old?	Says 5–15 words, uses jargon, communicates with gestures, points to 1–2 body parts on request, understands simple commands, listens to stories, points to designated pictures in a book
What social skills are typical for a 15 month old?	Shows functional understanding of objects (e.g., talks on toy phone), gives and takes toys, plays games with parents, tests parental rules or limits, communicates pleasure and displeasure

When do temper tantrums usually start? Why?	Common between 15 and 30 months. Tantrums occur as young children strive to become more independent, and are a normal way of expressing frustration.
How do you counsel parents about managing tantrums?	Encourage parents to praise desired behaviors, redirect, offer choices, warn the child in advance of transitions to other activities, remain calm during tantrums, and use time out.
What are typical motor skills for an 18 month old?	Walks quickly, may run, walks up stairs with 1 hand held, walks backwards, eats with spoon and fork, stacks blocks, and scribbles with crayons
What cognitive skills are typical for an 18 month old?	Knows location of objects that have been hidden, plays pretend games (e.g., drinking from empty cup, hugging a doll, talking on telephone)
What are the typical communication skills of an 18 month old?	Understands commands, points to body parts, may put two words together
What motor skills are typical for a 2 year old?	Runs, jumps in place, walks up and down stairs, throws ball overhead, opens doors, stacks blocks, imitates a vertical line, uses spoon and fork
What cognitive skills are typical for a 2 year old?	Begins to create means to accomplish a desired goal (pulls a chair to cabinet, climbs, retrieves hidden object)
What are the language skills of a 2 year old?	Has >50-word vocabulary, speaks several 2-word phrases, follows 1- and 2-step commands, listens to short stories, and uses pronouns
What are the typical social skills of a 2 year old?	Imitates adults, parallel play with other children, dresses and brushes teeth with help, and feeds self

When should toilet training begin?	It is best to wait for the child to show signs of readiness, such as awareness of impending urination or defecation, prolonged involuntary dryness, and ability to postpone briefly the urge to urinate or defecate.
At what age do signs of readiness usually occur?	Usually 18–30 months. By age 3 years, about 90% of children are bowel-trained, 85% are dry during the daytime, and 60–70% are dry at night.
What are some important considerations when counseling a parent about toilet training?	A child-size potty seat, modeling by parents and siblings, reward cooperation or success with praise, and avoid punishment or shame in dealing with accidents

PRESCHOOLERS

What are the typical motor skills of a 3 year old?	Jumps in place, kicks ball, pedals tricycle, walks up stairs with alternating gait, scribbles, copies a circle, puts on some clothing, stacks eight blocks
What are the typical social skills of a 3 year old?	Knows name, age, and sex; enjoys interactive play; participates in pretend play; may be oppositional or destructive
What communications skills are typical for a 3 year old?	Speech is at least 75% intelligible, uses short sentences, asks questions such as "what's that" and "why," understands prepositions and some adjectives
What motor skills are typical for a 4 year old?	Hops and balances on one foot, draws a circle and a cross, cuts with scissors, draws a person with 3–6 body parts
What language skills are typical for a 4 year old?	Extensive vocabulary, speech fully intelligible to strangers, uses full sentences with at least six words, asks questions such as "why" and "when," recognizes some letters of alphabet

What social skills are typical for a 4 year old?	Engages in interactive pretend play, may have an imaginary friend, may not differentiate reality from fantasy, brushes teeth, able to button and zip, and toilet trained
What are night terrors?	Children can cry inconsolably and appear terrified, confused, and glassy eyed, but cannot be awakened or comforted. Autonomic activity is common (sweating, tachycardia, tachypnea).
When do night terrors occur?	Commonly in preschool and early school-age children, during transition from stage IV nonrapid eye movement (NREM) sleep to rapid eye movement (REM) sleep, within about 2 hours of falling asleep.
How do night terrors differ from nightmares?	Children do not remember night terrors.

GENETIC DISORDERS

DOWN SYNDROME

What is Down syndrome?	A genetic disorder due to trisomy of chromosome 21
What are the three ways in which trisomy occurs?	By receiving three copies of a chromosome, a translocation, or a mosaicism
What is the major risk factor for having a child with Down syndrome?	Maternal age of >35 years
What are the common head and neck findings in a patient affected by Down syndrome?	Broad-bridged nose, flattened facies, upward slanted palpebral fissures, epicanthal folds, speckled iris, high arched palate, protruding tongue, webbing of neck

What is the most common neurologic/cognitive manifestation of Down syndrome?

Hypotonia and varying degrees of mental retardation

More than one third of individuals with Down syndrome have cardiac abnormalities. What are the common lesions?

Atrioventricular canal, ventricular septal defect, patent ductus arteriosus, atrial septal defect, tetralogy of Fallot

What are two notable gastrointestinal abnormalities associated with Down syndrome?

Duodenal atresia and Hirschsprung disease

What is the diagnostic test for Down syndrome?

Chromosomal analysis showing trisomy 21

What maternal serologic test supports the diagnosis of Down syndrome?

An abnormal triple screen with decreased α-fetoprotein, decreased unconjugated estriol, and increased human chorionic gonadotropin

Of all individuals with Down syndrome, 15% have thyroid dysfunction. How should this be followed?

Yearly thyroid screening

What is the recommended therapy for Down syndrome?

Children with Down syndrome should receive problem-directed therapy and intervention to ensure that they reach their full potential.

KLINEFELTER SYNDROME

What is Klinefelter syndrome?

A genetic condition of primary testicular failure; usually not evident until puberty

What is the incidence of Klinefelter syndrome?

1 in 1000 live-born male newborns

What are the manifestations of Klinefelter syndrome?

Mental retardation, psychosocial or learning problems, and delayed puberty

What causes Klinefelter syndrome?

The presence of an extra X chromosome. The classic form is 47,XXY.

How does Klinefelter syndrome present?

Often as psychosocial, learning, or school adjustment problems when child begins school. May present with delayed puberty.

What are the physical features of Klinefelter syndrome?

Patients tend to be tall, slim, and underweight with relatively long legs. Testes are small for age, phallus is smaller than average.

What organ systems does Klinefelter syndrome affect?

Most adults have gynecomastia, sparse facial hair, azoospermia, and infertility.

What kinds of cancers are increased in patients with Klinefelter syndrome?

Breast cancer and mediastinal germ cell tumors

What is the role of mosaicism in Klinefelter syndrome?

Mosaicism is common; presence of XX or XY cell lines in addition to XXY is associated with less severe features. However, individuals with a larger number of X chromosomes (e.g., XXXY) have more significant intellectual and social deficits.

How does Klinefelter syndrome affect mental development?

IQ usually in normal range, but verbal often lower than performance IQ. Reading problems in about 50% of patients, requiring special education.

How is the diagnosis of Klinefelter syndrome made?

Perform karyotype analysis in all boys with mental retardation and psychosocial or learning problems.

What other diagnostic test results are useful?

Abnormally high gonadotropin levels (luteinizing hormone, follicle-stimulating hormone) and low levels of testosterone. Elevated estradiol levels result in a high estradiol-to-testosterone ratio, and development of gynecomastia during puberty.

What treatment modalities are available for males with Klinefelter syndrome?

Replacement therapy with a long-acting testosterone preparation starting at 11–12 years of age

TURNER SYNDROME

What is Turner syndrome?

A genetic condition that is a common cause of short stature in females

What is the incidence of Turner syndrome?

1 in 2500 live-born female newborns

What are the manifestations of Turner syndrome?

Primary amenorrhea, sterility, and sparse pubic-axillary hair

What causes Turner syndrome?

Turner syndrome is due to the absence or abnormality of an X chromosome, the classic form being 45,XO (60%)

How does Turner syndrome present?

By early childhood, marked short stature with progressive deviation of height away from normal growth curve. Also may present in late adolescence as failure to develop secondary sex characteristics.

What are the physical features of Turner syndrome?

Webbing of neck, cubitus valgus, low hairline, low-set ears, micrognathia, shield chest with widespread nipples, short fourth metacarpals, lymphedema of feet or hands (especially in newborns)

What is the most common cardiac abnormality associated with Turner syndrome?

Coarctation of the aorta (20%)

What other organ systems are affected by Turner syndrome?	The kidneys and reproductive tract, with an infantile uterus and ovaries consisting of strands of connective tissue
How does Turner syndrome affect mental development?	Mental development usually normal, but average full-scale IQ may be somewhat lower than general population; difficulty with spatial orientation (e.g., map reading)
How is the diagnosis of Turner syndrome made?	Perform karyotype analysis, G-banded chromosome study, in any girl presenting with short stature of unknown cause
What other diagnostic tests are helpful?	Abnormally high gonadotropin levels (luteinizing hormone, follicle-stimulating hormone), indicating ovarian failure
What treatment is available for females with Turner syndrome? What is its goal?	Sex steroid replacement therapy during adolescence, to assist with development of secondary sex characteristics and stimulate menses
Are treatments available to assist with growth?	Growth hormone therapy (alone or with low-dose oxandrolone) has shown limited success in increasing height, but safety and efficacy are under investigation.

GASTROENTEROLOGY

COLIC

Define colic.	Crying during the first 3 months of life, for 3 or more hours a day, on 3 or more days a week, in infants without other conditions that may cause prolonged crying
How common is colic?	About 10% of babies have colic.
How is colic diagnosed?	Clinical history of long crying spells and lack of central nervous system disorder or intrinsic developmental difficulties in a normal infant with normal growth patterns

What are the exam findings of a child during a paroxysm?	Loud crying, facial flushing, hands clenched, legs drawn up, abdomen distended and tense
What other signs may occur?	Circumoral pallor, passage of flatus or feces, which may seem to provide relief
What is the cause of colic?	Unknown, despite many hypothesis and studies
Can formula allergy or intolerance present as colic?	Yes, but rarely
How can the clinician distinguish formula allergy from colic?	Formula allergy usually is accompanied by vomiting or diarrhea.
What is the earliest age at which colic might be seen?	Usually after first or second week of life
When does colic usually resolve?	Almost always by 12th week of life
Are there any universally effective "cures" for colic?	No
Name the three main management strategies for the clinician caring for an infant with colic.	Behavioral management, supportive counseling, and parental reassurance
What is a good initial behavioral management strategy to try to soothe a crying infant (who is not hungry and does not need a diaper change)?	Carry and cuddle the baby.
What are some strategies for carrying and cuddling the baby?	Cuddle in a rocking chair; rock baby in a cradle; place baby in an infant carrier or sling; use a windup or electric swing or vibrating chair; a stroller ride (indoors or out)

Does colic have any long-term detrimental effects?	No
If a parent is exhausted, is it OK to let the baby cry?	Yes, if the baby has been fed, changed, and cuddled for more than 30 minutes, it is OK to let the baby cry by himself for up to 15 minutes.
What is the role of medication in management of colic?	Currently no safe and effective medications

DIARRHEA/GASTROENTERITIS

What are the risk factors?	Sick contacts, contaminated water, house pets, undercooked meat or chicken, and recent travel to endemic areas
What is the most common cause?	Viruses (70–80%)
Which virus is more common in the summer?	Enterovirus
Which virus is more common in the winter and spring?	Rotavirus (65%)
What additional viruses can cause it?	Adenovirus and Norwalk virus
Which bacterial organisms are most likely to cause it?	*Salmonella, Shigella, Yersinia, Campylobacter*, and enteroinvasive *Escherichia coli*
Which bacterial organisms are less likely to cause it?	*Staphylococcus* and *Clostridium difficile*
What is a strong risk factor for *C. difficile* infection?	Long-term or multiple antibiotic use

How does viral gastroenteritis often present?	Vomiting before or with diarrhea
How does bacterial gastroenteritis often present?	Diarrhea and blood or mucus in stool; vomiting uncommon
Which bacterial organism produces both vomiting and diarrhea?	*Staphylococcus*
What physical exam findings suggest dehydration?	Tachycardia, tachypnea, weight loss, and dry mucous membranes
What basic lab tests should be considered?	Complete blood cell (CBC) count with differential, electrolytes, and blood cultures
What are the diagnostic tests of choice?	Stool culture and Gram stain, fecal polymorphonuclear leukocyte (PMN) count, and fecal occult blood test
What are the associated lab findings for bacterial organisms?	Positive fecal occult blood with numerous PMNs
What additional tests can confirm a viral cause?	Rotazyme assay (if rotavirus suspected, winter), enzyme-linked immunosorbent assay (ELISA) test for suspected virus
What is the treatment strategy for both viral and bacterial gastroenteritis?	Supportive; oral rehydration as needed
When is antibiotic use indicated?	*Shigella* infections; if conservative treatment fails in other bacterial gastroenteritis
What antibiotic is recommended to treat *Shigella* and many other bacterial infections causing gastroenteritis?	Ciprofloxacin or Bactrim

Are antidiarrheal medications (e.g., Lomotil, Imodium) recommended?	No

INTUSSUSCEPTION

What is intussusception?	Telescoping of part of the intestine into a segment distal to itself
What does this lead to, and why?	The intestine pulls the mesentery along, constricting it. This leads to venous pooling and edema of the mucosa, followed by bleeding.
What causes intussusception?	Usually, no cause is found. Associated with adenoviruses, gastroenteritis, Meckel diverticulum, intestinal polyps, and Henoch-Schönlein purpura
How does a lead point such as a Meckel diverticulum cause intussusception?	Possibly, the lead point (e.g., a Meckel diverticulum), stimulates the ileum to contract in an attempt to extrude the mass, thus causing an intussusception.
What is the usual age of presentation?	3 months to 6 years; two thirds occur before age 1 year.
How does intussusception usually present?	The triad of colicky abdominal pain, emesis, and bloody, mucoid stools
What causes the abdominal pain?	Peristalsis pulling on the intussusceptum
Describe the abdominal pain.	Because peristalsis is an on-and-off phenomenon, the pain initially comes and goes, and children are fine between episodes. Young children with pain usually pull up their knees and strain.
What is the nature of the emesis?	Initially clear. As swelling of the intussusceptum leads to bowel obstruction, it becomes bile stained.

What is the classic description of stools?	Currant jelly stool
Are patients usually febrile?	Not initially, but if untreated, children become shocky and febrile.
What is the characteristic physical finding?	In 65% of children, a sausage-shaped mass palpable in the right upper quadrant or midepigastric area
What is the primary site of intussusception?	95% of cases are ileocolic, beginning just proximal to the cecum.
What are the plain x-ray findings?	Occasionally a soft tissue mass displaces the gas-filled bowel; may also be evidence of bowel obstruction.
Does a normal x-ray rule out intussusception?	No
How is the definitive diagnosis made?	An air or barium enema done under fluoroscopic guidance shows a filling defect at the distal end of the intussusception. A "coiled spring" appearance is described, as contrast fills the space between the intussusceptum and the intussuscipiens.
How is intussusception treated?	The pressure of the enema is usually sufficient to reduce it.
What is the recurrence rate for idiopathic cases?	After radiologic reduction: 8–12% After surgical reduction: <3%

PYLORIC STENOSIS

What is pyloric stenosis?	Gastric outlet obstruction at the level of the pylorus
What causes pyloric stenosis?	Hypertrophy of the circular muscle of the pylorus
At what age does pyloric stenosis usually present?	1–10 weeks

What is the incidence?
3 per 1000 live births

Is there a gender bias?
Yes. Males are affected 4 times as often as females.

Is there a racial bias?
Yes. Whites are most frequently affected, followed by blacks. Orientals and Indians are rarely affected.

Does birth order play a role?
Yes. First-born children are the most frequently affected.

How does it usually present?
Emesis, often described as "projectile." However, the term is overused by families and useless in making the diagnosis.

Is the emesis bilious?
No, because the pylorus stands between the stomach and the biliary outlet.

What are the physical findings?
The hypertrophied pylorus is felt as a firm, 1–2-cm "olive," either midline or slightly to the right, 2–3 cm above the umbilicus. A peristaltic wave is also seen over the epigastrium.

Are there any associated laboratory abnormalities?
If vomiting persists, hypochloremic, hypokalemic metabolic alkalosis secondary to gastric fluid loss

What is the study of choice in making a diagnosis of pyloric stenosis?
Abdominal ultrasound picks up 90–100% of cases. If negative, perform upper GI x-ray series to evaluate for other causes of vomiting.

What is the treatment of choice?
Surgical correction, specifically pylorotomy

Is this curative?
Yes

INFECTIOUS DISEASES

RESPIRATORY SYNCYTIAL VIRUS (RSV)

What is viral bronchiolitis?
Inflammation and edema of the small airways, resulting in necrosis of respiratory epithelium with obstruction of airway lumen

What are the causes of viral bronchiolitis?
Most commonly, RSV; less commonly, influenza, parainfluenza, and adenovirus

How do RSV infections occur in the northern hemisphere?
In yearly epidemics between October and April

What age groups are most susceptible to RSV bronchiolitis?
Children <2 years of age

What are the symptoms of viral bronchiolitis?
Rhinorrhea, fever, poor feeding, coughing, irritability, lethargy, apnea, difficulty breathing, and wheezing

What are the signs of viral bronchiolitis?
Tachypnea, tachycardia, nasal flaring, retractions, cyanosis, decreased air entry, prolonged expiratory phase, wheezing, and crackles

What lab tests are useful in the initial workup?
CBC count with differential, chest x-ray, and oxygen saturation

What is the diagnostic approach for RSV bronchiolitis?
Immunofluorescent or enzyme immunoassay detection of RSV antigen in clinical specimens; highly sensitive and specific, rapid, and inexpensive

What abnormalities are seen on chest x-ray?
Hyperinflation, peribronchial thickening, atelectasis, bilateral interstitial infiltrates, and lobar infiltrate

What are the complications of RSV bronchiolitis?
Respiratory failure, pneumonia, apnea, and atrial tachycardia

What is the management of mild RSV bronchiolitis?	Most children can be treated at home with supportive treatment, oral hydration, and nasal suctioning.
Who should be admitted to hospital with RSV bronchiolitis?	Children with dehydration, poor oral intake, significant respiratory distress, hypoxia, and apnea.
What are the treatment options in the hospital?	Administer oxygen, hydrate, and observe for apnea and respiratory failure. Try inhaled bronchodilators, but stop if no beneficial response.
Are corticosteroids and antibiotics helpful?	No
What are the risk factors for severe RSV bronchiolitis?	Premature birth, chronic lung disease, bronchopulmonary dysplasia, cystic fibrosis, congenital heart disease, immunodeficiency, and age <6 weeks
What control measures should be taken to minimize spread of RSV infection to susceptible children in the hospital?	Contact isolation and strict hand washing
How could RSV bronchiolitis be prevented?	To prevent infection, give either RSV Immune Globulin Intravenous (RSV-IGIV) or Palivizumab once a month during RSV season for total of five treatments.
Who should be given RSV-IGIV or Palivizumab?	Children <24 months old at high risk for infection (i.e., premature birth, chronic lung or cardiac disease, bronchopulmonary dysplasia, immunodeficiency)

CHICKENPOX

What causes chickenpox?	The herpes varicella-zoster virus
What is the main risk factor?	Sick contact exposing child to varicella in the past 1–3 weeks

How does chickenpox present?	Constitutional symptoms (fever, headache, malaise) followed by pruritic vesicular rash on an erythematous base; vesicles break and crust over; rash begins on trunk or face and spreads to extremities
How can the diagnosis be confirmed?	Tzanck smear
What are the dreaded sequelae of varicella infection?	Reye syndrome and meningoencephalitis
What is the treatment?	Generally supportive with diphenhydramine (pruritus) and acetaminophen (fever); in severe cases, acyclovir

CROUP

What is croup?	A viral infection of upper and large airways (hence, "laryngotracheobronchitis"), causing swelling of the subglottic space, the narrowest part of the airway in young children
What are the causative organisms?	Most commonly, human parainfluenza type 1 virus (HPIV-1). Other agents: influenza, RSV, parainfluenza type 3, adenovirus, and mycoplasma
What are the symptoms of croup?	Usually preceded by upper respiratory tract infection; fever; loud, brassy, barking cough; hoarseness; inspiratory stridor. In severe cases: develop tachypnea, air hunger, cyanosis, and retractions
What time of day do symptoms usually worsen?	At night
What is the epidemiology and seasonal pattern?	Males are more affected than females. Mostly occurs in first 3 years of life with peak in second year. Major outbreaks are caused by HPIV-1 in late fall and winter.

How is the diagnosis made?	Clinical diagnosis is based on history and examination. Anterior view of upper airway may show narrowed subglottic space ("steeple sign"). Lateral neck film may rule out other causes of obstruction (e.g., epiglottitis).
What is the differential diagnosis?	Infection: bacterial tracheitis, epiglottitis, peritonsillar abscess, retropharyngeal abscess Aspiration: foreign body Congenital malformations: vascular ring, vocal cord paralysis, Arnold-Chiari malformation, tracheoesophageal fistula, laryngeal web, hemangioma Allergy: angioneurotic edema Other: trauma of larynx; tumors of upper airways
What is the treatment of mild cases?	Most are mild; patients generally improve spontaneously or with exposure to cold night air.
What is the treatment of moderate and severe cases?	Oxygen for hypoxia. Nebulized racemic epinephrine quickly relieves airway obstruction. Nebulized (beclomethasone) and systemic (dexamethasone) steroids decrease hospital admissions and need for intubation. Mixture of helium and oxygen may be tried before intubation. Humidified air (cool mist tent) is widely used, but has no proven benefit.
Can a child be discharged safely from the emergency room?	Yes, if dexamethasone was given and the patient was observed for 3–4 hours after racemic epinephrine.
What is the prognosis?	Excellent. Croup is usually a self-limited condition lasting a few days with no permanent airway damage or stenosis.

EPIGLOTTITIS

What is epiglottitis?	An infection of the larynx leading to inflammation of the epiglottis and supraglottic tissues, usually acute in onset and leading to upper airway compromise
What causes epiglottitis?	Classically, *Haemophilus influenzae* type B; use of vaccine greatly decreased incidence. *Streptococcus* and *Staphylococcus* species now cause a larger percentage of cases.
What is the usual age range for epiglottitis?	2–7 years
What is the peak age?	3.5 years
How does epiglottitis present?	Rapid (few hours) onset of fever, sore throat; patient complains of trouble swallowing, breathing, or speaking.
How is the presentation distinguished from that of croup?	Usually an associated upper respiratory infection in croup, but not in epiglottitis
How do patients look when they present?	Moderate to severe respiratory distress. Child is usually sitting up and leaning forward with hands on knees, tripoding to use accessory muscles.
What else might you notice in an affected child?	Neck is hyperextended to open airway as much as possible. Child is drooling; has inspiratory stridor.
What is the diagnostic physical finding?	A swollen, cherry red epiglottis, either by direct inspection or laryngoscopy
What precautions should be taken before this evaluation?	Laryngospasm is a potentially fatal complication of irritation of the posterior oropharynx during inspection; thus, inspect only in a controlled setting where airway management is possible.

What other diagnostic test can be done to assess the epiglottis?	Lateral neck x-ray shows "thumbprint sign" of a swollen epiglottis.
What is the mainstay of therapy?	Prompt airway control: insertion of artificial airway
Is there a role for antibiotics?	Yes; usually an associated bacteremia. Start children on intravenous cefuroxime for 7–10 days.
How long is the usual course of illness?	2–3 days

FEVER OF UNKNOWN ORIGIN

What is fever of unknown origin (FUO)?	Fever persisting beyond 7–10 days after careful history, physical, and preliminary lab testing
Name three aspects of the history that are important to pursue in evaluating children with FUO.	Travel history, exposure to pets, and transfusion history
What basic tests should be considered after a complete history and physical shows no obvious source of fever?	CBC count with differential; erythrocyte sedimentation rate; chest x-ray; urinalysis; blood culture; urine culture
What findings on history and physical might indicate the need for a more aggressive evaluation, potentially in the hospital?	Ill appearance and weight loss
What are the three most common broad categories of illness causing FUO?	Infectious diseases, connective tissue diseases, and malignancies
What category of illness is the most common cause of FUO in children in the United States?	Infectious diseases

After the initial assessment, what basic principles should be followed in the ongoing evaluation?

Observation and reexamination

What is the role of lumbar puncture in FUO?

Should be considered in all cases, but is not required in all cases.

How often might FUO occur without reaching a definitive diagnosis?

Up to one quarter of cases may go undiagnosed; most resolve spontaneously.

What is factitious fever?

Fever "fabricated" by a caretaker or the child, by altering temperature measurement or injecting child with infectious or noxious materials.

What are the risks of empiric antibiotics in the therapy of FUO?

May alter signs of occult infection or delay appropriate diagnosis.

IMMUNIZATIONS

Name the seven routine childhood immunizations.

Hepatitis B vaccine (HBV), diphtheria, tetanus, and acellular pertussis (DTaP), *Haemophilus influenzae* type B (HIB), polio, measles, mumps, rubella (MMR), pneumococcal vaccine (Prevnar), and varicella

When is the HBV vaccine given?

Birth, 1 month, and 6 months

What additional treatment to the infant is required after birth if the mother is HBV positive?

Hepatitis B immunoglobulin (HBIG)

When is the DTaP vaccine given?

2, 4, 6, 15–18 months, and 4–6 years

What side effects shortly after initial vaccination are contraindications for future doses of pertussis vaccine?

Immediate anaphylactic reaction or development of encephalopathy within 7 days

When is tetanus, diphtheria without pertussis (Td) vaccine given?	Once between ages 11 and 16 years
When is the HIB vaccine given?	2, 4, and 6 months
When is the polio vaccine given?	2, 4, and 12–18 months
What two forms of polio vaccine exist?	Live oral polio vaccine (OPV) and inactivated polio vaccine (IPV)
Which type of polio vaccine is routinely used in the United States?	IPV
Why is IPV used routinely in the United States?	No wild-type polio exists in the United States; all infections are caused by the vaccine strain.
When should the MMR vaccine be given?	12–15 months and 4–6 or 11–12 years
What possible side effect may occur in children with an allergy to eggs?	Anaphylactic shock
What test should be performed before vaccinating in children suspected of egg allergy?	Skin patch testing with egg allergens
When is the varicella vaccine given?	12–18 months
What are contraindications to the varicella vaccine?	Immunosuppression
What is Prevnar?	A 7-valent protein conjugate vaccine against invasive pneumococcal disease

How does Prevnar differ from Pneumovax?	Pneumovax contains 23 different serotypes and is a polysaccharide vaccine. It is given only to children older than 2 years who have specific medical conditions (e.g., sickle cell disease)
Is Prevnar useful in preventing ear infections caused by *Streptococcus pneumoniae*?	Possibly. Ear infections caused by strains covered in the vaccine decrease, but those caused by other strains tend to increase.
Which children are at high risk to develop invasive pneumococcal disease?	Children with sickle cell disease, congenital or acquired asplenia, splenic dysfunction, or human immunodeficiency virus (HIV) disease

KAWASAKI DISEASE

What is Kawasaki disease?	Febrile illness associated with vasculitis of the coronary arteries
Two of the criteria for diagnosis of Kawasaki disease are febrile illness for at least 5 days, not explained by another disease process. What is the third diagnostic criterion for Kawasaki disease?	4 of the following five symptoms: conjunctivitis, mucus membrane changes, cervical lymphadenopathy, rash, and swelling or desquamation of hands or feet
What are additional clinical findings in Kawasaki disease?	Irritability, abdominal pain, diarrhea, vomiting, uveitis, arthritis, aseptic meningitis, pericardial effusion, arrhythmias, carditis, and perineal rash
Kawasaki disease is divided into acute (1–11 days), subacute (11–21 days), and convalescent (21–60 days) phases. When do the coronary arteries become affected?	The subacute phase
What age is most at risk for Kawasaki disease?	Children 5 years and younger

What racial group is most often affected?	Japanese
What are the common lab findings in Kawasaki disease?	Leukocytosis with left shift, elevated C-reactive protein, elevated sedimentation rate, thrombocytosis, anemia, sterile pyuria, and elevated liver function tests
What is the recommended initial cardiac evaluation for Kawasaki disease?	Chest x-ray, electrocardiogram, and echocardiogram
What is the differential diagnosis for Kawasaki disease?	Scarlet fever, toxic shock, leptospirosis, Epstein-Barr virus, juvenile rheumatoid arthritis, measles, Rocky Mountain spotted fever, drugs, and Stevens-Johnson syndrome
How is acute Kawasaki disease treated?	Intravenous gamma globulin and salicylates
If Kawasaki disease is untreated, what are the consequences?	Up to 25% of patients with untreated disease develop dilated coronary arteries, which can become acutely thrombosed or chronically stenosed.
What is the recommended follow up for Kawasaki disease?	Serial echocardiograms at diagnosis, then 6–8 weeks and 6–12 months later

MEASLES (RUBEOLA)

What causes measles?	*Paramyxoviridae*, genus *Morbillivirus*
How is it transmitted?	Respiratory secretions
What classic triad do patients often present with?	Conjunctivitis, cough, and coryza
What physical exam finding is pathognomonic for measles?	Koplik spots (small red spots with bluish centers on buccal mucosa early in disease)

Describe the morbilliform rash that appears in measles.

Confluent, erythematous maculopapular rash that starts on the head and progresses caudally to trunk and extremities

How is the diagnosis made?

History and presentation

How could the diagnosis be confirmed?

ELISA test (rarely done)

What is the treatment?

Supportive (rest, oral rehydration, and acetaminophen for fever)

What are patients with measles at risk for?

Pneumonia, myocarditis, and subacute sclerosing panencephalitis (rare)

MENINGITIS

What is meningitis?

Inflammation of the meninges, usually caused by viral or bacterial infections

Which organisms commonly cause bacterial meningitis in neonates?

Streptococcus agalactiae (group B streptococcus), *Escherichia coli*, and *Listeria monocytogenes* acquired from passage through birth canal

Which organisms commonly cause bacterial meningitis in infants and in children older than 2 months of age?

S. pneumoniae, Neisseria meningitidis, and *H. influenzae* type B. With widespread use of HIB vaccine, incidence of *H. influenzae* type B meningitis has greatly decreased.

What pathogen is most commonly responsible for aseptic meningitis?

Viral infections of the meninges (mostly enteroviruses)

What are the risk factors for pneumococcal meningitis in children?

Basilar skull or cribriform fracture, cerebrospinal fluid leak, anatomic or functional asplenia, and HIV infection

What immune systems defects are associated with increased risk of *N. meningitis*?

Defects of the complement system (C5–C8) and properdin

What age group is most likely to get bacterial meningitis?	Infants and young children

How does meningitis present?	Depends on patient's age.
	   Infants: irritability, lethargy, poor feeding
	   Children older than 2 years: headache, photophobia, neck pain

What physical findings are suggestive of the diagnosis?	In an infant, bulging fontanel indicates increased intracranial pressure. Altered mental status and reduced level of sensorium common in infants between 12 and 18 months old. Nuchal rigidity, Kerning and Brudzinski signs more common in older children. Generalized or focal seizures in 20–30%.
What is the significance of a petechial or purpuric rash in a patient with meningitis?	Usually associated with meningococcal infections
What entities should be considered in the differential diagnosis?	Encephalitis, brain abscess, subdural or epidural abscess. Noninfectious illnesses: Kawasaki disease, collagen vascular disease, other vasculitides, hypersensitivity to drugs, and Reye syndrome
How is the diagnosis confirmed?	Perform lumbar puncture when bacterial meningitis is suspected, unless there are specific contraindications.
What cerebrospinal fluid (CSF) findings are suggestive of meningitis and how can they help differentiate bacterial from aseptic meningitis?	CSF leukocyte count in bacterial meningitis usually elevated with predominance of neutrophils, low glucose, and high protein. In viral meningitis, CSF leukocyte count usually slightly elevated with predominance of lymphocytes, normal to slightly decreased glucose, and normal to slightly elevated protein.
What empiric therapy is recommended for bacterial meningitis in children?	Infants younger than 2 months old: ampicillin and cefotaxime or gentamicin to provide coverage for group B streptococci, *E. coli*, and *L. monocytogenes*

Infants older than 2 months old: Ceftriaxone or cefotaxime to target *S. pneumoniae* and *N. meningitidis* and vancomycin for penicillin-resistant pneumococci

What are the potential complications of bacterial meningitis?

Neurologic sequelae: sensorineural hearing loss (most common); mental retardation, seizures, behavioral problems, speech delay, and visual impairment

What preventive strategies are available for *H. influenzae* type B bacterial meningitis in children?

Rifampin prophylaxis is given to close contacts. HIB conjugate vaccine is included in the routine childhood immunization schedule.

What preventive strategies are available for pneumococcal bacterial meningitis in children?

Protein conjugated pneumococcal vaccine is now available for children <2 years old as part of routine childhood immunizations.

What preventive strategies are available for *N. meningitidis* meningitis in children?

Antibiotic prophylaxis (usually Rifampin) recommended for all close contacts. Meningococcal quadrivalent vaccine recommended for high-risk patients older than 2 years of age (anatomic or functional asplenia, terminal complement component deficiency, and properdin deficiency).

MUMPS

What infectious agent causes mumps?

Paramyxovirus

What is the main risk factor?

Unimmunized child

How is paramyxovirus transmitted?

Nasopharyngeal secretions

How does it present?

Often asymptomatic, but may present with moderate fever, malaise, headache, abdominal pain, and swollen salivary glands (especially parotid, unilateral, or bilateral)

How is it diagnosed?	History and physical exam
How can the diagnosis be confirmed?	ELISA test for paramyxovirus
What are children with mumps at risk for?	Pancreatitis, meningitis, encephalitis, hearing loss, and orchitis (in pubescent males)
What is the treatment for mumps?	Supportive (oral rehydration and acetaminophen as needed)

PHARYNGITIS

What is pharyngitis?	Inflammation of pharyngeal and tonsillar mucous membranes and underlying structures
What are the common causes of pharyngitis?	Viral and bacterial infections
What are some of the most common viruses that can cause pharyngitis?	Adenovirus (most common); coxsackievirus, Epstein-Barr virus (EBV), influenza A and B, rhinovirus, parainfluenza
What are the most common bacterial agents that can cause pharyngitis?	Most common, group A β-hemolytic streptococci (GABHS) (*Streptococcus pyogenes*); group G and C streptococci, *Neisseria gonorrhoeae*, and meningitides
What are some of the risk factors and causative organisms for pharyngitis?	Overcrowding: streptococci Sexual activity: *N. gonorrhoeae*, *Treponema pallidum*, EBV Swimming in an inadequately chlorinated pool: adenovirus Eating undercooked meat: tularemia Incomplete immunization: diphtheria Immunodeficiency: fungus Use of antibiotics: candidiasis (thrush)
What are the common symptoms of pharyngitis?	Fever, sore throat, hoarseness of voice, rhinorrhea, cough, conjunctivitis, and cervical lymphadenopathy

What are some physical signs of infectious mononucleosis viral pharyngitis?

Pharyngeal erythema, tonsillar exudates, enlarged tonsils, lymphadenopathy, and hepatosplenomegaly

What are some of the signs of streptococcal pharyngitis?

Rapid onset of fever, pharyngeal erythema and petechiae, tonsillar exudates, tender cervical adenopathy, headache, abdominal discomfort, and absence of significant cough or rhinorrhea

How do you diagnose S. pyogenes pharyngitis?

Throat culture (diagnostic) or rapid streptococcal antigen detection tests (RADTs)

What is the sensitivity and specificity of RADTs?

Sensitivity, 60–95%; specificity, >95%. A negative RADT does not rule out streptococcal infection; throat culture may be required to confirm diagnosis.

What are some signs of enteroviral pharyngitis?

Pharyngeal or oral nodules or ulcers, conjunctivitis, and skin rash

What do you expect to see in the peripheral smear of a patient with infectious mononucleosis?

>10% atypical lymphocytes

What other lab tests are used in the diagnosis of EBV infection?

Monospot (heterophil antibodies) can be falsely negative in children <5 years. A more definitive test is EBV serology (detecting IgM antibodies to the viral capsid antigen).

What is the treatment of viral pharyngitis?

Symptomatic: analgesics and antipyretics

What are drugs of choice for GABHS pharyngitis?

Oral penicillin V for 10 days or 1 dose of intramuscular benzathine penicillin G; oral erythromycin for 10 days for penicillin-allergic individuals

What other drugs can be used instead of penicillin for GABHS pharyngitis?

Amoxicillin, clindamycin, first-generation cephalosporins, or azithromycin

When can a child with GABHS pharyngitis return to school or day care?	24 hours after starting antibiotics
What is the treatment failure rate of GABHS after 10 days of penicillin?	6–23%
What are some possible local complications of severe pharyngitis?	Peritonsillar abscess, airway obstruction, and retropharyngeal abscess
What are some long-term nonsuppurative complications of GABHS?	Acute rheumatic fever, streptococcal toxic shock syndrome, and acute glomerulonephritis

PNEUMONIA

What is pneumonia?	Inflammation of lungs due to infection by viral, bacterial, or other organisms. Classified anatomically as lobar pneumonia or bronchopneumonia.
What is the annual incidence?	In developed nations, 2–5%; in developing countries, 5–30%. Preschool children are at higher risk.
What are the causative organisms?	Viral, bacterial, mycobacterial, *Mycoplasma*, *Chlamydia*, *Rickettsia*, *Pneumocystis*, and *Legionella*
What is the most common cause of pneumonia?	Viral agents, including RSV, influenza, parainfluenza and adenovirus
What are the bacterial pathogens of pneumonia?	Vary according to age and immune status of patient. Newborns: group B streptococci, gram-negative bacilli, and *Chlamydia* 3 months to 5 years: *S. pneumoniae*, *H. influenzae* >5 years: *S. pneumoniae*, *Mycoplasma pneumoniae* Hospitalized and immunocompromised patients: gram-negative bacilli, *Pneumocystis carinii*, fungal agents

What are some risk factors?	Young age, malnutrition, overcrowding, day care attendance, exposure to airway irritants, immunodeficiency, chronic lung disease, congenital heart disease, and aspiration syndromes
How does pneumonia often present in children?	Febrile tachypnea
What are the symptoms of pneumonia?	Fever, chills, nausea, vomiting, diarrhea, abdominal pain, coughing, chest pain, and sputum production
What are the signs of pneumonia?	Lethargy, irritability, tachypnea, retractions, cyanosis, and grunting. On chest exam: dullness to percussion, decreased air entry, crackles, abnormal tactile or vocal fremitus. Pleural rub heard in pleurisy.
What is the differential diagnosis?	Atelectasis, asthma, foreign body aspiration, congenital malformations of lung, congestive heart failure, cystic fibrosis, interstitial lung disease, trauma, pulmonary hemosiderosis, and abdominal pathology
How is the diagnosis made?	Mainly clinical. Chest x-rays in severely affected and immunocompromised patients or in cases of recurrent pneumonias.
How are the pathogens isolated?	Sputum specimens not reliable; nasopharyngeal swabs (viral stains and cultures) may be useful. Blood cultures may be positive in 10–15% of bacterial pneumonias. Bronchoalveolar lavage fluid or lung biopsy may be needed in immunocompromised patients. Aspirate pleural fluid for Gram stain and culture if effusion is present.
What is the treatment of bacterial pneumonias?	Uncomplicated cases: treat with oral antibiotics (e.g., penicillin, amoxicillin, cephalosporins or macrolides). Neonates, severely affected, and immunocompromised patients: admit and treat with IV antibiotics.

What is the treatment of nonbacterial pneumonias?	Antituberculous agents for tuberculosis; antifungal drugs for mycotic infections; macrolides for mycoplasma, legionella, and chlamydia; ganciclovir for cytomegalovirus; trimethoprim-sulfa for *Pneumocystis carinii*
What are the complications of pneumonia?	Empyema, necrotizing pneumonia, pneumatocele formation, pneumothorax, septicemia, distal infection of other organs, and respiratory failure

RETROPHARYNGEAL ABSCESS

What is retropharyngeal abscess?	A suppurative infection of the retropharyngeal space and its contents
What age group is most often affected?	Preschool children
What and where is the retropharyngeal space?	A potential space located behind the pharynx and upper esophagus. It extends from the skull base to the superior–posterior mediastinum.
What are its components?	2 paramedial anatomically separate chains of lymph nodes that drain the nasopharynx, middle ear, eustachian tube, adenoids, and paranasal sinuses
What causes the retropharyngeal abscess?	In the first 2 years of life, bacterial infection of the structures can lead to suppurative infection of the draining nodes and abscess formation.
What causes the infection in an older child?	Usually, penetrating injury of posterior pharynx, chest or neck trauma
What are the causative organisms?	Usually β-hemolytic streptococci, and *Staphylococcus aureus*
What is the differential diagnosis?	Pharyngitis, peritonsillar abscess, cervical lymphadenitis, and epiglottitis

What are the symptoms?	Fever, stiff neck, dysphagia, drooling, dyspnea, stridor, and muffled voice
What are the signs of retropharyngeal abscess?	Palpable and tender cervical lymphadenopathy, neck fullness, and tenderness. In a cooperative child, oral exam may reveal unilateral and generalized swelling or bulging of posterior pharyngeal wall.
What is seen in a lateral neck radiograph?	The diagnosis is suspected if any of the following is present: retropharyngeal soft tissues greater than half of the adjacent vertebral body, retropharyngeal space of >7 mm, retrotracheal space of >14 mm, presence of free air or air-fluid levels in the retropharyngeal space.
What other imaging studies can be used in the patient with retropharyngeal abscess?	Computed tomography scan with contrast or magnetic resonance imaging may help distinguish abscess, cellulitis, and lymphadenitis, and delineate extent and proximity to major cervical vessels.
What is the initial therapeutic approach?	Immediate hospital admission and consultation with an otolaryngologist or pediatric surgeon. Start intravenous (IV) antibiotics (broad-spectrum semisynthetic penicillins or clindamycin).
Should the retropharyngeal space be explored?	Surgical drainage is required if an abscess is identified or if the patient is moderately to severely affected.
What are the complications of retropharyngeal abscess?	Extension of infection to mediastinum, rupture and aspiration of purulent material, erosion of major blood vessels, and airway obstruction
What is the prognosis?	Excellent with supportive care, IV antibiotics, and timely drainage of abscess

RUBELLA

What is another name for rubella?	German measles

What infectious agent causes it?	Togavirus
How is it transmitted?	Airborne droplets of nasopharyngeal secretions or transplacental passage to fetus
Who is at greatest risk?	Fetuses of unimmunized pregnant women in first and second trimester
What increases the risk in adolescents and adults?	Inadequate MMR vaccination as a child
How does it often present in neonates of unimmunized mothers?	Congenital anomalies ($>50\%$) with risk of hydrops fetalis
Will rubella vaccination at time of exposure prevent congenital anomalies?	No; contraindicated during pregnancy
How does it present in children?	Prodrome of low-grade fever, cough, conjunctivitis, coryza, malaise, headache, and lymphadenopathy 1–5 days before rash appears
Describe the rash.	Erythematous maculopapular rash that starts on the head and progresses caudally to trunk and extremities
How is it different from the rash seen in rubeola (measles)?	The rash does not coalesce.
Is rubella contagious?	Yes, for 7 days before and after onset of rash
What additional physical exam findings may be found in adolescent and adult patients?	Arthritis and arthralgias (rare)
How is a tentative diagnosis made?	History (especially missed MMR vaccination) and presentation

How is the diagnosis confirmed?	Increase in serum antibodies to rubella virus
How is it treated?	Supportive (most spontaneously resolve); acetaminophen for fever
What additional measures should be taken?	Rubella is contagious; do not expose patient to unimmunized individuals (especially pregnant women) 1 week before or after onset of rash.

NEPHROLOGY

ENURESIS

Define enuresis.	Involuntary passage of urine at age after most children have reached continence (girls, 5 years; boys, 6 years)
When do most children achieve bladder control?	24–36 months, but many normal children take significantly longer
What is the difference between primary and secondary enuresis?	Primary enuresis: child has never been continent for a period of at least 6 months. Secondary enuresis: prolonged periods of bladder control, then enuretic behavior.
What hormone, if inadequate during sleep, can cause enuresis?	Antidiuretic hormone (rare)
What associated conditions can cause enuresis?	Diabetes mellitus (DM), urinary tract infections (UTI), obstruction, sickle cell disease, chronic stool retention, and developmental delay
How does it often present?	Bedwetting (most common), but daytime enuresis can occur.
What lab tests should be performed?	Urinalysis (detects UTI, DM) and culture

What is the initial treatment?	Correct underlying cause if present, then behavior modifications such as counseling, charting, night awakening by parents 1.5 hours after sleep onset, and use of a buzzer alarm.
What is the next step if the above treatment fails?	Consider medical therapy with imipramine (tricyclic antidepressant)or intranasal desmopressin acetate (an endogenous vasopressin analog).
What risks are associated with imipramine therapy?	Arrhythmias, conduction blocks, accidental overdose, and death
What study should be ordered before starting a child on imipramine?	Electrocardiogram

REYE SYNDROME

What is Reye syndrome?	An acute syndrome of encephalopathy and fatty degeneration of the liver
What is Reye-like syndrome?	A group of primarily metabolic disorders producing a clinical picture similar to Reye syndrome
With what illnesses is Reye syndrome associated?	Influenza A and B, varicella, and other viruses
With what medication is Reye syndrome associated?	Aspirin. Epidemiologic studies have identified aspirin consumption during infection with the above viruses to be the initiating factor in Reye syndrome.
What is the usual age of presentation?	4–12 years; mean age 6 years
How does Reye syndrome usually present?	Illness is biphasic. Initially, a prodromal period consists of initiating viral illness. Apparent convalescence lasts about 1 week, and then the child develops intractable vomiting. Some develop delirium, combativeness, seizures, and coma, and may die.

What are the physical exam findings?	Mild liver enlargement; usually no jaundice, fever, or focal neurologic findings
What are the laboratory findings?	Elevated serum aminotransferase, creatinine kinase, and lactic dehydrogenase levels. Elevated ammonia is associated with likely progression to coma. Prolonged prothrombin times can lead to coagulopathy. Hypoglycemia is common.
How is Reye syndrome distinguished from other causes of fulminant hepatic failure?	Bilirubin levels are normal in Reye syndrome.
What causes the neurologic changes?	Cerebral edema leads to increased intracranial pressure.
What must be ruled out?	Reye-like syndrome, the causes of which are more frequent than Reye syndrome itself
How is Reye syndrome treated?	Therapy is symptomatic. Administer glucose to all patients initially. Observe mildly affected patients; restrict fluid to those with cerebral edema. Treat coagulopathies with transfusions of platelets and fresh frozen plasma and vitamin K.
How long do the mental status changes last?	24–96 hours

CHILD ABUSE

What types of child abuse exist?	Physical, emotional, sexual, and neglect
Are physicians legally obligated to report suspected child abuse?	Yes, social services must be notified; physicians are liable if they fail to do so.

What is the most common cause of abuse?	Neglect, defined as failure to provide for a child's basic needs (food, clothing, shelter, medical care, education, safety, nurturing)
What physical signs may indicate neglect?	Dehydration, poor weight gain, malnutrition, poor hygiene, inadequate clothing, and depression
What behavioral signs may indicate neglect?	Developmental delay, poor school attendance, lack of supervision (repeated episodes of ingestion), and exploitation (excessive home chores)
What should raise suspicion of physical child abuse?	History of multiple injuries, injuries not adequately explained by mechanism of injury, inconsistencies in the history, and delay in seeking medical treatment
What is Munchausen syndrome by proxy?	An illness inflicted on a child by a caregiver. The child may have repeated medical assessments and procedures, yet the caregiver claims not to know the cause of illness and the child improves in the caregiver's absence.
Name some common physical child abuse injuries.	Burns, fractures, head (shaken baby syndrome), abdominal and genital trauma
What physical finding is characteristic of shaken baby syndrome?	Retinal hemorrhage
What constitutes child sexual abuse?	Nonconsensual sexual activity: exposure (physical contact not required), genital manipulation, oral sex, and intercourse
How might a sexually abused child present?	Recurrent abdominal pain, enuresis, encopresis, urinary tract infection, vaginal discharge or bleeding, and depression
Does a normal genital exam rule out sexual abuse?	No

What sexually transmitted disease tests should be ordered?

Gonorrhea, chlamydia, syphilis, and HIV

How is child abuse diagnosed?

History, physical exam, x-rays (complete skeletal survey), and social work report

How is child abuse managed?

Do not allow child to return home until it is safe; make full report to child protective services; treat injuries; and arrange counseling for child and family.

What is the most common cause of death in abused children?

Intracranial injury

11 ___ Psychiatry

PSYCHOSIS

SCHIZOPHRENIA

What is the common age of onset of schizophrenia?

Late teens to early 30s

What causes it?

Unknown; dopamine hyperactivity is implicated (dopamine hypothesis)

What factors are involved in causing schizophrenia?

Genetic and environmental

What is the dreaded outcome of schizophrenia?

Suicide

Describe the classification of schizophrenia symptoms:
    Positive symptoms?

Delusions, hallucinations, disorganized speech or behavior, catatonia

    Negative symptoms?

Flat affect, apathy, anhedonia, inattentiveness

How is it diagnosed?

Positive and negative symptoms, with social and occupational deterioration for ≥6 months

Describe the five subtypes of schizophrenia:
    Paranoid?

Paranoid delusions, auditory hallucinations, nonflat affect (best prognosis)

    Catatonic?

Psychomotor disturbance (excessive increase or decrease in activity), echolalia, mutism

    Disorganized?

Disorganized speech and behavior, flat or inappropriate affect (worst prognosis)

Undifferentiated?	Criteria not met for paranoid, catatonic, or disorganized
Residual?	Persistent negative or mild positive symptoms after one acute schizophrenic episode

What is the first-line treatment for positive symptoms?

Antipsychotic medications:
    Haloperidol (higher potency for severely agitated or disruptive behavior) or
    Chlorpromazine (lower potency)

What is the mechanism of action for haloperidol and chlorpromazine?

Dopamine receptor antagonists

What are the side effects?

Akathisia (restlessness), tremors, rigidity, tardive dyskinesia, acute dystonia, neuroleptic malignant syndrome

What is an alternative medication for patients with negative symptoms?

Risperidone

What medication is prescribed if patients fail first-line agents?

Clozapine

What is the dreaded side effect of clozapine?

Agranulocytosis (1%)

DISORDERS ORIGINATING IN CHILDHOOD

ATTENTION DEFICIT HYPERACTIVITY DISORDER (ADHD)

What is ADHD?

A disorder characterized by inattention, impulsiveness, and hyperactive behavior in young children

What causes it?

Unknown; possibly depletion of neurotransmitter dopamine, prenatal substance abuse

Is it usually a lifelong condition?

No; most patients improve with age.

In which sex is it more common?	Males (4:1)
What are patients at risk for in adulthood?	Personality disorders

How do the behaviors of ADHD present?

Inattention	Inability to finish tasks (often in school, where they are labeled "troublemakers"); easy distractibility, forgetfulness
Impulsiveness	Impatience, often interrupts
Hyperactivity	Excessively talkative, restless, fidgety

How is ADHD diagnosed?	Age <7 years; symptoms in two separate locations (e.g., school, home)
What is the treatment strategy?	1. Behavior management techniques 2. Psychostimulants [e.g., methylphenidate (Ritalin)] if needed
What are the side effects of Ritalin?	Insomnia, depressed mood, irritability, tics, decreased growth rate (higher doses)

ANXIETY

GENERALIZED ANXIETY DISORDER (GAD)

What are the main clinical features of GAD?	Excessive, persistent, uncontrollable anxiety or apprehension about most daily events
What secondary symptoms may be present?	Difficulty concentrating, restlessness, easily fatigued, sleep disturbance, muscle tension
What lab tests are used to rule out anxiety secondary to a medical condition?	Thyroid function; complete blood cell (CBC) count; levels of glucose, electrolytes, calcium
What basic cardiac study should be considered?	Electrocardiogram
How is GAD diagnosed?	Persistent anxiety that occurs most days for ≥6 months with three or more secondary symptoms

What is the first-line therapy?	Psychotherapy, relaxation techniques
What is the second-line therapy?	Anxiolytics (e.g., benzodiazepines, buspirone)
Which anxiolytic is best for acute anxiety?	Benzodiazepines
What risk is associated with benzodiazepine use?	Drug tolerance, dependence
Which anxiolytic is better for chronic dosing?	Buspirone

OBSESSIVE-COMPULSIVE DISORDER (OCD)

What condition may accompany OCD?	Tourette syndrome
Define an obsession.	Persistent intrusive thoughts, impulses, ideas, or images that cause significant anxiety and cannot be controlled
Define a compulsion.	Repeated mental or motor behavior performed to lessen anxiety; often follows obsession
What are some examples of compulsions?	Repeated checking, washing, and counting
How is OCD diagnosed?	Recurrent obsessions and compulsions that cause significant distress Patient is aware these do not make sense.
What is the first-line medical therapy?	Selective serotonin reuptake inhibitors (SSRI) (e.g., fluvoxamine)
What is the next medical therapy available?	Tricyclic antidepressants [TCAs (e.g., clomipramine)]
What additional therapy should be considered?	Behavior modification techniques (e.g., systemic desensitization, flooding)

PANIC DISORDER

What sex is at greater risk for panic disorder?	Females
In what age range does it often present?	20–30 years
What medical conditions may be found in patients with panic disorder?	Mitral valve prolapse, thyroid disorders
How does panic disorder present?	Recurrent, unexpected, discrete periods of intense fear or discomfort; >4 panic symptoms; constant worry about another attack
Name some common panic attack symptoms.	Palpitations, accelerated heart rate, sweating, shaking, shortness of breath, choking feeling, chest discomfort, nausea, dizziness, fear of losing control or dying
How is it diagnosed?	Recurrent attacks (>4 symptoms) with ≥1 month of associated anxiety
What other disorder may occur with panic disorder?	Agoraphobia
Define agoraphobia.	Intense fear of places or situations in which escape might be difficult or help unavailable if panic symptoms occur
What medical treatments are used to treat panic attacks?	TCAs (desipramine), monoamine oxidase inhibitors [MAOIs (phenelzine)], SSRIs (fluoxetine), benzodiazepines (alprazolam)
What additional therapy should be considered?	Cognitive-behavioral therapy (e.g., relaxation exercises, desensitization)
What is the treatment for agoraphobia?	Exposure therapy

POSTTRAUMATIC STRESS DISORDER (PTSD)

What is the main risk factor for PTSD?	Traumatic events (e.g., rape, assault, combat, natural disasters)
How does it present?	Re-experience (recurrent hallucinations, illusions, flashbacks) Increased arousal (anxiety, sleep disturbance, hypervigilance) Avoidance of stimuli associated with the trauma
How is it diagnosed?	Presenting symptoms lasting >1 month in which patient must have experienced severe fear, hopelessness, or horror
What is the treatment?	Psychotherapy and medication, including some antidepressants [TCAs (e.g., imipramine) and SSRIs (e.g., fluoxetine)] and anticonvulsants (carbamazepine and valproate)
What is an alternative drug for imipramine?	Phenelzine (an MAOI)

SOCIAL PHOBIA

How does social phobia present?	Excessive, persistent fear of social or performance situations
How is it diagnosed?	History
What is the first-line treatment?	Behavioral therapy (desensitization, rehearsal)
What is the second-line therapy?	SSRI (e.g., fluoxetine) or MAOI (e.g., phenelzine)
What medication is useful if taken 30 minutes before performance situations?	Propranolol

MOOD DISORDERS

BIPOLAR DISORDER

What disorders constitute bipolar disorder?	Mania (or hypomania) and major depression
Describe the following features of a manic episode:	
Self-esteem?	Highly elevated; grandiosity
Sleep?	Decreased need
Speech?	Pressured
Thoughts?	Racing; flight of ideas
Attention?	Easily distracted
Activity?	Increased goal-directed activity or psychomotor agitation
Hedonism?	Excessive involvement in pleasurable activities (e.g., sex, spending, travel)
How is a manic episode diagnosed?	Three to four features, lasting 1 week or severe enough to require hospitalization
Define bipolar I disorder.	At least one episode of mania with or without a major depressive episode (see Major Depressive Disorder)
Define bipolar II disorder.	One or more hypomanic episodes plus major depressive episodes (no history of manic episode)
What medications are used for rapid treatment of manic episodes?	Benzodiazepines or antipsychotics
What is the long-term treatment strategy?	Psychotherapy, cognitive therapy, lithium (monitor levels closely due to toxic potential)
What are the side effects of lithium?	Gastrointestinal (GI) distress, weight gain, fatigue, tremor, hypothyroidism
What are the toxic side effects of lithium?	Vomiting, diarrhea, ataxia, confusion, seizure, coma

What second-line drugs are available to treat mania?	Carbamazepine and valproic acid

ADJUSTMENT DISORDER WITH DEPRESSED MOOD

What are common identifiable stressors?	Marital problems, divorce, moving, financial hardship, criminal victim
How does it present?	Depressed or anxious mood within 3 months of identifiable stressor, lasting <6 months Mood change is excessive; impairs social and occupational function
How is it diagnosed?	History and presentation
What is the first-line therapy?	Psychotherapy
What is the treatment for severe anxiety?	Short-term use of benzodiazepines
What is the treatment for depressed mood?	Antidepressants (controversial)

COMPLICATED BEREAVEMENT

What are some risk factors for complicated bereavement?	Sudden or traumatic death; death of a child; concurrent stress; insecure personality
How does it present?	Sudden or delayed onset (up to 1 year) of depressive symptoms after death; symptoms last >2 months
What are patients at risk for?	Major depression and suicide
What is the first-line therapy?	Bereavement therapy
What is the treatment for disturbed sleep or anxiety?	Short course of benzodiazepines

When should antidepressant medication be considered?	Impaired social and occupational functioning or symptoms present for >2 months
What is the treatment for psychotic symptoms?	Antipsychotic medication
When should hospitalization be considered?	If patient is suicide risk

CYCLOTHYMIC DISORDER

How does cyclothymic disorder present?	Hypomanic symptoms and depressive symptoms for ≥2 years; symptom free for <2 months at a time
How is it diagnosed?	History and presentation
What is the treatment?	Group and individual psychotherapy
What medications are helpful?	Mood-stabilizing medications (e.g., lithium, anticonvulsants) and antidepressants

DYSTHYMIC DISORDER

What is dysthymic disorder?	Chronic, mild depression
How does it present?	Almost continuous depressed mood; symptoms most of time for ≥2 years
Name some common depressive symptoms.	Appetite change, sleep disturbances, fatigue, low self-esteem, decreased concentration, hopelessness
How is it diagnosed?	History and presentation
What is the treatment?	Psychotherapy, antidepressants

MAJOR DEPRESSIVE DISORDER

In what age range does major depression typically appear?	20–50 years

What two neurotransmitters are implicated in major depression?	Norepinephrine and serotonin
Describe the following criteria for major depression:	
Mood?	Depressed mood most of day, nearly every day
Sleep?	Insomnia or hypersomnia
Interest?	Marked decrease in interest and pleasure in most activities
Guilt?	Feeling worthless or inappropriate guilt
Energy?	Fatigue or low energy nearly every day
Concentration?	Decreased concentration or increased indecisiveness
Appetite?	Increased or decreased; weight gain or loss
Psychomotor?	Psychomotor agitation or retardation
Suicidality?	Recurrent thoughts of death, suicidal ideation, suicide plan or attempt
How is major depression diagnosed?	Five or more criteria for ≥2 weeks; must include depressed mood or loss of interest or pleasure
What lab tests are done to rule out major depression secondary to a medical condition?	CBC count, electrolytes, liver function, urinalysis, thyroid function, drug screen
What radiographic studies can exclude intracranial causes?	Computed tomography scan or magnetic resonance imaging
What is the treatment for milder cases?	Psychotherapy
What additional treatment is available?	Pharmacotherapy (e.g., SSRIs, TCAs, MAOIs)
What determines which medication is prescribed?	Medication history and side-effect profile of the medication
What is considered an adequate trial of a medicine?	4 weeks at maximum recommended dose

In which patients are SSRIs especially useful? Why?

Patients with
  Cardiac disease (minimal risk of cardiac complications)
  Suicide risk (overdose less likely to be fatal)

What are the common side effects of SSRIs?

GI effects, sexual dysfunction, appetite suppression

Name some commonly prescribed TCAs.

Amitriptyline, nortriptyline, imipramine, desipramine, doxepin

What are the side effects of TCAs?

Anticholinergic (e.g., dry mouth, constipation), sexual dysfunction, potential for fatal overdose

Name some MAOIs.

Phenelzine, tranylcypromine, isocarboxazid

In which patients are MAOIs useful?

Those with anxiety syndromes (including panic symptoms) or atypical depression (e.g., increased sleep and appetite)

What is the main side effect of MAOIs?

Hypotension

What are patients taking MAOIs at risk for if they eat foods containing tyramine?

Tyramine hypertensive crisis, which could lead to death

What foods contain tyramine?

Aged cheese, red wine, aged or processed meats

When should electroconvulsive therapy be considered?

If pharmacotherapy fails
Acutely suicidal patients

When should a patient be hospitalized?

If patient has significant risk of harming self or others (e.g., those with command auditory hallucinations), or patient whose physical well-being is at significant risk because of mental disorder

POSTPARTUM DEPRESSION

Describe the three mood disorders that occur postpartum.

Postpartum blues? — Mild depressive symptoms that develop in first week postpartum and resolve in second week; very common—up to 85% of postpartum women

Postpartum depression? — Major depressive episode occurring within 4 weeks of childbirth; common—up to 15% of postpartum women

Puerperal psychosis? — Psychotic disorder developing postpartum, usually within 6 weeks; usually presents as mood episode with psychotic symptoms; rare—1 in 1000–1500 postpartum women; medical emergency

What are the causes? — Combined:
  Genetic predisposition
  Physiologic changes (decreased estrogen, progesterone, cortisol)
  Psychosocial factors

What are the major risk factors for postpartum depression? — Previous mood disorder, particularly postpartum
  Social stresses (e.g., unemployment, marital conflict, limited social support)
  Infant health problems or irritability

What is the treatment for postpartum depression? — Psychotherapy (interpersonal or cognitive-behavioral) and medication
  Electroconvulsive therapy for severe symptoms

What medications are used to treat postpartum depression?
1. SSRIs
2. TCAs (frequent second choice)

What specific concerns exist with postpartum drug therapy? — All psychoactive medications are secreted into breast milk; effect on infant is unclear.
  Breast-feeding contraindicated with lithium.

How is the mother at risk?	Poor parenting skills Other risks of depression
How is the infant at risk?	Increased risk of retarded cognitive, behavioral, and emotional development Child abuse, neglect, infanticide

SOMATOFORM DISORDERS

BODY DYSMORPHIC DISORDER

How does body dysmorphic disorder present?	Gradual onset of excessive preoccupation with imagined defect in appearance that causes significant distress and psychosocial impairment
How is it diagnosed?	History and presentation
What is the treatment strategy?	Noninvasive treatment of any medical disorder Psychotherapy, medication trial
What medications may be useful?	Fluoxetine (first-line); clomipramine (second-line) If refractory, try pimozide (an antipsychotic)
When is hospitalization required?	Severe depression with suicide risk

CONVERSION DISORDER

What is thought to cause conversion disorder?	Redirection of unconscious psychologic conflict into physical symptoms
How does it present?	Loss or alteration of physical functioning, usually neurologic (e.g., paralysis, seizures); acute stressor precedes symptoms
How is it diagnosed?	Presence of symptoms causing significant impairment without medical explanation, with inciting psychologic stress
What is the treatment?	Psychotherapy and reassurance

FACTITIOUS DISORDER

What is another name for factitious disorder?	Munchausen syndrome
How does it present?	Intentionally produced or feigned signs and symptoms of medical or psychiatric illness without obvious motive; often resulting in multiple hospitalizations
How is this different from malingering?	In malingering, patient assumes sickness for external reward (usually money)
How is it diagnosed?	History, presentation, evidence of feigned or self-induced illness
What is the treatment?	No effective therapy known Avoid unnecessary procedures and hospitalizations

HYPOCHONDRIASIS

How does hypochondriasis present?	Preoccupation with fear of having a serious disease; preoccupation causes significant distress or impairs functioning.
How is it diagnosed?	Preoccupation persists for >6 months despite medical evaluation and reassurance.
What is the treatment?	Regular office visits followed by psychotherapy

PAIN DISORDER

How does pain disorder present?	Pain causing disability or distress, with psychologic factors as major cause of pain
How is it diagnosed?	History, presentation, negative medical workup

How is it treated?

Multidisciplinary approach focusing on patient functioning:
    Manage medical disorders
    Treat pain with minimal surgery or
        opiates
    Psychotherapy (group, individual)

SOMATIZATION

How does somatization present?

Multiple medical complaints requiring treatment or impairing functioning, starting before 30 years old, persisting for several years

Name some common medical complaints.

Pain, GI disturbance, menstrual irregularities, sexual, pseudoneurologic

How is it diagnosed?

History of pain in four sites plus symptoms in three areas: GI (two symptoms), sexual, and neurologic, without medical explanation; some symptoms develop before age 30 years

What is the treatment?

Regular office visits
No lab tests or procedures without clear indications
Psychiatry consultation if patient amenable (usually not)

EATING DISORDERS

What are eating disorders?

Syndromes characterized by marked abnormalities in eating behavior

Name the eating disorders and their subtypes.

Anorexia nervosa:
    Restricting type
    Binge-eating/purging type
Bulimia nervosa:
    Purging type
    Nonpurging type

ANOREXIA NERVOSA (AN)

How does AN present?	Abnormally low weight, amenorrhea
What are the psychologic criteria needed to diagnose AN?	Extreme fear of gaining weight or getting fat Distorted perception of one's weight (e.g., claiming to be overweight) or body (e.g., claiming that emaciated areas, such as abdomen or thighs, are too fat)
What are risk factors for AN?	Female; family history; industrialized society
What physical symptoms are often present in patients with AN?	Constipation, abdominal pain, cold intolerance, lethargy or excess energy
What physical signs are often present in patients with AN?	Severe cachexia, hypotension, hypothermia, xerosis, lanugo, bradycardia, parotid gland swelling, edema, dental enamel erosion, calluses on dorsum of hand
What lab test abnormalities are seen in patients with AN?	Anemia, leukopenia, hypokalemia, hypochloremic metabolic alkalosis, hypercholesterolemia, hypoalbuminemia, low plasma estradiol levels, high plasma cortisol levels
What medical complications are associated with AN?	Cardiac arrhythmias; prolonged QT intervals; decreased left ventricular mass; gastric/intestinal dilatation; osteoporosis; sick euthyroid syndrome; cognitive dysfunction (e.g., poor long-term recall, reaction time, motor speed)
What associated psychiatric conditions develop in patients with AN?	Depression; anxiety, often with obsessive-compulsive features
How is AN managed?	Manage medical complications (hospitalize if severe) Family and behavioral psychotherapy Medicine (e.g., chlorpromazine, cyproheptadine, fluoxetine)

What is the prognosis?	Full recovery, up to 50%
	No substantial improvement, 25%; increased mortality due to medical complications or suicide, 5–18%

BULIMIA NERVOSA (BN)

How does BN present?	Recurrent binge eating followed by inappropriate behaviors to prevent weight gain
What are some behaviors used to prevent weight gain in BN?	Self-induced vomiting, laxative abuse, fasting, excessive exercise
What psychologic symptom is necessary to diagnose BN?	Self-esteem excessively influenced by body shape or weight
What physical signs are associated with BN?	Normal weight
	With vomiting: eroded dental enamel, scars/calluses on hand used to induce vomiting, enlarged parotid gland
What lab abnormalities are associated with BN?	Electrolyte disturbances
	Metabolic alkalosis, elevated serum amylase with vomiting
	Metabolic acidosis with laxative abuse
What medical complications are associated with BN?	Acute dilatation or rupture of stomach
	Esophageal tears
	Cardiac arrhythmias
	Ipecac intoxication
What psychiatric syndromes are associated with BN?	Depression; anxiety; substance abuse or dependence; personality disorders
How is BN managed?	Psychotherapy, especially cognitive-behavioral
	Antidepressants
	Hospitalize for acute medical complications

COGNITIVE DISORDERS

AMNESTIC DISORDER

What is an amnestic state?	Clinical syndrome characterized by memory loss
What is retrograde amnesia?	Inability to recall events preceding onset of amnestic state
What is anterograde amnesia?	Inability to learn new information
What is confabulation?	Unintentionally untrue responses to questions by patients with acute amnestic disorder, seemingly to fill gaps in their memory
What is the pathophysiology of the amnestic state?	Usually, damage to the limbic system
What are some causes of the amnestic state?	Stroke, head injury, tumors, herpes encephalitis, Korsakoff encephalopathy
What is Wernicke encephalopathy?	Syndrome of ataxia, ophthalmoplegia, and confusion secondary to thiamine deficiency
What is Korsakoff psychosis (syndrome)?	Chronic amnestic disorder associated with heavy alcohol use; often follows acute episode of Wernicke encephalopathy
What is transient global amnesia?	Amnestic state usually seen in late middle age Presents as acute disorientation with anterograde amnesia Usually resolves in 24–48 hours Cause often unknown

DELIRIUM

What is the definition of delirium?	Clinical syndrome of cognitive deficits (e.g., disorientation, confusion) or perceptual disturbances (e.g., illusions, hallucinations) in the presence of clouded consciousness

Name some common causes of delirium.	Head injury, drug intoxication or withdrawal, infections, metabolic and endocrine disorders
What are some predisposing factors to delirium?	Increasing age, underlying brain disease, increasing severity of physical illness, hypoalbuminemia
What are the major differences between	
Delirium?	Onset—hours-days Course—often fluctuating Consciousness/attention—decreased
Dementia?	Onset—usually months to years Course—usually stable or slowly progressive Consciousness/attention—alert
What are the associated features of delirium?	Mood changes (e.g., depression, euphoria, irritability), anxiety, psychosis symptoms (e.g., hallucinations, delusions), psychomotor retardation, agitation, impaired judgment
What are the nursing approaches to a delirious patient?	Quiet environment—decreased stimulation, frequent orientation, reassurance by family and staff Observe closely for agitation, impaired judgment Minimal use of physical restraints
What are the medical approaches to management?	Identify and correct contributing factors Nutritional support Sedation with high-potency antipsychotics

DEMENTIA

What is dementia?	Syndrome of acquired and persisting memory impairment and other cognitive deficits in presence of preserved consciousness
What is the main pathologic process responsible?	Neurodegenerative process leading to loss of cortical or subcortical neurons

How is dementia classified?	1. Cortical—cortical dysfunction: amnesia, apraxia, agnosia, aphasia (e.g., Alzheimer's disease) 2. Subcortical—slowed thought processes, movement disorders (e.g., Huntington's disease, progressive supranuclear palsy, Parkinson's disease); often accompanied by personality change, mood disorder
What are the major causes of dementia?	Alzheimer's disease [AD (>50%)], vascular disease, diffuse Lewy body disease (demential with Lewy bodies)
What are potentially reversible causes of dementia?	Pseudodementia (depression), normal-pressure hydrocephalus, adverse drug effects, syphilis, subdural hematoma, tumors, thyroid disorders, B_{12} and thiamine deficiency
What are the pathologic hallmarks of AD?	Intracellular neurofibrillary tangles, neurotic (β-amyloid) plaques
What are some risk factors for AD?	Increasing age, family history, female gender, head injury, lower education level
Are there identifiable genetic factors in AD?	Yes. Familial cases have been mapped to chromosomes 1, 14, 19, and 21.
How is the diagnosis of dementia made?	History and physical exam, including cognitive function screening test [e.g., mini-mental state examination (MMSE)]
What does the MMSE test?	Orientation, attention, memory, language
What are some noncognitive symptoms seen in AD?	Depression, anxiety, hallucinations, delusions, agitation, sleep disturbances
What drug treatment may improve cognitive symptoms in AD?	Cholinesterase inhibitors (e.g., donepezil)

What nonpharmacologic treatments are useful in AD?	Establish daily routine with familiar surroundings Support services for caregiver (e.g., social services, education, counseling)

PERSONALITY DISORDERS

What is a personality disorder (PD)?	Chronic pattern of behavior that is not due to another medical or psychiatric condition (e.g., mood disorder that causes mental distress to patient and impairs social interaction and occupational functioning)

CLUSTER A PERSONALITY DISORDERS: ODD OR ECCENTRIC

How does paranoid PD present?	Extensive and excessive suspiciousness, distrust of others
How does schizoid PD present?	Socially isolated, emotionally cold
How does schizotypal PD present?	Odd thinking, eccentric behavior, social discomfort

CLUSTER B: DRAMATIC, EMOTIONAL, OR ERRATIC

How does antisocial PD present?	Frequent disregard for social norms and interests of others; often lacks remorse
What other terms are often used to describe persons with antisocial PD?	"Psychopaths" or "sociopaths"
How does borderline PD present?	Unstable with mood swings, rocky relationships, anger- and impulse-control problems
How does histrionic PD present?	Excessive attention-seeking and dramatic behavior
How does narcissistic PD present?	Self-centered, insensitive to others

CLUSTER C: ANXIOUS OR FEARFUL

How does avoidant PD present?	Inhibited with low self-esteem, excessive fear of rejection
How does dependent PD present?	Passive and submissive, difficulty making decisions, fear of being left on one's own
How does obsessive-compulsive PD present?	Perfectionist, preoccupied with order and control
How is a PD diagnosed?	Assess patient's behavior over time
What psychologic tests may be helpful in assessing personality?	Objective personality test (e.g., Minnesota Multiphasic Personality Inventory) Personality test (e.g., Rorschach test or thematic apperception test)
Are PDs treated?	Most are not, because the behaviors are generally ego-syntonic: The patient is comfortable with them; therefore, they do not cause the patient distress.
When are PDs treated?	When they result in patient distress. For example: 　Avoidant and dependent PDs can be associated with anxiety. 　Borderline and narcissistic PDs can be associated with behaviors leading to job or relationship problems.
What treatments are available for PD?	Psychotherapy and medication
How are medications used in PD?	Treat target symptoms 　Antipsychotics—psychosis and near-delusional thinking 　Antidepressants—depression and anxiety 　Mood stabilizers—emotional lability, impulsivity, aggression

INFECTIOUS DISEASES

PNEUMONIA

What are the two major mechanisms of pathogen transmission in pneumonia?	Aspiration of bacteria colonizing the oropharynx (most organisms) and inhalation of infected aerosols (*Legionella*, influenza)
What is the usual presentation of a "typical" pneumonia?	Sudden onset of fever, cough productive of purulent sputum, shortness of breath; pleuritic chest pain may be present
What are the two most common organisms that cause typical community-acquired pneumonia?	*Streptococcus pneumoniae* and *Haemophilus influenzae*
What is the usual presentation of an "atypical" pneumonia?	Gradual onset of dry cough, fevers, prominent extrapulmonary symptoms such as headaches, myalgias, sore throat, nausea, vomiting, and diarrhea
What are the most common organisms that cause atypical community-acquired pneumonia?	*Mycoplasma pneumoniae, Chlamydia* species, *Legionella pneumophila*, influenza
What is the usual presentation of a lung abscess?	Indolent course (>2 weeks) of cough, purulent putrid sputum, dyspnea, fevers and chills (without rigors), night sweats, weight loss. Mimics tuberculosis.
What are two important risk factors for aspiration pneumonia?	Impaired consciousness, esophageal or intestinal abnormalities

What organisms must be considered potential causes of aspiration pneumonia or lung abscess?

Anaerobic bacteria

What are risk factors for nosocomial pneumonia?

Acute illness (e.g., shock); comorbidity (e.g., smoking, pulmonary disease, diabetes, renal failure); poor nutrition; endotracheal or nasogastric tubes; sedation; histamine (H_2) blockers

What are the most common organisms that cause nosocomial pneumonia?

Enteric gram-negative bacilli, *Pseudomonas aeruginosa*, *Staphylococcus aureus*

What are the most common organisms that cause pneumonia in patients with human immunodeficiency virus (HIV)?

Streptococcus pneumoniae, *Pneumocystis carinii*, *Haemophilus influenzae*

What are typical findings on physical exam?

Rales, dullness, increased fremitus, egophony, bronchial breath sounds

What tests should be performed?

Chest x-ray, complete blood cell (CBC) count with differential, sputum Gram stain and culture
Arterial blood gas (ABG) levels if severely dyspneic
Blood cultures if hospitalized

What are characteristic chest x-ray findings in
  Typical pneumonia?
  Atypical pneumonia?

Alveolar consolidation and pleural effusion
Reticulonodular infiltrates

What is the typical chest x-ray finding in anaerobic lung infection?

Cavity with air-fluid level

Which other organisms should be considered if a cavity is present?

Enteric gram-negative bacilli, *S. aureus*, certain fungi (*Histoplasma*, *Coccidioides*). If upper lobe, think *Mycobacterium tuberculosis* or *Nocardia* species.

Which lobes of the lung are commonly affected in aspiration pneumonia?

If supine during aspiration, right lower lobe

If prone, right upper lobe or superior segment of lower lobe

What characteristics on a sputum Gram stain indicate it may be useful in the differential diagnosis of the pneumonia?

On a low-power field, >25 polymorphonuclear (PMN) and <10 epithelial cells

When should hospitalization be considered?

Age >60 years, comorbidity (e.g., heart disease, diabetes), respiratory rate >30, pulse >140, hypotension, altered mental status, hypoxemia

Which antibiotics are used to treat outpatient community-acquired pneumonia?

Macrolide (e.g., erythromycin, azithromycin) or a fluoroquinolone (e.g., levofloxacin)

What is the usual treatment for inpatient community-acquired pneumonia?

A third-generation cephalosporin (e.g., ceftriaxone) with or without a macrolide

Why a third-generation cephalosporin instead of a penicillin?

Because of the increasing resistance of *S. pneumoniae* to penicillins

Which antibiotic should be considered for an aspiration pneumonia?

Clindamycin

Which antibiotics should be considered for a nosocomial pneumonia?

Higher generation cephalosporins (e.g., ceftazidime, cefepime) or higher generation penicillins with a β-lactamase inhibitor (e.g., ticarcillin with clavulanate). Add an aminoglycoside if *Pseudomonas* infection highly suspected.

What are common complications of pneumonia?

Parapneumonic effusions and empyema, meningitis, sepsis

TUBERCULOSIS (TB)

What causes TB and how is it transmitted?	*Mycobacterium tuberculosis* (MTB), via respiratory droplets

Which medical groups are at high risk for TB?	Patients who are
	    Immunosuppressed (drugs, HIV)
	    Age <5 or >65 years
	    Diabetic
	    Receiving dialysis

Which social groups are at high risk for TB?	Immigrants from countries with high infection rates Residents of long-term care facilities Medically underserved persons Prison populations
Define and describe MDR-TB.	Multiply drug-resistant TB: resistance of MTB to at least two primary drugs, usually isoniazid and rifampin
What causes MDR-TB?	Inadequate treatment: either failure to finish treatment course or treatment with just one drug

What is the most common pulmonary site of involvement
  In reactivation TB?
 	
  In primary TB?
	
	Upper lobes (apical and posterior segments)
	Middle to lower lung zones

What extrapulmonary sites can be involved in TB?	Most commonly lymph nodes, pleura, genitourinary tract, bones and joints, and meninges, but can affect all organs.
How does TB present?	Productive cough (often with blood streaking) associated with fevers and night sweats, malaise, anorexia, and weight loss
What is the classic pathologic feature of TB?	Caseating granuloma

What are the radiographic findings?	Upper lobe infiltrates with cavitation
What is a Ghon lesion?	Small calcified nodule, indicating a healed primary TB infection. The lesion may have an associated enlarged lymph node.
What tests should be performed?	Sputum sample for acid-fast bacillus (AFB) stain and mycobacterial culture; purified protein derivative (PPD) skin test
What additional test can be performed if the diagnosis is not clear?	Bronchoscopy with bronchoalveolar lavage and biopsy, if sputum is negative but suspicion is high
How much induration is needed for a positive PPD?	The risk of infection determines the degree of induration for a positive test. High risk (e.g., HIV, close contact): 5 mm Moderate risk (e.g., high-risk medical condition; immigrants; health care workers): 10 mm Low risk (all others): 15 mm
Which groups always need prophylactic therapy for a positive PPD?	Close contacts, persons with HIV, recent PPD conversion to positive, high-risk medical conditions, health care workers
Which groups need prophylaxis if <35 years old?	Immigrants from high-risk areas, medically underserved persons, residents of long-term care facilities
Which antibiotics are usually used for prophylaxis?	Isoniazid and rifampin
What are the two major treatment principles for TB?	1. Never treat with fewer than two drugs. 2. Prolonged therapy is standard.
What are the two standard treatment regimens for TB?	1. Isoniazid, rifampin, and pyrazinamide for 2 months, followed by isoniazid and rifampin for 4 months 2. Isoniazid and rifampin for 9 months

What is the standard regimen for drug-resistant TB?	Initially, add one to two additional antibiotics to the above three drugs (usually ethambutol, streptomycin, or both). Drug regimen is tailored based on results of susceptibility testing.
What are common side effects of isoniazid?	Hepatitis and peripheral neuropathy
What drug can be given to prevent peripheral neuropathy?	Pyridoxine
How can MDR-TB be prevented?	Directly observe therapy of patients at high risk for poor compliance with medication instructions.

PNEUMOCYSTIS CARINII PNEUMONIA (PCP)

What are the risk factors for PCP?	Immunocompromised patients (e.g., transplant recipients) Patients with acquired immunodeficiency syndrome (AIDS) and a CD4 cell count of <200 Chronic use of steroids (often when tapering dose), particularly in lymphoma patients and transplant patients
How does PCP present initially?	Usually subacute (1–3 weeks) with exertional dyspnea and dry cough
What additional features may present later?	Progressive dyspnea, fever, and fatigue
What is a possible complication of PCP?	Pneumothorax
What is the risk factor for pneumothorax in PCP patients?	Aerosolized pentamidine prophylaxis
What findings on physical exam support the diagnosis of PCP?	Bilateral crackles although the lungs may be clear

What are the associated lab findings?	Increased lactate dehydrogenase (LDH) level and hypoxia
What are the associated radiographic findings?	Diffuse interstitial infiltrates on chest x-ray; however, chest x-ray may be normal in 10% of patients with PCP.
How is it diagnosed?	Positive identification of the organism using a silver or Giemsa stain of collected respiratory secretions (bronchoalveolar lavage or induced sputum)
What is the treatment?	Trimethoprim-sulfamethoxazole (TMP-SMZ) for 21 days
What is the major side effect of TMP-SMZ?	Rash occurs in up to 30% of HIV-infected patients
What alternative drug may be substituted when patients are allergic to TMP-SMZ?	Pentamidine. Atovaquone can be used for mild to moderate disease.
What additional treatment should be considered in severe cases with a partial pressure of oxygen (PaO$_2$) of <70 or an alveolar-arterial (A-a) gradient of >35?	Steroids
When is prophylactic therapy with TMP-SMZ indicated?	In AIDS patients with a CD4 cell count of <200

OBSTRUCTIVE AND RESTRICTIVE DISEASES

ASTHMA

What is asthma?	A reversible disease characterized by hyperresponsiveness and bronchoconstriction of the airways to specific and nonspecific stimuli

What factors are associated with asthma?	Allergens (pollen, dust), irritants (fumes, smoke), chronic sinusitis, viral infection, exercise, cold weather, gastroesophageal reflux disease, and possibly aspirin (especially in patients with nasal polyps)
How can it present?	Intermittent episodes of shortness of breath, cough, and chest tightness. No respiratory complaints between episodes.
What should patients be asked during the history?	Known triggers; family history of allergy or asthma; previous hospitalizations, ICU admissions, intubations; medication compliance
What physical exam signs are present in mild attacks?	Tachypnea, wheezing, and a prolonged expiratory phase
What additional signs present in more severe attacks?	Inability to speak more than a few words, accessory muscle use, pulsus paradoxus, and distant breath sounds
What test is key in the outpatient workup?	Pulmonary function tests (PFT) to look for evidence of obstruction, as shown by ratio of forced expiratory volume in 1 second to forced vital capacity (FEV_1/FVC) of $<70\%$
What outpatient test should be performed if obstruction is not present on PFTs?	Methacholine challenge test. A positive test supports the diagnosis of asthma; a negative test rules it out.
What tests should be included in the workup of a patient having an acute attack?	Chest x-ray, ABG, peak flows
What ABG result indicates impending respiratory failure?	A rising (or normal) carbon dioxide (CO_2) level

What are the associated radiographic findings?	Usually normal, but may reveal underlying pneumonia, pneumothorax, or atelectasis; hyperinflation during a severe attack
What PFT value can be used as a criterion for hospital admission?	FEV_1 value is <30–50% of predicted (or peak flow of <60–120 L/min)
What are the treatment goals?	Decrease airway inflammation and bronchial constriction
What is the treatment for mild acute attacks?	Bronchodilators (albuterol; nebulized or via metered dose inhaler) Increased dose of inhaled steroids or an oral steroid (usually tapered over 7 days) Oxygen to keep oxygen saturation in arterial blood (SaO_2) ≥90%
How is the therapy modified in severe attacks?	Steroids are usually given IV; can add anticholinergic agent (ipratropium).
What test is used to monitor response to therapy?	Peak expiratory flow. If peak flow in the emergency department improves to ≥70% of predicted, patient can be discharged home.
What is the outpatient maintenance therapy?	Inhaled steroids and as-needed β_2-agonist bronchodilators (albuterol)
When should an outpatient be treated with inhaled steroids?	If they use their β_2-agonist daily
What are the side effects of β_2-agonist bronchodilators?	Tachycardia, irritability, and tremor
When should an antileukotriene drug be started?	If patient still symptomatic with inhaled steroids and a bronchodilator

What are the two drawbacks to adding theophylline to the treatment regimen in patients refractory to the above therapy?	Narrow therapeutic index and side effects (nausea, vomiting, tremors, and cardiac arrhythmias)
What other measures are important in asthma treatment?	Patient education Pollen and dust control, avoidance of triggers Treat associated conditions, especially sinusitis and gastroesophageal reflux disease (GERD).

CHRONIC OBSTRUCTIVE PULMONARY DISEASE (COPD)

Which two clinical entities constitute COPD?	Chronic bronchitis and emphysema
Define chronic bronchitis.	Chronic productive cough for 3 months in each of 2 consecutive years after other causes of chronic cough have been excluded (a clinical diagnosis)
Define emphysema.	Abnormal permanent enlargement of the airspaces distal to the terminal bronchioles, accompanied by destruction of their walls and without fibrosis (a pathologic diagnosis)
What is the epidemiology of COPD in the United States?	14.1 million persons have chronic bronchitis; 1.8 million have emphysema. COPD is the fourth most common cause of death (>114,000 deaths in 1998).
What are the major risk factors for COPD?	Tobacco smoking (90% of cases), inherited α_1-antitrypsin (AAT) deficiency, family history, male gender, Caucasian ethnicity, and lower socioeconomic status
What is the natural history of COPD?	15% of smokers have a rapid decline of FEV_1 (150 mL/year compared to 30 mL/year in nonsmokers). Smoking cessation can slightly increase the FEV_1 and slow the rate of the decline to that of nonsmokers.

What are the pathologic findings of chronic bronchitis?

Enlargement of the bronchial mucus glands

Disproportionate increase in mucous versus serous glands

Accumulation of mucus in small airways, which become narrowed and inflamed

Which type of emphysema is more common in smokers?

Centrilobular emphysema, which begins in the respiratory bronchioles, spreads peripherally, and involves upper lobes

Which type of emphysema is more common with AAT deficiency?

Panacinar emphysema, which involves the entire alveolus, and predominates in lower lobes

What are the clinical features of mild COPD?

Cough productive of mucoid sputum, dyspnea on exertion (often insidious onset), wheezing

What are the clinical features of severe COPD?

Hypoxemia, cyanosis, hypercapnia, cor pulmonale

What are the physical exam findings in mild disease?

Barrel chest, hyperresonant lungs, decreased breath sounds, prolonged expiration, distant heart sounds, wheezes

What are the physical exam findings in severe disease?

Cachexia, pursed-lip breathing, accessory muscle use, cyanosis, accentuated P_2 heart sound, and peripheral edema

What is the definition of COPD exacerbation?

A sustained worsening of the patient's condition, from the stable state and beyond normal day-to-day variations, acute in onset and necessitating a change in regular medications. Exacerbations become more frequent as the disease progresses.

What are the associated chest x-ray findings in COPD?

Low and flat diaphragms, bullae, increased retrosternal lucency, narrow heart shadow, and attenuation of lung markings. Prominence of hila and right ventricle in pulmonary hypertension

What are the associated pulmonary function test findings?

Reduced FEV_1/FVC ratio, elevated total lung and functional residual capacities, increased residual volume, reduced diffusion capacity. Bronchodilator responsiveness is seen in 30%.

What preventive measures are important in COPD?

Smoking cessation, pneumococcal vaccine, and yearly influenza vaccinations

When is supplemental oxygen therapy warranted?

Hypoxemic patients (improves dyspnea and survival)

Which bronchodilators are used to treat COPD?

Ipratropium, an anticholinergic agent, and salmeterol, a long-acting β_2-agonist, are first-line therapies.
Short-acting sympathomimetic β_2-agonists (e.g., albuterol)
Theophylline (oral) is useful if patient still symptomatic on inhaled bronchodilators.

What are the benefits of combining ipratropium and a β_2-agonist?

Greater increases in FEV_1 compared to either agent alone

When is treatment with corticosteroids indicated?

Primarily in acute exacerbations. Long-term use should be limited to symptomatic and maximally treated patients who show improvement in airflow after a monitored trial of steroids.

What additional treatment options exist?

AAT supplementation in deficient individuals; lung volume reduction surgery and lung transplantation in selected patients. Pulmonary rehabilitation can improve exercise capacity and quality of life, and decrease number of hospitalizations.

What factors are used to predict mortality?

Advanced age, low FEV_1, severity of hypoxemia and hypercapnia

What is the long-term prognosis for most patients?

If the FEV_1 is <0.75 L, 1-year mortality is 30%. However, patients with severe disease survive for many years if complications are treated or prevented.

What is a chronic complication of COPD?	Pulmonary hypertension and cor pulmonale
How does pulmonary hypertension present?	Progressive decrease in exercise tolerance
What may be evident on physical exam?	Parasternal heave, loud P_2 heart sound, right-sided S_4 or S_3, tricuspid regurgitation, jugular venous distention, pulsatile liver, and lower extremity edema
What studies should be ordered to assess right ventricular function?	Electrocardiogram (ECG) and echocardiography with Doppler
What is the treatment?	Treat underlying COPD, particularly the hypoxemia.
What is the most common cause of pulmonary hypertension?	Left-sided heart failure from any cause
What are other causes of pulmonary hypertension?	Any pulmonary disorder with chronic, untreated hypoxemia; primary pulmonary hypertension (PPH); chronic thromboembolic disease

INTERSTITIAL LUNG DISEASE (ILD)

What is ILD?	A heterogenous group of lung diseases characterized by inflammation and fibrosis of the interalveolar septum
What causes it?	Idiopathic, sarcoidosis, occupational exposure, infection, radiation, drugs, collagen-vascular disease

Idiopathic Pulmonary Fibrosis (IPF)

How does IPF present?	Middle-aged patient with insidious onset of dyspnea on exertion and nonproductive cough

What signs may be evident on physical exam?	Bibasilar end-inspiratory (Velcro-like) crackles and clubbing of the digits
What radiographic studies are included in the workup?	Chest x-ray and thoracic CT scan
What radiographic findings are associated with IPF?	Diffuse bilateral reticular infiltrates, predominantly at bases; honeycombing in end-stage disease
What are the associated PFT findings in IPF?	Restrictive pattern, reduced lung compliance, and decreased carbon monoxide diffusion capacity (DLCO)
What are the associated ABG findings?	Mild respiratory alkalosis with a normal or reduced PaO_2
How is it diagnosed?	Bronchoscopy with transbronchial biopsy to rule out more common disorders (e.g., sarcoidosis) Open-lung biopsy for definitive diagnosis
What are the treatment options?	Corticosteroids, cytotoxic therapy (cyclophosphamide or azathioprine), interferon gamma
What surgical treatment is available if medical therapy fails?	Lung transplant

Occupational Lung Diseases

What inorganic dusts are commonly associated with occupational ILD?	Asbestos (steel workers, shipyard workers), silica (sandblasters), coal dust (coal miners)
What are two occupations commonly associated with organic dusts that cause ILD?	Farming (thermophilic actinomyces, fungal species); bird breeding (avian proteins)

How does inorganic dust ILD present?

Insidious onset of dyspnea and nonproductive cough, usually 25–30 years after occupational exposure

How does organic dust ILD (or hypersensitivity pneumonitis) present?

Acute onset of fever, cough, and dyspnea 3–6 hours after inhaling dust, with improvement in 24 hours if no repeated exposure. Can progress to chronic dyspnea and fatigue with repeated dust exposure.

What chest x-ray findings are associated with asbestosis?

Diffuse linear opacities in lower lung fields; pleural plaques; pleural effusions

What chest x-ray findings are associated with silicosis?

Multiple small nodules (usually upper lobe) and calcification of the hilar lymph nodes

What chest x-ray findings are associated with hypersensitivity pneumonitis?

Interstitial and alveolar infiltrates, predominantly lower lobes; often fleeting; fibrosis and honeycombing in chronic disease

How is the diagnosis made?

Careful occupational or hobby history in a patient with ILD. Symptom-free periods outside of job or hobby suggest hypersensitivity pneumonitis.

What is the treatment of inorganic dust ILD?

Prevention of infections (influenza, pneumococcal vaccines), oxygen when needed

What is the treatment of hypersensitivity pneumonitis?

Avoid exposure to offending dust; administer steroids if chronic disease develops.

What infection is associated with silicosis?

Tuberculosis

SARCOIDOSIS

What is sarcoidosis?	A mononuclear, noncaseating granulomatous inflammatory process usually characterized by a heightened T-helper lymphocyte immune response at the involved sites
What is the etiology and pathogenesis?	Unknown. Theorized as immune hyperresponsiveness to external or autologous antigens. The antigens may be acquired through exposure, heredity, or both.
Who gets it	
Worldwide?	Diverse racial and ethnic groups
In the United States?	More common in African Americans
What organ is most frequently involved?	Lung: bilateral hilar adenopathy, pulmonary infiltrates, or both
What are the skin manifestations?	Erythema nodosum: bilateral tender red nodules on anterior shins (especially in acute disease with joint involvement); purple plaques; flat, waxy maculopapular lesions; lupus pernio: indurated, blue-purple shiny lesions on nose, cheeks, lips
What are common eye and nervous system manifestations?	Uveitis, optic nerve dysfunction (both with blindness), Bell (seventh nerve) palsy
What are the cardiac manifestations?	Cardiomyopathy, ventricular arrhythmias (including sudden death)
What other organs can be involved?	Joints: migratory arthralgias and arthritis Liver: granulomas with cholestasis Parotid gland enlargement: dry mouth Kidneys: hypercalciuria, hypercalcemia, nephrocalcinosis (related to overproduction of 1,25-dihydroxyvitamin D)
What are the presenting symptoms?	Fatigue, anorexia, weight loss, fever, malaise, dyspnea, retrosternal chest pain, and cough. Onset is usually insidious.

What are the four x-ray stages of sarcoidosis?

Type I: bilateral hilar adenopathy
Type II: bilateral hilar adenopathy with parenchymal involvement
Type III: diffuse parenchymal involvement without hilar adenopathy
Type IV (or type IIIb): fibrosis and upper lobe retraction

How is the diagnosis made?

Biopsy confirmation of noncaseating granulomas in affected organs (usually lung or skin). Other infectious or malignant causes must be ruled out.

What are the common pulmonary function test abnormalities?

A restrictive pattern [decreased FEV_1, FVC, total lung capacity (TLC) and DLCO] is the most frequent. Can show an obstructive pattern with a decreased FEV_1/FVC ratio.

What other lab abnormalities may be present?

Mild lymphocytopenia, increased serum angiotensin-converting enzyme (ACE), increased sedimentation rate, or hypergammaglobulinemia may be present but are not specific. Increased alkaline phosphatase if liver is involved.

Is treatment always needed?

No. May resolve spontaneously without treatment in 2–3 months, particularly with patients who present with adenopathy and erythema nodosum.

What is the current treatment protocol for unremitting or highly symptomatic disease?

Prednisone 1 mg/kg for 8–12 weeks, then gradually tapered to 10–20 mg every other day over 2–3 months

What drugs can be used for skin disease?

Plaquenil and topical steroids

What consults are needed?

Patients should see an ophthalmologist yearly for serial slitlamp evaluations and visual acuities for eye disease.

What is the prognosis?

Spontaneous resolution occurs in ~40% (Stage I with or without erythema nodosum, 60–80%; Stage II, 50–60%; Stage III, <30%)
~50% have chronic involvement.
Only 10–20% require chronic steroid treatment.

OTHER

RESPIRATORY FAILURE

Hypoxemic Respiratory Failure

Define hypoxemic respiratory failure.

PaO_2 of <55 mm Hg when patient is inspiring ≥60% oxygen

What are the three major mechanisms of hypoxemia? Give clinical examples of each.

Hypoventilation: drug overdose, stroke
Shunt: pulmonary edema, pneumonia
Ventilation-perfusion mismatch: asthma, COPD, interstitial lung diseases

What are some common causes of hypoxemic respiratory failure?

Pneumonia, acute respiratory distress syndrome (ARDS), congestive heart failure (CHF). Although asthma and COPD are associated with hypoxemia, respiratory failure in these patients is generally related to both hypoxemia and hypercapnia.

Name and define the equation used to calculate adequate alveolar ventilation.

The alveolar-oxygen equation predicts the partial pressure of oxygen in the alveolus (PAO_2). The equation is: $PAO_2 = PIO_2 - PaCO_2/0.8$, where PIO_2 is the partial pressure of inspired oxygen. At sea level and room air, $PIO_2 = 150$ mm Hg and $PAO_2 = 100$ mm Hg.

What is the alveolar-arterial gradient?

It is the difference between the alveolar and arterial oxygen partial pressure. An increased gradient indicates pulmonary parenchymal disease. Normal gradient in a 20–25-year-old person is 10–15 mm Hg. Gradient increases by 2.5 mm Hg per decade of life.

How is shunt differentiated from the other causes?	PaO_2 does not increase with 100% oxygen in shunt.
How is hypoventilation differentiated from the other causes?	If the hypoxemia is from hypoventilation alone, the alveolar-arterial gradient is normal.
What tests should be ordered?	ABG and chest x-ray (used to differentiate pneumonia from pulmonary edema)
How can ARDS and CHF be differentiated?	Clinical history (e.g., evidence of infection versus evidence of myocardial infarction). Measurement of pulmonary artery occlusion pressure (PAOP): a PAOP of <18 mm Hg is suggestive of ARDS; a PAOP of >18 mm Hg is suggestive of CHF.
What is the initial treatment?	Establish and maintain patent airway; administer supplemental oxygen to keep SaO_2 >90%; maintain adequate alveolar ventilation and treat underlying cause.
What additional treatment is required in severe hypoxemic respiratory failure?	Mechanical ventilation with settings adjusted to increase oxygen concentration and positive end-expiratory pressure

Hypercapnic Respiratory Failure

How is hypercapnic respiratory failure defined?	$PaCO_2$ >45 mm Hg
What are the two most common mechanisms of increased $PaCO_2$? Give examples of each.	Decreased minute ventilation (lack of central nervous system drive, neuromuscular disorders); increased dead space (asthma, COPD)
What are common causes of acute hypercapnic failure?	Drug overdose (particularly narcotics, benzodiazepines), stroke, asthma, and COPD exacerbations

What are common causes of chronic hypercapnic failure?

Obesity-hypoventilation syndrome, COPD, kyphoscoliosis, nervous system disorders (amyotrophic lateral sclerosis, myasthenia gravis), muscle disorders (muscular dystrophy)

What ABG lab values help you distinguish acute from chronic respiratory failure?

In chronic failure, decrease in pH will be less than in acute failure (0.03 pH unit decrease per 10 mm Hg increase $PaCO_2$ versus 0.08 pH unit) and bicarbonate will be elevated.

What workup should be done for acute hypercapnic failure?

ABG and chest x-ray
Suspected drug overdose: urine or serum drug screens
Suspected stroke or other neurologic insult: head CT

What workup should be done for chronic hypercapnic failure?

Careful history and physical exam
Pulmonary function tests: if obstructive, COPD likely; if restrictive, neuromuscular disorder or obesity
Electromyography and nerve conduction studies if neuromuscular disease suspected
Sleep study in obese patients

What is the treatment of acute hypercapnic failure?

Establish and maintain patent airway, instituting mechanical ventilation if hypercapnia is severe (pH <7.20, PCO_2 >60 mm Hg, patient cannot protect airway) and not immediately reversible. Supplemental oxygen as needed. Treat underlying cause.

What is the treatment of stable chronic hypercapnic failure?

Treat underlying condition; give supplemental oxygen as needed. Nocturnal noninvasive positive-pressure ventilation (NIPPV) appears to stabilize daytime $PaCO_2$ and PaO_2, and improve quality of life; indicated if $PaCO_2$ is >45 mm Hg.

ACUTE RESPIRATORY DISTRESS SYNDROME (ARDS)

What is ARDS?

A severe form of acute lung injury (ALI) clinically defined by bilateral infiltrates on chest x-ray, no evidence for elevated left atrial pressure (or pulmonary artery occlusion pressure of 18 mm Hg), and a PaO_2/FiO_2 of 200 mmHg for ARDS (300 mm Hg for ALI) regardless of positive end-expiratory pressure (PEEP).

What are the causes of ARDS?

Most common: sepsis, aspiration of gastric contents, pneumonia, and trauma with burns or shock requiring multiple transfusions

Other: inhalational injuries, fat emboli, drowning, drug overdose, pancreatitis, cardiopulmonary bypass, reperfusion injury, lung and bone marrow transplantation

What is the pathophysiology of ARDS?

The initiating event causes alveolar macrophages to secrete inflammatory cytokines [tumor necrosis factor (TNF); IL-1, IL-6, IL-8], which promote neutrophil chemotaxis and activation. In turn, neutrophils release oxidants, proteases, leukotrienes, and platelet-activating factor. The resulting injury to the alveolar-capillary barrier leads to influx of protein-rich fluid into the alveoli. Physiologic consequences include impaired gas exchange and compliance, and pulmonary hypertension.

What is the differential diagnosis of ARDS?

Pulmonary edema secondary to transient myocardial ischemia or cardiomyopathy, alveolar hemorrhage, lymphangitic spread of solid tumors, lung involvement with lymphoma, and leukemia may be clinically indistinguishable from ARDS.

What are important diagnostic considerations?

Decreased respiratory compliance is common. Invasive determination of PAOP is helpful, though not necessary for the diagnosis if heart failure is not clinically suspected. If in doubt, however, a PAOP of <18 mm Hg supports a diagnosis of ARDS.

What are the pathologic features of ARDS?

Marked by three phases:
1. Exudative phase—injury to the alveolar-capillary unit and diffuse alveolar damage; lasts about 1 week.
2. Proliferative phase—myofibroblast proliferation
3. Fibrotic phase—collagen deposition, fibrosis, and cysts

What are the radiographic features of ARDS?

Bilateral alveolar infiltrates, with atelectasis and consolidation particularly prominent in dependent areas. In fibrotic phase, interstitial and reticular opacities develop, with bullae and cysts. Barotrauma with pneumothorax may occur in about 10–13%.

What is the treatment of ARDS?

General supportive care: adequate nutrition, avoid nosocomial infection, antibiotics when indicated, support of cardiac output, and oxygen delivery

Fluid management to keep a low intravascular volume yet adequate systemic perfusion

Mechanical ventilation for most patients; low tidal volumes (6 mL/kg) are associated with reduced mortality compared to traditional tidal volumes (12–15 mL/kg). Recruitment of collapsed alveoli with PEEP can reduce the FiO_2 to <60% and avoid oxygen toxicity.

Steroids may reduce mortality in fibroproliferative ARDS.

What is the outcome of ARDS?

Better supportive care, ventilation methods, and treatments for sepsis have reduced mortality from 60% to 35%. Most deaths occur within 30 days, from sepsis and multiorgan dysfunction rather than respiratory failure. Therefore, indices of ventilation or oxygenation do not predict outcome. Dysfunction of extrapulmonary organs (in particular the liver), sepsis, and age >60 years adversely affect prognosis. In 75% of survivors, lung function is nearly normal 6–12 months later. Residual impairment relates to initial severity and prolonged ventilation.

HEMOPTYSIS

What is hemoptysis?

Expectoration of blood, ranging from blood-streaked sputum to gross blood without sputum

What is massive hemoptysis?

Life-threatening hemoptysis defined either by the volume of blood expectorated (100–600 mL of blood in 24 hours), or by the magnitude of the effect (e.g., hypoxemia, hypotension)

What are the most common causes of hemoptysis?

Airway diseases: bronchitis, bronchiectasis, neoplasms
Parenchymal infections: pneumonia, tuberculosis, aspergilloma, lung abscesses, septic emboli

What are other causes of hemoptysis?

Alveolar hemorrhage syndromes: Goodpasture syndrome, Wegener granulomatosis, cocaine use
Vascular: pulmonary embolism, hereditary hemorrhagic telangiectasia, mitral stenosis, aortic aneurysms

What are iatrogenic causes of hemoptysis?

Bronchoscopy, pulmonary artery catheterization

Which clinical features are useful?

Infections: fever, productive cough, prior infections, or lung disease
Hemorrhagic syndromes: epistaxis, skin rash, renal disease
Vascular: chest pain, leg trauma or prolonged inactivity
Medications: aspirin, nonsteroidal anti-inflammatory drugs (NSAIDs), anticoagulants

What features of the social and family history are helpful?

Neoplasms: smoking
Vascular: family history of telangiectasias or hemoptysis, gastrointestinal bleeding, or brain aneurysms

What features of the physical exam are helpful?	Lungs: crackles, rhonchi, egophony, chest bruits Heart: loud P_2, murmurs, gallops Skin: splinter hemorrhage, rash, needle tracks, telangiectasia Extremities: clubbing, cyanosis
What laboratory tests can be performed?	CBC with platelet count and cell differential, renal and liver function tests, prothrombin time/partial thromboplastin time (PT/PTT), urine microscopy for RBC casts. Sputum for culture, cytology. Serologies: anti–glomerular basement membrane (GBM) antibody, antineutrophil cytoplasmic antibody (ANCA), antinuclear antibody (ANA).
What differentiates lung from upper respiratory or gastrointestinal causes?	High pH, pus, and foamy appearance suggest pulmonary source.
Which diagnostic procedures should be performed first?	Chest x-ray, possibly with a CT scan, will indicate a neoplasm, pneumonia, or evidence of diffuse alveolar hemorrhage.
What other diagnostic tests may be helpful?	Bronchoscopy, especially during active bleeding. Echocardiography may detect valvular disease, pulmonary hypertension, and thoracic aneurysms. Ventilation/perfusion (V/Q) scan if embolism suspected Bronchial arteriography to localize source of bleeding
How is mild hemoptysis treated?	Control cough. Reverse coagulopathy if present. Treat underlying disease.
Which invasive procedures can be performed to treat hemoptysis?	Bronchoscopy with topical epinephrine, balloon tamponade, cautery Bronchial arteriographic embolization Surgical resection

What protective measures are needed in massive hemoptysis?	Protect the nonbleeding lung and maintain adequate oxygenation by placing the bleeding lung in dependent position, and intubating with large endotracheal tube; in severe hemoptysis, perform double-lumen endotracheal intubation.

PLEURAL EFFUSION

What is pleural effusion?	Accumulation of at least 10–20 mL of fluid in pleural space
What factors control production and absorption of pleural fluid?	Hydrostatic and oncotic pressures of the capillary intravascular and pleural space compartments
What are the two major types of pleural effusions?	Transudates and exudates
How are transudative and exudative effusions differentiated?	A pleural effusion is exudative if one of the following is present: pleural/serum protein of >0.5, pleural/serum LDH of >0.6, pleural LDH of more than two-thirds upper limit of normal serum LDH
What are the causes of transudate?	Congestive cardiac failure from any cause, hepatic cirrhosis, nephrotic syndrome, hypoalbuminemia, overhydration
What are the causes of exudative pleural effusion?	Infection, malignancy, pancreatitis, collagen vascular diseases, chylothorax, trauma, pulmonary embolism, drugs, and chemical and irradiation injury
What are the biochemical characteristics of parapneumonic and malignant effusions?	High LDH, low glucose, low pH
What is an empyema?	The accumulation of frank pus in the pleural space

What are the common symptoms of a parapneumonic effusion?

Fever, cough, chills, dyspnea, chest pain that is worse with inspiration, and tachypnea

What physical signs of pleural effusion are seen on chest exam?

Decreased chest excursion, dullness to percussion, decreased air entry, decreased tactile and vocal fremitus, and decreased egophony. A pleural rub may be heard initially.

What radiologic studies are often performed?

Upright posteroanterior and lateral chest x-rays initially. Lateral decubitus film with affected side down to show layering of a free-flowing effusion.

What other radiologic tests can be helpful?

Ultrasound and CT scans of the chest in loculated effusions and to identify underlying lung parenchyma

When should a thoracentesis be performed?

Always, if malignancy or TB suspected
In pneumonia: if pleural fluid layers to >10 mm on the decubitus film, or if fever and other symptoms do not resolve as expected

What serum biochemistries should be ordered?

Total protein, LDH, glucose, triglycerides, and amylase

What other lab tests should be performed, if exudative effusion?

WBC count, blood culture, erythrocyte sedimentation rate (ESR), serum ANA level, PPD skin test

What tests should be performed on aspirated pleural fluid?

pH, LDH, protein, glucose, triglycerides, amylase, Gram stain, culture
AFB stain and mycobacterium culture if TB suspected
Cytology if malignancy suspected

What other test is often needed to make a diagnosis?

Closed or open pleural biopsy for malignant or tuberculous pleural effusions

What is the treatment of transudative pleural effusion?

Treat the underlying medical condition.

When should a chest tube be placed if parapneumonic?	Frank pus or pH <7.1
What other interventions are required for loculated effusions?	Administer fibrinolytic agents (e.g., streptokinase and urokinase). Perform video-assisted thoracoscopic surgery for direct visualization of pleural space and lysis of adhesions.
Why is a chest tube placed in a malignant pleural effusion?	To perform pleurodesis, which prevents reaccumulation of fluid
When should a chest tube be placed if effusion is malignant?	Rapid reaccumulation of pleural fluid (<2 weeks) after adequate thoracentesis drainage

OBSTRUCTIVE SLEEP APNEA-HYPOPNEA SYNDROME (OSAHS)

What is OSAHS?	Recurrent complete (apnea) or partial (hypopnea) obstruction of the upper airway during sleep
What are the clinical manifestations of OSAHS?	Snoring, choking, or gasping during sleep, morning headaches, unrefreshing sleep, daytime sleepiness, impaired concentration
What are the risk factors for OSAHS?	Strongest risk factors: obesity and male gender Other: retrognathia or micrognathia, macroglossia, alcohol or sedative use, sleep deprivation In children: tonsillar or adenoidal hypertrophy
What are the cardiovascular consequences of OSAHS?	Increased risk of hypertension, ischemic or congestive heart disease, and cerebrovascular disease
What is the mechanism for those cardiovascular consequences?	Increased sympathetic nervous system activity from recurrent hypoxemia and arousals. Swings in intrathoracic pressure release renin, aldosterone, and atrial natriuretic factor.

What are the neurocognitive consequences of OSAHS?

Depression, irritability, poor performance, anxiety, excessive daytime sleepiness, impaired attention and learning, excess motor vehicle accidents

What is the mechanism for those neurocognitive consequences?

Fragmentation of sleep due to recurrent arousals

How is OSAHS diagnosed?

A polysomnogram (sleep study) showing five or more obstructed breathing events per hour of sleep, each lasting at least 10 seconds and associated with arousal or desaturation

What are the nonsurgical treatment options for OSAHS?

Weight loss, continuous positive airway pressure (CPAP), oral appliances (work by either anterior repositioning of mandible or forward pull of tongue)

What are the disadvantages of those nonsurgical options?

Weight loss may be difficult to achieve and maintain. CPAP may be poorly tolerated in some. Oral appliances are better tolerated but less effective.

When is CPAP indicated?

First-line therapy in all symptomatic patients

How is CPAP administered?

Through interfaces such as nasal pillows or masks

How does CPAP work?

A constant flow of pressurized room air is conducted to the airway via the interface (e.g., nasal pillow or mask) and splints the airway open.

How is the amount of CPAP determined?

A sleep study with CPAP is usually required. The level of CPAP is progressively increased until OSAHS resolves.

What are surgical treatment options for OSAHS?

Bariatric surgery, tonsillectomy, uvulopalatopharyngoplasty (UPPP), mandibular osteotomy-hyoid myotomy (MOHM), maxillary and mandibular advancement (MMO), tracheostomy

What are the disadvantages of those surgical options?

Bariatric surgery may not keep OSAHS reduced over time. UPPP works for only 50% of patients. Other procedures may be curative but have associated morbidity and are limited to a few centers.

When are surgical procedures indicated?

Tonsillectomy if tonsillar or adenoidal hypertrophy. Other procedures only if CPAP therapy fails. Best results in thinner patients with mild sleep apnea.

What is the mortality from OSAHS?

About 6% per 5–8 years

What are the causes of increased mortality in OSAHS?

Cardiovascular disease, motor vehicle and work-related accidents

SOLITARY PULMONARY NODULE

What is the definition of a solitary pulmonary nodule?

A radiologically visible opacity present within and surrounded by lung parenchyma, with no potentially associated pulmonary pathology such as pleural effusion or lymphadenopathy

What is the upper size limit of a solitary pulmonary nodule?

Usually ≤4 cm. Larger lesions are called masses.

What is the differential diagnosis of malignant solitary pulmonary nodules?

Bronchogenic carcinoma: squamous cell, large cell, small cell, adenocarcinoma
Metastatic cancers: breast, head and neck, melanoma, colon, kidneys, germ cell tumors
Carcinoid tumors

What is the differential diagnosis of infectious causes of solitary pulmonary nodules?

Abscess, septic embolus, filariasis, hydatid cyst, *Pneumocystis*, aspergilloma
Granulomas: mycobacteria, histoplasmosis, coccidioidomycosis, cryptococcosis, blastomycosis

What are other causes of solitary pulmonary nodules?

Benign tumors: hamartoma, fibroma, lipoma

Vascular or developmental: arteriovenous malformation, bronchial cysts

Inflammatory: Wegener granulomatosis, rheumatoid nodule, sarcoidosis

What radiographic features point to a benign cause?

Diffuse, central, laminated, or "popcorn" calcifications strongly suggest a benign lesion. Eccentric calcification does not exclude malignancy.

What other radiographic feature suggests a benign cause?

Stability of lesion size over at least 2 years.

What CT feature may indicate a benign process?

Fat attenuation within a lesion suggests hamartoma.

What clinical factors increase the likelihood of a malignant solitary pulmonary nodule?

Older age, smoking history, size >3 cm, lesion with irregular border

What is the first step in the evaluation?

Review old chest x-rays to determine if it is a new lesion or old and stable process.

What are the different biopsy techniques?

Fiberoptic bronchoscopy: washings and brushings for cytology and transbronchial biopsy

Percutaneous needle aspiration under fluoroscopic or CT guidance

Open-lung biopsy

What is the yield for each diagnostic technique?

Bronchoscopy: 5% in lesions of <2 cm, to 48% for lesions 3–4 cm

Percutaneous needle aspiration: 43–97%

Open-lung biopsy: high yield; can be both diagnostic and therapeutic

What is the role of positron emission tomography (PET)?

PET has a sensitivity of 95% and a specificity of 70% for diagnosis of malignancy. A conservative approach with follow-up chest x-rays is recommended with negative PET scan, whereas excision or biopsy should be performed with positive PET scan.

What approach can be adopted for nodules that cannot be shown to be benign?	Based on probability of cancer:
	    High—resectional surgery
	    Intermediate—diagnostic biopsy
	    Low—observation

LUNG CANCER

Where does lung cancer rank with regard to mortality compared to other cancers?	It is the most common cause of cancer deaths in the United States.
What is the number 1 risk factor?	Smoking causes >90% of all lung cancers.
How are lung cancers classified?	As small cell (rapid growing and virulent tumors) and non-small cell carcinomas
Name the four histologic cell types of lung cancer.	Squamous cell carcinoma, adenocarcinoma (most common), large cell carcinoma, and small cell carcinoma
What is the differential?	Metastatic cancer, hamartoma, and granuloma (tuberculosis or fungal)
What are the general symptoms of lung cancer?	Fatigue, weight loss, fever, and weakness
What are the respiratory signs and symptoms?	Cough, dyspnea, hemoptysis, chest pain, and wheezing
What metastatic signs and symptoms may be present?	Stridor, hoarseness, pleural effusion, bone pain, and neurologic abnormalities
What is superior vena cava (SVC) syndrome?	A syndrome caused by large lung tumors compressing the SVC; characterized by facial, neck, and arm swelling
What is a Pancoast tumor?	A lung tumor that arises in the superior pulmonary sulcus, and causes shoulder or arm pain (due to nerve compression) and Horner syndrome (ptosis, myosis and anhidrosis)

What paraneoplastic syndromes may arise from small cell carcinoma?	Syndromes characterized by adrenocorticotropic hormone (ACTH)-like (Cushing) or antidiuretic hormone-like activity [syndrome of inappropriate secretion of antidiuretic hormone (SIADH)]
What paraneoplastic syndromes may occur with non-small cell carcinoma?	A syndrome characterized by parathyroid hormone (PTH)-like activity (hypercalcemia; usually squamous cell)
What radiographic tests are included in the workup?	Chest x-ray and CT scan of chest (helps with staging)
What are the associated radiographic findings?	Pulmonary nodule, mass or infiltrate, mediastinal widening, atelectasis, hilar enlargement, and pleural effusion
Which lung tumors are centrally located on the chest x-ray?	Squamous cell carcinoma and small cell carcinoma
Which lung tumors are peripherally located on chest x-ray?	Adenocarcinoma and large cell carcinoma
What additional radiographic tests are usually included in the staging workup?	Bone scan for bone pain; head CT for neurologic abnormalities
What basic lab tests should be ordered, and why?	CBC count (look for anemia suggesting anemia of chronic disease), liver function tests, PT, PTT, and platelet count (abnormalities suggest liver metastasis)
How is lung cancer diagnosed?	Lung biopsy
What biopsy procedures are commonly used to obtain lung tissue?	Transbronchial biopsy, fine needle aspiration biopsy, thoracentesis (with or without pleural biopsy), and thoracotomy

What is the nonsurgical treatment?

Radiation therapy, chemotherapy, and pain relief when applicable

When is surgery indicated?

In non–small cell lung cancer with chance of curative resection

What two tests must be ordered for preoperative evaluation?

ABG levels and PFT

What PFT results prohibit surgical resection?

Preoperative FEV_1 of <1 L, or a diffusion capacity of <35%

Is chemotherapy or radiation useful in patients with curative resection?

No

When is chemotherapy indicated?

In small cell lung cancer (used in combination with radiation therapy)

13

Nephrology

ACID-BASE DISORDERS

What is the difference between acidosis and acidemia?

Acidosis is a process that tends to produce an excess of acid; acidemia is a blood pH in the acidic range (pH 7.38). Similarly, alkalosis produces an excess of base; alkalemia is a blood pH 7.42. A patient may have multiple acidoses and alkaloses simultaneously, but blood pH can only be acidic, normal, or alkaline. Thus, a normal pH may obscure a complex acid-base situation.

What is a simple acid-base disorder?

Characterized by one process (metabolic or respiratory, acidosis or alkalosis) with the expected compensation

What is a mixed acid-base disorder?

Simultaneous occurrence of two or more disorders

What are causes of, and what is the usual compensation for, metabolic alkalosis?

Causes: loss of acid [vomiting, nasogastric (NG) suction], bicarbonate ingestion (including bicarbonate precursors, e.g., citrate), diuretic use, volume contraction, aldosterone excess (primary or secondary)
Compensation: decreased minute ventilation, so that pCO_2 rises by 0.7 mm Hg for each mEq/L increase in serum bicarbonate

What are the causes of, and compensation for, respiratory alkalosis?

Causes: hypoxia, sepsis, congestive heart failure (CHF), liver failure, anxiety, central nervous system (CNS) disorders, pregnancy, pulmonary embolism (PE)
Compensation: renal excretion of bicarbonate is increased, and acid excretion is decreased, so serum

bicarbonate falls by 2–5 mEq/L for a 10 mm Hg fall in pCO_2. Acute fall is 2 mEq/L. Chronic compensation begins within hours and peaks within days and ranges 4–5 mEq/L per mm pCO_2 fall.

What are the causes of, and compensation for, respiratory acidosis?

Causes: CNS depression (of respiratory center), sleep apnea, compromise of diaphragmatic excursion (e.g., flail chest, neuromuscular disorders), severe asthma, salicylates

Compensation: renal acid excretion increases, leading to a rise of serum bicarbonate by 1–4 mEq/L for each 10 mm Hg rise in pCO_2. Acute compensation is 1 mEq/L. If respiratory acidosis persists, chronic compensation occurs over several days to raise serum bicarbonate by 4 mEq/L.

What are the causes of, and compensation for, metabolic acidosis?

Causes: loss of bicarbonate [diarrhea, proximal renal tubular acidosis (RTA)]; inability of tubules to acidify urine (distal RTA), excess endogenous acid production (lactate, ketone bodies); intoxication with exogenous acids or precursors (salicylates, methanol, ethylene glycol)

Compensation: minute ventilation increases, so that pCO_2 falls by 1.2 mm Hg for each mEq/L fall in HCO_3^-

What is the anion gap?

Serum Na − (HCO_3 + Cl). It normally is 8–12 mEq/L, and represents the excess of unmeasured (in the usual set of "lytes") anions (albumin, PO_4, urate) over unmeasured cations (Ca, Mg). Of course, total anions equal total cations, to achieve electroneutrality.

How is the anion gap used?

In metabolic acidosis, if anion gap is normal, look for gastrointestinal (GI) or renal loss of alkali; if elevated, look for endogenous or exogenous acid excess.

Is it true that acidosis invariably raises serum K?

No. Nonorganic acidoses [e.g., HCl ingestion, sulfate and phosphate accumulation in chronic renal failure (CRF), and diarrhea] do raise K (although K rise in diarrhea is mitigated by its loss in stool). However, the common organic acidoses [lactic, diabetic ketoacidosis (DKA)] do not raise K per se. Hyperkalemia in those cases is due to other mechanisms (tissue necrosis, osmotically driven shifts).

What equation describes the relationship of H^+ concentration (or pH), serum bicarbonate, and arterial CO_2 tension?

The Henderson-Hasselbalch equation, as applied to carbonic acid: $[H^+] = 24 \times pCO_2/[HCO_3^-]$

Is the compensation in acid-base disorders ever complete, to normalize pH?

No. A normal pH in a known acid-base disorder implies the existence of an "opposite" process; in other words, overcompensation beyond predicted values implies a second primary disorder. An example: a patient with DKA, with a pCO_2 lower than predicted for the HCO_3^- (so the pH is higher than expected). This might be due to primary respiratory alkalosis from sepsis or hypoxia.

What is a useful rule of thumb for expected compensation in metabolic acidosis?

$pCO_2 \approx$ last two digits of pH

Which acid-base disorder is self-sustaining (i.e., may persist after original cause has resolved)?

Metabolic alkalosis. Volume contraction depletes Cl^- and raises aldosterone; these factors stimulate renal acid excretion, perpetuating alkalosis. Similarly, hypokalemia exacerbates alkalosis.

What is the role of urinary chloride (Cl^-) in metabolic alkalosis?

Predicts response to treatment with NaCl. Chloride-responsive alkaloses (urinary Cl^- of <10 mEq/L): vomiting, NG suction, posthypercapnia, villous adenoma, and diuretic use (urinary Cl^- of >10 until diuresis abates)

Chloride-resistant alkaloses (urinary Cl^- of >20 mEq/L): disorders of excess mineralocorticoid, including primary hyperaldosteronism (Conn syndrome), Cushing syndrome, secondary hyperaldosteronism, Bartter syndrome (a rare cause)

What is the urinary anion gap?

A method of calculating unmeasured cations; in urine, the principal one is the ammonium ion NH_4^+, which is given by $(U_{Na}^+ + U_K^+) - U_{Cl}^-$. Useful in evaluating normal anion gap metabolic acidosis.

What does a negative urinary anion gap indicate?

A negative value indicates significant ammoniagenesis, as seen in GI loss of bicarbonate.

What does a positive urinary anion gap indicate?

A positive value suggests impaired renal ammoniagenesis, as seen in distal renal tubular acidosis (RTA) or aldosterone deficiency.

What is the treatment for respiratory alkalosis?

Treat underlying cause (sepsis, hypoxia); reduce minute ventilation (respirator patients)

What is the treatment for respiratory acidosis?

Secure the airway and ensure adequate oxygen delivery, but avoid excess FIO_2 in CO_2 retainers.

What is the treatment for metabolic alkalosis?

Stop ingestion of alkali.
Chloride responsive: volume expansion with normal saline if dehydrated, otherwise, KCl; in any case, correct K depletion.
Chloride resistant: K replacement with KCl; spironolactone as indicated for hyperaldosteronism; in severe cases, 0.1 N HCl via a central line

What is the treatment for type I (distal) RTA?

Bicarbonate or citrate, 1–2 mEq/kg per 24 hours, as the sodium or potassium salts based on serum potassium; correction of acidosis with sodium bicarbonate or citrate will reduce potassium wasting, so K replacement might not be necessary

What is the treatment for type II (proximal) RTA?

Bicarbonate, 10–20 mEq/kg per 24 hours, mainly as $NaHCO_3$, but potassium citrate needed as well; unlike in distal RTA, potassium supplementation is always required in proximal RTA

What is the treatment for the acidosis of DKA?

If arterial pH is >7.10, treatment of DKA will suffice

If arterial pH is <7.10, many clinicians treat with bicarbonate as a temporizing measure, using caution to avoid overshoot.

What is the treatment for lactic acidosis?

Treat underlying cause; although bicarbonate therapy may worsen lactic acidosis, it may be needed to avoid severe acidemia (pH <7.10). Calculate bicarbonate deficit as approximately $0.5 \times$ weight (kg) $\times$ (target serum HCO_3^- − current serum HCO_3^-); infuse and reassess. Note that target serum bicarbonate should be 10–12 mEq/L, as that would bring blood pH to 7.20 (out of the danger zone). Overcorrection has no benefit and may cause harm (metabolic alkalosis). As acidemia worsens, volume of distribution of bicarbonate goes up; some authors use 0.7 as factor instead of 0.5 for that reason. Regardless of calculation used, close monitoring of patient's response is critical.

What is the treatment for acidosis due to diarrhea?

Treat underlying cause; if refractory, replace sodium and potassium bicarbonate using estimate of bicarbonate deficit, as above.

A patient in the emergency department has a high anion gap metabolic acidosis with no obvious cause (renal failure, DKA, shock). What next?

Calculate serum osmolar gap. If elevated, obtain toxicology studies for ethylene glycol and methanol.

Which is more harmful, acidemia or alkalemia?	Although the causes of severe acidemia are often quite worrisome (e.g., lactic acidosis or DKA), the effects of even moderate alkalemia may be worse (tetany and seizures, altered sensorium, hypoxia, and cardiac arrhythmias).

ACUTE RENAL FAILURE (ARF)

Into what three groups are cases of ARF typically divided?	**Prerenal**: inadequate perfusion (volume depletion, CHF, decreased effective blood volume) **Renal**: acute tubular necrosis (ATN); acute interstitial nephritis; acute glomerulonephritis **Postrenal**: obstruction—bladder outlet or bilateral ureteral or intratubular (uric acid, methotrexate, oxalate, acyclovir)
How is ARF further characterized based on urine output?	**Anuric**: <100–150 mL/24 hours **Oliguric**: <400 mL/24 hours **Nonoliguric**: >400 mL/24 hours
What are key history features to obtain in evaluating ARF?	History of cardiac events, hypotension (including relative to patient's baseline) Recent decompensation of CHF, cirrhosis Drug history, including over-the-counter (OTC) drugs, especially potential nephrotoxins [radiocontrast materials, nonsteroidal anti-inflammatory drugs (NSAIDs)]; recent changes in prescriptions Recent angiography (cholesterol embolization risk) Urinary symptoms: hematuria, retentive symptoms, flank pain, changes in output (anuria, polyuria, nocturia) Trauma, myalgia, rashes, fever, recent infections History of renal disease, urinary tract infection (UTI), hypertension History of malignancy, especially those with retroperitoneal spread

What are key physical findings to elicit?

Volume status: overload—hypertension, rales, gallop, edema, jugular venous distention (JVD); depletion—orthostatics, dry mucosae, poor skin turgor

Bladder percussion

Rash, muscle tenderness, flank tenderness

Bruits

Evidence of liver disease

Evidence of infection anywhere

Signs of cholesterol embolization

How is the urinalysis helpful?

In general, a bland sediment suggests prerenal azotemia or obstruction. ATN sediments typically show amorphous debris, pigmented coarse granular casts, and tubular cells. Red blood cell (RBC) casts are strongly suggestive of glomerulonephritis. White blood cells (WBCs) and WBC casts, with eosinophils on Hansel stain, suggest acute interstitial nephritis. Dipstick positive for heme, without RBCs in sediment, implies pigmenturia (hemoglobin or myoglobulin). In practice, there may be considerable overlap and variability in sediment findings.

How is urinary sodium (UNa) interpreted?

As a measure of tubular integrity and avidity for sodium retention. A low UNa (<20 mEq/L) suggests functional tubules stimulated to retain sodium. Thus, a low UNa in a hypertensive overloaded patient implies a pathologic stimulus to Na retention [e.g., acute glomerulonephritis (GN)]; a high UNa in a hypotensive patient implies failure of the tubules to retain Na despite appropriate stimulus.

What is FENa?

Fractional excretion of sodium is a refinement of UNa, by adjusting for urinary concentration: FENa = (UNa/PNa)/(UCr/PCr) × 100%. A FENa of <1% implies tubular retention of Na.

What other lab findings suggest prerenal azotemia?

Blood urea nitrogen (BUN)/creatinine of >20–40
Urine specific gravity 1.025

Does a stable creatinine prove stable renal function?

No. A patient with oligoanuric renal failure in an intensive care setting may be getting enough fluids to dilute daily production of urea and creatinine, so as to cause "stable" reading of BUN and creatinine despite total renal failure.

How quickly can creatinine rise in severe renal failure?

Depends on muscle mass (source of creatinine production). Usually 1–2 mg/dL per 24 hours, but may be considerably higher in rhabdomyolysis and other hypercatabolic states.

Name four ways in which ultrasound is useful in evaluating ARF.

Sensitive (>95%) screen for obstruction
Small kidneys prove underlying CRF
Asymmetric size of kidneys implies preexisting urologic abnormality or vascular compromise
Large kidneys in amyloidosis, some cases of human immunodeficiency virus-associated nephropathy, acute renal vein thrombosis

What additional tests are indicated in ARF?

Depends largely on results thus far:
Nephritic sediment calls for antistreptolysin titer (ASO) and/or streptozyme test, antineutrophil cytoplasmic antibody (ANCA), complements, antinuclear antibody (ANA), hepatitis serologies, and possible renal biopsy.
Findings for interstitial nephritis prompt a careful review of all drug (including OTC and herbal) exposure.
Bland sediment not in a prerenal setting calls for rigorous exclusion of obstruction.

What is the treatment for ARF?

Based on cause:
Prerenal: ensure adequate volume; maximize cardiac output

Obstruction: relieve obstruction with Foley or percutaneous nephrostomy, as indicated

Renal: acute GN and rapidly progressive glomerulonephritis (RPGN)—see discussions later

Acute intersitial nephritis—remove offending agents, consider steroids

ATN—optimize cardiac output, volume status; loop diuretics to convert oliguric to nonoliguric ATN, if possible; restrict Na, K, protein (0.8 g/kg per 24 hours, unless on dialysis)

Adjust medication dose, as indicated, for impaired glomerular filtration rate (GFR)

Avoid further nephrotoxin exposure

Dialysis as indicated

What are the indications for dialysis?	Volume overload, hyperkalemia, acidosis refractory to medical measures Uremic platelet dysfunction with bleeding Uremic syndrome (encephalopathy, pericarditis) Expectantly, if ARF not likely to reverse soon, to prevent uremic syndrome "Early" vs. "late" dialysis still controversial To protect kidneys in acute urate nephropathy (tumor lysis syndrome), ethylene glycol intoxication
What is the prognosis for ARF?	Mortality up to 70%, which hasn't improved over past decades (however, ARF occurs in sicker patients now) Better prognosis for nonoliguric ATN, reflecting less severe insult Prognosis ultimately linked to underlying causes, coexisting system failures If patient survives ATN, renal prognosis generally good

CHRONIC RENAL FAILURE (CRF)

What are the most common causes of CRF in the United States?	Diabetes (40%) and hypertension [25% of incident end-stage renal disease (ESRD) cases]

What is the annual mortality rate of adult dialysis patients in the United States?

About 20%

Dialysis provides partial replacement of kidney function. Approximately what percent of normal kidney function is provided by dialysis?

10–15%

What hormone is markedly increased in CRF as an adaptive response?

Parathyroid hormone increases in an attempt to maintain normocalcemia.

How is anemia related to CRF?

Due to inadequate erythropoietin production by the diseased kidneys, and some reduction in red cell survival in advanced CRF, hemoglobin falls progressively as GFR falls. Interstitial diseases (e.g., chronic pyelonephritis) produce the greatest fall; polycystic kidney disease, the least.

How is anemia of CRF treated?

Exclude other factors (vitamin deficiencies, bone marrow disorders), then prescribe therapy with recombinant human erythropoietin, with a target hemoglobin of 10–12 g/dL. Maintain adequate iron stores with oral or intravenous (IV) iron supplements as indicated.

How is secondary hyperparathyroidism controlled?

Limit dietary phosphate, and prescribe phosphate binders (e.g., calcium acetate or sevelamer) to keep PO_4 below 5.5 mg/dL. Add active vitamin D analogues (calcitriol, doxercalciferol) to keep intact parathyroid hormone (iPTH) $<3\times$ upper limit of normal.

How can progression of CRF be prevented or slowed?

Aggressive blood pressure control has long been known to be beneficial. Recent studies of diabetic patients, extended to other causes of CRF, showed a benefit to using ACE inhibitors, despite initial upswing in serum creatinine. Studies of severe protein restriction have been disappointing, but moderate restriction of 0.8 g/kg per 24 hours is prudent.

Must acidosis of CRF be treated?

Chronic metabolic acidosis of CRF exacerbates calcium loss from bone, and may contribute to GI symptoms of nausea and anorexia. $NaHCO_3$ should be given (650 mg tid to start with) and titrated to maintain serum HCO_3 of 18–20 mEq/L.

Is potassium restriction necessary in CRF?

The kidney has great adaptive abilities, and single-nephron potassium excretion increases many fold to compensate for lost renal mass. Most patients adapt to normal potassium intakes, but may have problems with acute surges in intake. As renal function falls toward ESRD, potassium restriction (2 g/day) is generally necessary. Some patients develop hyperkalemia much earlier in their course, with only mild loss of renal function. See discussion in Hyperkalemia section of this chapter.

What is ESRD?

End-stage renal disease is the point in CRF at which renal replacement therapy (dialysis or transplant) is necessary to sustain life. Slightly better renal function is termed "advanced CRF" or "near-ESRD."

How is renal function measured?

Inulin clearance is the gold standard, but is impractical for clinical use. Measured creatinine clearance is useful, but limited by collection errors, and by the fact that it overestimates GFR, particularly in advanced CRF. Urea clearance always underestimates GFR, so many authorities now recommend measuring both C_{Cr} and C_{urea}, and using the average of the two. For a quick estimate, the Cockcroft-Gault nomogram has largely withstood the test of time: $C_{Creat} = (140 - age) \times$ lean body mass [kg]/72 × serum creatinine. (Multiply result by 0.85 for females.) Formula requires steady state level of creatinine, and ability to measure or estimate lean body mass.

What common drugs and conditions affect creatinine measurement?

Cimetidine and trimethoprim block tubular secretion of creatinine, raising serum levels. Cefoxitin and acetoacetate (in DKA) will cause spurious elevations of creatinine when measured by the Jaffe (picric acid) reaction.

What are the symptoms of uremia?

Fatigue, anorexia, metallic or ammoniacal taste, sleep cycle disturbances, pruritus, dyspnea

What are the signs of uremia?

Asterixis, peripheral neuropathy, serositis (especially pericarditis), dry skin, prurigo, signs of volume overload

When should dialysis be initiated?

When GFR, as discussed above, is 5–10 mL/min per 1.73-m^2 body surface area. Start earlier (10–12 or even higher) in diabetic or elderly patients, who can ill tolerate uremic symptoms. Uremic signs or symptoms in patients with borderline GFR merit initiation, as does falling albumin (sign of malnutrition or inflammation). Also, start for hyperkalemia, volume overload, acidosis, or hypertension refractory to medical measures.

What drugs should be avoided in CRF?

Nephrotoxins (e.g., radiocontrast, aminoglycoside) or drugs with significant renal effects (e.g., NSAIDs). Adjust dose of drugs with renal excretion, and drugs whose metabolites are renally excreted (e.g., procainamide). Avoid some drugs entirely (e.g., meperidine).

When should angioaccess be placed?

Timing is key to an orderly transition to renal replacement therapy. The renal team (nephrologist, transplant surgeon, dietitian, social worker) should see the patient early enough to present therapy options, plan for appropriate access surgery, and ensure adequate medical therapy of CRF in the months and years before onset of ESRD.

HYPONATREMIA

What does serum sodium tell you about a patient's volume status?

Nothing. Volume status is determined by history and physical. Serum sodium gives the ratio of body sodium to body water, not absolute lack or excess. Any combination of volume excess or depletion or euvolemia and hypernatremia or hyponatremia or normonatremia is possible.

Does the kidney sense hyponatremia and try to conserve sodium?

No. Unlike with potassium and magnesium, the kidney does *not* act to conserve sodium to maintain normonatremia. The kidney conserves sodium in response to a perceived need to conserve *volume*. Hypernatremia and hyponatremia are generally disorders of renal handling of water, not sodium.

What is pseudohyponatremia?

Apparent hyponatremia with normal or high serum osmolality. In severe hyperglycemia, high extracellular glucose causes Na-poor intracellular water to efflux from cells, by osmotic force. This dilutes serum Na, but serum osmolality is normal (or high due to hyperglycemia). In hyperlipidemia (>1200 mg/mL) or severe hyperproteinemia (e.g., myeloma), plasma water (with a presumably normal sodium level) is displaced in vitro by lipids or proteins, so the sodium concentration in the aliquot of serum falls.

What is the approach to hyponatremia?

Establish volume status by history and physical exam. Measure Na and osmolality of serum and urine. History gives clues to recent Na and water intake and losses. Note drugs that affect renal water handling. Rule out pseudohyponatremia. Further evaluation based on volume status.

What else should one look for in hypovolemic hyponatremia?

Rule out adrenal insufficiency. Review diuretic use. A high urine Na suggests renal disease (salt-wasting), diuretic effect, or adrenal insufficiency.

Why is volume overload (CHF, cirrhosis, nephrosis) commonly associated with hyponatremia?

Despite pathologic sodium retention, even greater amounts of water have been retained, resulting in dilution of the excess sodium; hence the term "dilutional hyponatremia" often applied here. CHF and decreased *effective* plasma volume stimulate antidiuretic hormone (ADH), causing water retention. The renal diluting mechanism may be impaired, due to decreased GFR and distal Na delivery. In hospital, sodium restriction is enforced more successfully than free water restriction.

What is appropriate ADH release?

Release due to either volume depletion (real or perceived by baroreceptors) or hypertonicity. In case of conflicting stimuli [e.g., volume depletion (to turn ADH release on) and hypotonicity (to turn it off)], volume wins.

What is syndrome of inappropriate secretion of antidiuretic hormone (SIADH)?

Normovolemic hyponatremia (i.e., net free water accumulation) in a patient lacking known pathophysiologic stimuli to ADH release, such as CHF, cirrhosis, pain, nausea. Must rule out endocrine disorders (thyroid, adrenal). Urine shows ADH effect: less than maximally dilute.

What is SIADH usually associated with?

Intrathoracic processes: lung cancer (primary or metastatic to lung), bronchiectasis, tuberculosis
Intracranial events: hemorrhage, meningitis, encephalitis, tumors

Why is serum uric acid low in SIADH?

Volume expansion decreases proximal Na and urate reabsorption. May also be an associated tubular defect.

What drugs may produce a SIADH-like picture?

Chlorpropamide, narcotics, phenothiazine, tricyclics, selective serotonin reuptake inhibitors (SSRIs), carbamazepine, vincristine, cyclophosphamide (Cytoxan), clofibrate. NSAIDs potentiate ADH effect.

What's the difference between SIADH and syndrome of reset osmostat?

Given a free water load, SIADH patients become more hyponatremic; reset osmostat patients can excrete the excess water to maintain a stable, albeit low, serum tonicity.

How can you distinguish SIADH from psychogenic polydipsia?

SIADH—low urine volumes and concentrated urine
Psychogenic polydipsia—very high urine outputs, with low urine osmolalities

Why is urine Na high in SIADH?

There is no volume stimulus for Na retention, so 24-hour urine Na balances 24-hour sodium intake.

What are symptoms of hyponatremia?

If it develops slowly, often none. More rapid or severe hyponatremia can cause headache, lassitude, seizure, and coma.

How is hypovolemic hyponatremia treated?

Volume replacement with saline; monitor serum sodium.

How is SIADH treated?

Fluid restriction is key, but often difficult to achieve. High protein intake may help, by increasing daily osmotic load to be excreted. Demeclocycline, to deliberately produce nephrogenic diabetes insipidus, has been used in difficult cases. Very low Na (120 mEq/L or less) requires admission to intensive care unit for administration of 3% hypertonic saline.

How is hypervolemic hyponatremia treated?

Fluid restriction is vital. Treat underlying disease (CHF, cirrhosis). Administer diuretics, and carefully monitor electrolytes.

What are the risks of too-rapid correction of hyponatremia?

Central pontine myelinosis may occur if rate of correction is >1–2 mEq/L per hour, or if total increase is >25 mEq/L over 48 hours. In mild, less symptomatic cases, correction should be limited to 0.5 mEq/L per hour, or 12 mEq/L per 24 hours.

HYPERNATREMIA

What does the presence of hypernatremia tell you about a patient's volume status?

Nothing. A hypernatremic patient may have high, normal, or low volume (total body sodium).

What typically causes hypernatremia and volume overload?

Excess administration of normal saline or sodium bicarbonate; usually occurs in hospital.

What are some causes of hypernatremia with normal body sodium?

Impaired thirst mechanism; excess loss of free water, as could occur with fever and tachypnea; lack of access to free water (as in a desert, but note that sweating also causes sodium losses). Pathologic renal loss of free water is pathognomonic of diabetes insipidus, which can be central or nephrogenic.

How can one get hypernatremia with volume depletion?

Loss of both salt and water, as in sweating, vomiting, diarrhea, in a patient lacking thirst or the ability to act upon it. Typical scenario: a cerebrovascular accident patient with tube feedings in nursing home, who lacks access to salt and free water.

What is central diabetes insipidus?

Inability of the pituitary to respond normally to hypertonicity by releasing ADH. Lack of ADH release may be complete or partial.

What are the causes of central diabetes insipidus?

Idiopathic, seen in childhood. In adults, usually due to head trauma, tumors, encephalitis.

What is nephrogenic diabetes insipidus?

Lack of response (partial or complete) of concentrating segment of collecting tubules to ADH.

What are the causes of nephrogenic diabetes insipidus?

In adults, hypercalcemia; toxins (e.g., lithium, demeclocycline); hypokalemia; obstructive nephropathy. May be congenital in children. Tubulointerstitial nephritis may reduce corticomedullary gradient, thereby impairing concentrating mechanism, but not to the degree in true nephrogenic diabetes insipidus.

What are the symptoms of hypernatremia?

Depending on severity and rapidity of rise, may see irritability, nausea, confusion, obtundation, fasciculations, seizures

What is the treatment for hypernatremia?

Treat volume depletion with saline, volume excess with diuretics. Calculate free water deficit = $0.6 \times$ weight (lean) $\times$ [Na − 140)/140]. Replace with D5W slowly, to lower Na by 1–2 mEq/L per hour in acute hypernatremia. In chronic hypernatremia (present >48 hours), lower by 0.5 mEq/L per hour.

How is central diabetes insipidus treated?

With ADH or synthetic ADH analogues (e.g., DDAVP). Ensure adequate access to free water.

How is nephrogenic diabetes insipidus treated?

Paradoxically, thiazides reduce urine output by blocking the tubular diluting segment. This works best with moderate Na restriction. Ensure free water access. NSAIDs and amiloride may also help reduce urine output, the latter in cases due to chronic lithium use.

How is diabetes insipidus confirmed?	Water deprivation test, with administration of aqueous pitressin to differentiate central from nephrogenic diabetes insipidus.

HYPOKALEMIA

What are typical clinical manifestations of hypokalemia?	Paralytic ileus, muscle weakness, cardiac arrhythmias and digitoxicity, glucose intolerance, polyuria
Why does hypokalemia predispose to exercise-induced rhabdomyolysis?	Local release of K in muscle beds during exertion allows for local vasodilatation and muscle oxygen delivery; K depletion doesn't allow this, so active muscles become ischemic and may progress to rhabdomyolysis.
What are the two major causes of hypokalemia?	Renal: abnormal losses GI: inadequate intake, excess loss, or both
Are there other causes?	Redistribution into cells can occur, as with β_2-agonists, insulin, refeeding/anabolism, alkalosis. Rare causes: thyrotoxicosis and paroxysmal familial hypokalemia.
What factors suggest GI losses?	History of diarrhea, finding of urinary K conservation (K <20 mEq/L), and normal anion gap metabolic acidosis. Vomiting/NG suction would produce metabolic alkalosis, which itself would increase renal losses of potassium. Laxative abuse may be hard to diagnose.
What are six common renal causes of hypokalemia?	1. Diuretics (acetazolamide, loop, and thiazide). As with laxatives, surreptitious use may be difficult to diagnose conclusively. 2. Tubulointerstitial renal disease may cause hyperkalemia or hypokalemia. 3. Hypomagnesemia, if severe, may contribute to renal K wasting.

4. Renal tubular acidosis, proximal or distal
5. Hyperaldosteronism, primary or, more commonly, secondary
6. Drug effects: cisplatin, amphotericin, ticarcillin, glucocorticoids

What are three uncommon renal causes of hypokalemia?

1. Licorice ingestion (natural, not artificially flavored), including licorice-flavored chewing tobacco
2. Bartter and Gitelman syndromes
3. Due to lysozymuria in acute myelomonocytic leukemia

What are typical ECG changes in hypokalemia?

Lowering of T-wave height, and appearance of U waves

How is hypokalemia treated?

1. Identify cause and estimate severity of depletion; serum K doesn't always correlate well with body stores, due to transient shifts.
2. Treat reversible causes.
3. Oral replacement by diet or supplements is safer than IV.
4. IV may be needed in severe depletion, ongoing losses, and inability to take orally.
5. Identifying and correcting Mg depletion may be very helpful.

Does it matter which K salt is used orally for correction?

Yes. In hypochloremic metabolic alkalosis, as seen with loop and thiazide diuretics, KCl is preferred because the patient is also Cl depleted, and use of K citrate would perpetuate alkalosis and K loss. In hypokalemia with metabolic acidosis (GI losses or RTA), it is rational to use K citrate to replace alkali losses.

Is there any role for K-sparing diuretics?

Yes, they are useful in chronic situations provided the patient's K can be adequately monitored. Spironolactone is of particular value in cases of secondary hyperaldosteronism (e.g., cirrhosis and CHF).

HYPERKALEMIA

What is the distribution of K in the body?	98% intracellular, with only 2% extracellular
What hormones affect K distribution?	K influx into cells is produced by insulin, aldosterone, and β_2-agonist
How much K excretion is via the GI tract?	Normally, <10%. May increase to 30% in ESRD.
What is the usual range of dietary K intake?	50–150 mEq/day (2–6 g)
What is pseudohyperkalemia?	High K readings in blood specimens, which do not reflect true potassium level in vivo. May be seen in thrombocytosis, due to release of platelet K in the clot formed in a red-top tube; the rise of serum K has been estimated to be 0.15 mEq/100,000 platelets per mm^3. Other causes include leukocytosis, difficult venipuncture, and hemolysis.
What are the ECG findings in hyperkalemia?	Peaked T waves, with a short QT interval, followed by widened QRS complexes and loss of the P wave, culminating in a "sine wave" pattern that leads rapidly to ventricular fibrillation or asystole. This progression may occur rapidly.
What drugs commonly cause hyperkalemia?	β-Blockers (inhibit renin release, block cellular uptake of K if nonselective), ACE inhibitors (block angiotensin II production), angiotensin receptor blockers, spironolactone (inhibits aldosterone). Heparin blocks adrenal synthesis of aldosterone. NSAIDs reduce renin release. Amiloride and triamterene block renal K excretion, as does high-dose trimethoprim, as well as cyclosporin and tacrolimus (various mechanisms involved).

Is urinary K helpful in the diagnosis of hyperkalemia?

Much less so than in workup of hypokalemia. High serum or plasma K means renal excretion is inadequate. A very high urinary K might suggest a large exogenous K load, an endogenous source, or both.

What is the transtubular K gradient (TTKG)?

TTKG is given by the formula $[U_K/(U_{osm}/P_{osm})]/P_K$. It estimates the urine-to-plasma K gradient at the end of the distal tubule, prior to the concentrating segments of the nephron, and as such corrects for effects of urinary concentration on interpreting urinary K. A normal value is 6–9; a lower value in hyperkalemia suggests hypoaldosteronism or impaired renal response to aldosterone. The test is not useful if the urine is dilute or if urinary Na is low.

What are some endogenous sources of hyperkalemia?

GI bleeding, rhabdomyolysis, tumor lysis syndrome, hypercatabolic states

What is type IV RTA?

Hyperkalemia with inadequate renal K excretion despite only mild to moderate CRF (also called tubular hyperkalemia); overlaps with hyporeninemic hypoaldosteronism. Seen in diabetes, chronic interstitial nephritis, systemic lupus erythematosus (SLE), sickle cell disease, and obstructive uropathy. May be due to combination of low renin production, reduced aldosterone synthesis, and impaired tubular response to aldosterone; the last cause is most common.

How is symptomatic (i.e., with ECG changes) hyperkalemia treated?

Calcium gluconate 10% 10 mL. Repeat as needed to reverse ECG changes. This does **not** lower serum K. Repeat as needed to reverse EKG changes, pending other measures to lower serum K.

How can K be shifted into cells to quickly (but transiently) lower serum K?

Insulin and glucose, 5–10 U regular with 25–50 mL D50, followed by drip. $NaHCO_3$ is less useful in renal failure and more likely to cause other electrolyte derangements. Albuterol (β-agonist) by inhalation may be used.

How can K be removed from the patient (rather than just shifted)?

Kayexalate removes up to 1 mEq K per gram. Can be given orally (in sorbitol, to ensure catharsis) or by enema. Start with 30–60 g; total dose limited only by patient tolerance and sodium load. Hemodialysis is effective and needed in renal failure, but initiate medical measures pending availability of dialysis treatment.

What is total body potassium in DKA, and why?

DKA patients are usually potassium depleted, due to:
1. Decreased intake of food and potassium
2. Osmotic diuresis due to glycosuria, with resulting kaliuresis
3. Distal delivery of nonreabsorbable anions (e.g., acetoacetate) further augments kaliuresis and negative K balance.

If DKA patients are usually potassium depleted, then why is serum potassium elevated?

1. Hyperglycemia raises extracellular osmolality. This engenders shift of K-rich water out of cells, leading to hyperkalemia.
2. Diabetics lack insulin needed to shift glucose and potassium into cells.
3. Diabetic autonomic neuropathy may play a role, by decreasing $β_2$-agonist effect of shifting K into cells. K usually falls to low levels soon after initiating treatment of DKA.

Isn't the acidosis per se a cause of hyperkalemia in DKA?

No. This is a common misconception. Only *mineral* acids (e.g., HCl) produce a significant shift of K out of cells. Organic acids (e.g., lactate and acetoacetate) do not, because of their greater diffusivity across cell membranes.

NEPHRITIC SYNDROME

What is nephritic syndrome?	Acute or subacute glomerulonephritis manifesting with hematuria and RBC casts
Are RBC casts pathognomonic of GN?	No. They may be seen in acute interstitial nephritis and, rarely, after vigorous exercise. In the correct clinical setting, however, they are very strong evidence for GN.
Are RBC casts always seen in GN?	No. After formation in the tubular lumen, they degenerate fairly quickly, forming pigmented coarse granular casts. RBC casts are always accompanied by free RBCs, which, to the trained observer, are dysmorphic, suggesting glomerular origin. Often, several urine specimens must be examined to demonstrate RBC casts.
Does proteinuria accompany the nephritic sediment?	Yes. Because GN implies glomerular injury, some proteinuria is expected (1–2+), whereas gross hematuria from urologic causes also shows proteinuria due to the admixture of blood. In some cases, nephritic and nephrotic syndromes coexist (e.g., in diffuse proliferative lupus nephritis).
What is the workup for a patient with nephritic sediment?	Determine current renal function; if abnormal, try to obtain prior creatinine values, to assess acuity of the problem. Renal ultrasound to estimate kidney size, assist in distinction between acute and chronic renal disease Careful history and physical exam for systemic illness History of recent infection, especially with streptococci
What usually causes poststreptococcal GN? What infections are seen?	Nephritogenic strains of group A β-hemolytic streptococcus. The infection may be pharyngitis, or, more commonly worldwide, impetigo.

What are the usual signs and symptoms of poststreptococcal GN?	Gross hematuria (described as "Coca-Cola urine"), edema, hypertension
What blood tests are useful?	ASO or other streptococcal antigens to confirm recent infection. C_3 component of complement usually low.
How does nephritic edema differ from nephrotic edema?	In acute GN, decreased blood flow to tubular capillaries promotes Na retention by the functionally intact tubules, leading to intravascular volume overload, which then distributes to the interstitium. In nephrotic edema, decreased effective plasma volume leads to Na retention by the kidney.
What is the prognosis for poststreptococcal GN?	Most children recover without sequelae. Adults have slower, less complete recovery. Small numbers, usually those with severe poststreptococcal GN, go on to chronic GN.
What other infections cause postinfectious GN?	*Staphylococcus epidermidis* infections of ventriculoperitoneal shunts; acute or subacute bacterial endocarditis, various organisms; infectious mononucleosis
What is Goodpasture syndrome?	Pulmonary-renal syndrome mediated by anti–glomerular basement membrane antibody, manifest by acute GN and pulmonary involvement, often with frank hemoptysis
What are the demographics for Goodpasture syndrome?	Males affected more than females by 2:1 ratio, peak ages in 20s and in 60s
What is the treatment and prognosis?	Plasmapheresis, followed by prednisone and cyclophosphamide. Remission usually accomplished, unless late presentation delays therapy.
What parameters are followed?	Renal function, chest x-ray, and anti–glomerular basement membrane antibody levels

What is Wegener granulomatosis? How does it commonly present?	Small vessel necrotizing vasculitis of kidneys, lungs, and upper respiratory tract. Epistaxis, sinusitis are common presentations.
What is the spectrum of renal involvement?	May insidiously follow prominent upper airway disease, or present as RPGN
What are the demographics for Wegener granulomatosis?	Middle aged and elderly, no gender difference
What blood test is useful to support diagnosis?	Cytoplasmic antineutrophil cytoplasmic antibody (C-ANCA), which can be used to follow response to treatment
What is the treatment and prognosis for Wegener granulomatosis?	Steroids and cyclophosphamide. Plasmapheresis is not well established. High rate of remission, although one third will relapse.
How does chronic hepatitis affect the kidney?	Chronic hepatitis can be associated with membranous GN (a nephrotic syndrome), and with membranoproliferative GN (nephritic and nephrotic). Although there is overlap, hepatitis B is more commonly associated with the former, and hepatitis C with the latter.
What is IgA nephropathy? How does it present?	Also known as Berger disease, a common cause of chronic GN worldwide. Male predominance up to threefold. May present with classic loin pain and gross hematuria shortly after pharyngitis (viral), with spontaneous resolution until next episode. Others present with sustained microhematuria, often with varying degrees of proteinuria, unrelated to upper respiratory infection. Children may present with Henoch-Schönlein purpura variant, with GI involvement and purpuric rash.

How is IgA nephropathy diagnosed?	Although serum IgA levels are elevated in 50% of cases, serum IgA lacks specificity and sensitivity. Renal biopsy confirms diagnosis.
What is the treatment and prognosis for IgA nephropathy?	In United States, most cases follow indolent course with slow progression to CRF. Use ACE inhibitors if hypertension develops, or, perhaps, even in its absence. Some studies suggest fish oil, for its omega-3 fatty acid content. Steroids and cytotoxic agents are reserved for cases with nephrotic syndrome or progressive azotemia.
What is pauci-immune RPGN?	RPGN in which the immune deposits are not found on renal biopsy. Includes Wegener, Churg-Strauss disease, and microscopic polyarteritis nodosa.
What serologic test is helpful?	ANCA. C-ANCA is almost always positive in Wegener, whereas other paucimmune RPGN cases usually demonstrate elevated P-ANCA levels.
What is the treatment and prognosis for P-ANCA positive RPGN?	Untreated, renal prognosis is poor. Treatment with pulse methylprednisolone (often with cyclophosphamide or azathioprine) results in sustained improvement in renal function in about half of cases. Response and prognosis depends on early diagnosis, often defined as serum creatinine <6 mg/dL.

NEPHROLITHIASIS

Name the four major types of kidney stones.	Calcium oxalate, uric acid, struvite, and cystine
What is the most common type?	Calcium oxalate
What endocrine disorder is a risk factor for developing calcium oxalate stones?	Hyperparathyroidism

Which type of stone is associated with urea-splitting bacteria (*Pseudomonas*, *Proteus*, *Klebsiella*) and high urinary pH?	Struvite
How does the patient with stones typically present?	With renal colic, characterized by severe, intermittent, unilateral flank pain lasting 20–60 minutes that radiates to the groin or testicle; dysuria, frequency, nausea, vomiting, and gross hematuria may also be present. Stones may be entirely asymptomatic, however, particularly so-called "first stones."
What basic diagnostic tests are included in the workup?	Urinalysis, BUN, creatinine, serum calcium, x-ray of kidneys, ureter, and bladder (KUB), and complete blood cell (CBC) count (if febrile). Further metabolic workup, including urine collections, is deferred until patient has recovered from acute episode, and returned to usual diet.
What type of stone is not seen on x-ray?	Uric acid stones
What additional diagnostic test may be ordered if suspicion is high in patient with normal renal function and KUB?	Intravenous pyelogram, which has been the gold standard, although computed transaxial tomography (CTT) scanning may replace it.
What test may be useful if obstruction is suspected?	Renal ultrasound, which may also detect radiolucent stones missed on KUB.
What is the treatment for stones?	Hydration (oral or IV) and analgesics (narcotics or NSAIDs) as needed for pain
What additional treatment is required if infection is present?	IV antibiotics and aggressive workup for obstruction

What treatment should be considered if an upper tract stone does not pass?	Extracorporeal shock wave lithotripsy to break stone into smaller fragments, which then will be able to pass
What treatment may be useful if the stone is located in the lower urinary tract?	Surgical extraction per cystoscopy

NEPHROTIC SYNDROME

What is meant by "nephrotic range proteinuria"?	Urinary protein excretion in amount of 3.5 g/24 hours per 1.73-m^2 body surface area. To meet the definition, the protein should be predominantly albumin (i.e., normal plasma protein); excretion of large amounts of paraprotein (e.g., Bence-Jones protein) does not count as nephrotic proteinuria.
What is a nephrotic urinary sediment?	Sediment containing oval fat bodies, free fat droplets, and fatty casts. Refractile bodies (Maltese cross appearance) may be seen. Sediment may also contain nephritic (q.v.) elements.
What are some of the symptoms of nephrotic syndrome?	The patient complains of swelling, and may note foaming of the urine. Nonspecific findings may include fatigue. The underlying illness (e.g., diabetes mellitus, SLE) may produce additional symptoms.
What are commons signs of nephrotic syndrome?	Hallmark sign is edema, which may be only dependent (ankles at end of day) or generalized anasarca, including periorbital edema. Ascites and pleural effusions may be present. Additional signs may be attributable to underlying disorder.
What are common complications of the nephrotic syndrome?	Venous thrombosis, including deep vein thrombosis, renal vein thrombosis, and pulmonary embolism; poor wound healing; susceptibility to infection, malnutrition; ARF; hyperlipidemia

Is there a unifying mechanism leading to these phenomena?

Loss of albumin through the pathologically leaky glomerular basement membrane leads to hypoalbuminemia. The resulting fall in plasma oncotic pressure leads to increased hepatic synthesis of cholesterol, sodium retention by the kidneys, and development of edema. The kidneys also lose other proteins (e.g., opsonins) and clotting factors, with the net balance of procoagulant and anticoagulant proteins favoring the former.

What are some causes of the nephrotic syndrome?

Diabetes is one of the most common. SLE very commonly involves the kidneys; typically produces a combined nephritic and nephrotic syndrome. Certain infections, including hepatitis B and C, HIV, syphilis, and malaria, are frequently associated with nephrotic syndrome. Chronic bacterial infections of skin or viscera may result in amyloidosis. Malignancies also have been associated with nephrotic syndrome (Hodgkin lymphoma with minimal change disease; solid tumors of breast, lung, and colon with membranous nephropathy).

Which drugs can produce nephrotic syndrome?

Penicillamine and gold have been linked to membranous glomerulopathy. NSAIDs have produced cases of minimal change disease. In intravenous drug abusers, heroin abuse results in focal glomerulosclerosis and amyloidosis ("skin-popping"), but these are epiphenomena of abuse, not direct drug effects.

What is the usual workup for nephrotic syndrome?

Urinary protein (24-hour or spot urinary protein to creatinine ratio) to confirm diagnosis. Renal ultrasound for kidney size and echogenicity. Serologic tests for common causes, including hepatitis B, hepatitis C, HIV, C_3, C_4, ANA. Immunoelectrophoreses if myeloma is suspected.

What are the four major histologic types of idiopathic nephrotic syndrome?

Minimal change (also called nil) disease
Focal segmental glomerulosclerosis
Membranous glomerulopathy
Membranoproliferative glomerulonephritis

What is the treatment for nephrotic syndrome?

Specific measures for SLE, minimal change disease, and other select cases (glucocorticoids and cytotoxic agents)
General measures: salt restriction, moderate protein restriction (0.8 g/kg per day), judicious use of diuretics. ACE inhibitors or angiotensin III receptor blockers for antiproteinuric and renoprotective effects. Support hose for legs.

What is the role of anticoagulation?

Not used preemptively, but maintain high index of suspicion for deep or renal vein thrombosis or pulmonary embolism, and treat as indicated.

What is the prognosis?

Significant morbidity from infection, malnutrition, lipid abnormalities, hypercoagulable state. Most eventually progress to ESRD, with resolution of nephrotic syndrome as GFR falls.

14 Rheumatology

GENERAL MUSCULOSKELETAL PROBLEMS

FIBROMYALGIA (FIBROSITIS, FIBROMYOSITIS)

Define fibromyalgia.	A common nonarticular musculoskeletal disease consisting of muscle pain and stiffness, fatigue, and nonrestorative sleep; seen mostly in women
Name three disorders commonly associated with it.	Irritable bowel syndrome, tension headache, and dysmenorrhea
How do patients typically describe the pain?	Worse in the morning, poorly localized, spares the joints
Describe the physical exam findings.	Bilateral tender points over the trapezius ridge, posterior cervical musculature, upper gluteal area, and trochanteric bursae
What are the associated lab findings?	Normal white blood cell (WBC) count and erythrocyte sedimentation rate (ESR)
How is the diagnosis made?	Clinical history and physical exam
What is the treatment strategy?	Low-dose tricyclic antidepressants at bedtime for disturbed sleep; physical therapy and aerobic exercise for muscle aches; no role for nonsteroidal anti-inflammatory drugs (NSAIDs)

LYME DISEASE

What is Lyme disease?	A tick-borne inflammatory disorder caused by the spirochete *Borrelia burgdorferi*

What months is Lyme disease most prevalent?	Between May (early spring) and August (late summer)
What are the risk factors?	Recent travel or residence in endemic areas (i.e., Northeastern coastal states, the upper Midwest, northern California); exposure to tick bites
What signs and symptoms are often present 7–10 days after the tick bite?	An erythematous annular rash (Erythema chronicum migrans) at least 5 cm in diameter (bull's-eye) and mild constitutional symptoms (influenza-like symptoms)
What are common manifestations weeks to months later in the following body systems:	
Rheumatologic?	Monoarticular or asymmetric oligoarticular arthritis that most commonly affects the knees
Neurologic?	Peripheral neuropathies, meningoencephalitis, seventh cranial nerve palsy
Cardiac?	Atrioventricular block, myopericarditis
How is the diagnosis often made?	Strong clinical suspicion (endemic area, tick bite if reported, and rash)
What laboratory test is commonly ordered first?	Enzyme-linked immunosorbent assay (ELISA)
What additional test should be ordered if the ELISA is positive?	A Western blot to confirm (ELISA often false positive)
Can ELISA and Western blot distinguish between active and previous infections?	No
What is the initial therapy?	Oral doxycycline or amoxicillin and probenecid

What is the next therapy if the first fails?	Parenteral ceftriaxone
How is therapy monitored?	Antibody studies

POLYMYALGIA RHEUMATICA (PMR) AND TEMPORAL ARTERITIS (TA)

Why are these diseases discussed together?	Because they frequently coexist
Who is at risk for PMR and TA?	Persons over the age of 50 years
What is PMR?	A chronic, intermittent, inflammatory disease of the large arteries
What is TA?	A progressive inflammatory disorder that affects mainly large cranial arteries, primarily the temporal artery
What is TA also known as?	Giant cell arteritis
How does PMR present?	Fever, malaise, weight loss, and fatigue, with difficulty climbing stairs, getting out of bed in the morning, and combing hair due to proximal muscle (shoulder and pelvic girdle) pain and stiffness
How does TA present?	Unilateral throbbing temporal headaches, scalp tenderness, difficulty chewing, visual disturbances (including blindness), and stroke; fever, malaise, and weight loss may be present; physical exam may reveal a nodular, enlarged, tender, or pulseless temporal artery.
How is PMR diagnosed?	Clinically, based on pain and stiffness (not weakness) in the shoulder and pelvic girdle; fever, malaise, and weight loss may be present.

How is TA diagnosed?	Typical clinical presentation with an elevated ESR suggests the diagnosis; unilateral or bilateral temporal biopsy confirms it.
What lab tests support the diagnosis of both PMR and TA?	Anemia with an elevated sedimentation rate
How is PMR without TA treated?	Low-dose prednisone (10–15 mg/day PO) with gradual tapering to 5–10 mg/day PO when ESR returns to normal and symptoms improve Question diagnosis if steroids do not slightly improve symptoms within 72 hours Continue steroids for at least 1 year to minimize risk of relapse NSAIDs may be used to facilitate tapering of steroids Consider weekly dose of methotrexate if unable to taper prednisone
What is the TA treatment strategy?	Start high-dose oral prednisone (1–2 mg/kg per day PO qd) immediately without biopsy results to prevent irreversible blindness Taper steroids gradually to 10–20 mg PO qd after symptoms have resolved and ESR returns to normal (usually 1–2 months) Long-term low-dose prednisone may be required; consider azathioprine or methotrexate if prednisone fails

POLYMYOSITIS AND DERMATOMYOSITIS

What is polymyositis?	An inflammatory systemic disease of the muscles causing weakness and occasional tenderness
How is dermatomyositis different from polymyositis?	Dermatomyositis exhibits a concomitant heliotrope skin rash (bilateral raccoon eyes); otherwise, they are identical.

What presenting feature is shared by both polymyositis and dermatomyositis?	Difficulty climbing stairs or combing their hair due to proximal muscle weakness (shoulder and pelvic girdle)
What presenting feature distinguishes dermatomyositis from polymyositis?	Heliotrope skin rash on physical exam
How is polymyositis diagnosed?	Clinical presentation; elevated muscle enzymes (creatine phosphokinase and aldolase) and abnormal EMG patterns suggest the diagnosis; muscle biopsy confirms it.
How is dermatomyositis diagnosed?	Identical to polymyositis, with additional clinical evidence of heliotrope skin rash
What else must be included in any adult workup?	Screening for internal malignancy, because these patients are at higher risk for it
Describe the treatment strategy for polymyositis and dermatomyositis.	Start with high-dose oral prednisone (40–60 mg/day); adjust dose according to muscle enzyme levels If resistant or intolerant to prednisone, may attempt therapy with azathioprine or methotrexate Long-term use of steroids may be needed

SCLERODERMA

What is scleroderma?	A chronic disease of unknown etiology characterized by diffuse fibrosis of the skin and internal organs
Who is at the greatest risk of developing the disease?	Women 20–50 years old
How do patients commonly present early in the disease?	Thick, tight, shiny skin, Raynaud phenomenon, and polyarthralgia

Name and describe the syndrome associated with the limited type of systemic scleroderma.	CREST syndrome (**C**alcinosis, **R**aynaud phenomenon, **E**sophageal dysmotility, **S**clerodactyly, **T**elangiectasia)
How is diffuse systemic scleroderma different from the limited type?	More severe skin disease involving the trunk, a greater risk of pulmonary hypertension (which may precipitate a renal crisis), and an overall worse prognosis
What other signs or symptoms could the patient present with?	Angina (from coronary artery vasospasm), heart failure or arrhythmias (from myocardial fibrosis), or pulmonary hypertension (from pulmonary fibrosis)
How is the diagnosis made?	Strong clinical suspicion, anticentromere antibodies (CREST syndrome), and anti-Scl 70 antibodies (diffuse scleroderma)
What problems are associated with the antibody tests?	Lack of sensitivity and (usually) specificity decreases their effectiveness in making the diagnosis.
What is the treatment strategy?	Symptomatic and supportive. No definitive treatment is available.
What is the treatment for the following:	
Severe Raynaud phenomenon?	Vasodilating drugs (calcium channel blockers or prazosin)
Skin and periarticular changes?	Physical therapy
Gastrointestinal hypomotility?	Aggressive gastroesophageal management, antibiotics for intestinal bacteria overgrowth, and prokinetic agents (e.g., cisapride and metoclopramide) if significant gastroparesis develops
Hypertension and renal involvement?	Angiotensin-converting enzyme (ACE) inhibitors to decrease risk of renal crisis (a poor prognostic sign)

SYSTEMIC LUPUS ERYTHEMATOUS

What is systemic lupus erythematous?	A multisystem disease of unknown etiology (autoantibodies to nuclear and other autoantigens are suspected) that primarily affects women of childbearing age
What are the most common symptoms?	Fever, fatigue, malaise, malar ("butterfly") skin rash, and photosensitivity
Describe the disease course.	Waxing and waning of symptoms is most common

Name the most common associated manifestations of the following organ systems:

Musculoskeletal?	Arthralgias, myalgias, and arthritis
Central nervous system?	Seizures, psychosis, anxiety, and depression
Cardiac?	Pericarditis, myocarditis, endocarditis, and arrhythmias
Gastrointestinal?	Nausea, vomiting, anorexia, and abdominal pain
Vascular and hematologic?	Anemia, thrombocytopenia, lymphadenopathy, splenomegaly
Immune?	Lymphadenopathy and splenomegaly
Renal?	Impairment due to associated vasculitis

When should the diagnosis be considered?	When a young women presents with multisystemic findings
What serologic markers are commonly used to make the diagnosis?	Antinuclear antibody (ANA), anti–double-stranded DNA, and anti–Smith antibodies
Which serologic tests are more specific?	Anti–double-stranded DNA and anti–Sm
What other lab tests may support the diagnosis?	White blood cell count revealing leukopenia, a false positive Venereal Disease Research Laboratory (VDRL)

test (due to antiphospholipid antibodies), a positive direct Coombs test, and low serum complement levels (C3, C4, and CH50)

What lab tests are commonly used to monitor disease activity?

Serum complement levels and anti–double-stranded DNA

What is the treatment strategy?

Decrease number of active episodes. Minimize end-organ damage.

What is the first line of treatment?

NSAIDs for musculoskeletal symptoms, fever, and serositis

In what patients are NSAIDs contraindicated?

Patients with active nephritis

When is hydroxychloroquine often used?

For dermatologic and musculoskeletal manifestations

When are steroids indicated?

For severe systemic symptoms (e.g., glomerulonephritis, severe CNS involvement, thrombocytopenia, and hemolytic anemia) and debilitating manifestations unresponsive to conservative treatment

What medication is used for patients who fail to respond to steroids or who become dependent on them?

Immunosuppressive agents (e.g., methotrexate, azathioprine, and cyclophosphamide)

DISORDERS OF THE BACK, SPINE, AND BONE

ACUTE LOWER BACK PAIN

Name the three most common causes of lower back pain.

Strain, lumbar disk disease, and vertebral fractures

Name three common aggravating factors.	Heavy lifting, trauma, and forceful coughing or sneezing
How does a patient with a strain present?	Localized lower back pain without radiation (i.e., nerve root not involved)
What is appreciated on physical exam?	Regional tenderness, severe restriction of movements, and paraspinal muscle spasms
How does lumbar disk disease present?	Back pain with decreased mobility and compensatory posture; pain radiates to the groin or leg (usually unilateral) if nerve root is compressed.
What is the most common disk space affected?	L5–S1
What is often found on physical exam if L5–S1 is affected?	Paresthesias in the posterior lateral calf, heel, and lateral foot; impaired tendon reflexes
What level is involved if bowel or bladder symptoms are present?	Conus medullaris or cauda equina
How does a patient with vertebral fractures present?	Sudden onset of excruciating pain
Name some common risk factors for vertebral fractures.	Osteoporosis, metastatic bone disease, multiple myeloma, Paget disease, chronic steroid use
How is the diagnosis made?	Clinical presentation and radiograph or computed tomography (CT) scan
What is the treatment strategy for acute lower back pain?	NSAIDs, bed rest, muscle relaxants Surgical consult if radiographic studies reveal underlying pathology

OSTEOMYELITIS

What is osteomyelitis?	An infection of the bone, usually caused by direct or hematogenous spread of bacteria from a wound or local infection
What bones are affected most commonly?	The long bones (femur, humerus, tibia) and vertebrae
What are the risk factors?	Coexisting infections, age, diabetes, intravenous drug abuse, and immunodeficiency
Name the two most common bacterial organisms	*Staphylococcus aureus* and coagulase-negative staphylococci
What organisms are typically found in patients with diabetes?	Polymicrobial infections with gram-negative rods and anaerobes
How does the patient with osteomyelitis present?	Usually incapacitated or with a limp, and complaining of dull pain in the affected limb (long bones)
What might the physical exam reveal?	Systemic fever, point tenderness, swelling, warmth, erythema, effusion, decreased range of motion, and regional muscle spasms in the affected area
How is the diagnosis made?	Bone biopsy and culture of specimen
What diagnostic test strongly suggests the diagnosis?	Culture of needle-aspirated pus from the bone
What lab tests should be ordered?	White blood cell count, ESR, C-reactive protein, and blood cultures
What radiographic studies may be helpful?	Radiograph, radionucleotide bone scanning, CT scan, and magnetic resonance (MR) imaging

When would radiographic findings reveal possible pathology?	Not until at least 10 days after infection; 2–6 weeks are needed to reveal lytic lesions.
What are the common radiographic signs?	Destruction of normal bony architecture (bone erosion, periosteal elevation) with evidence of soft tissue swelling
What are the advantages and disadvantages of radionuclide bone scanning?	Can reveal positive finding within 2 days of infection. Cannot distinguish between infection of soft tissue and bone.
How does MR scanning compare with bone scan?	MR scanning has equal sensitivity and greater specificity.
What is the medical treatment?	4–6 weeks of antibiotics after the causative organism is identified
What is the treatment for a *Staphylococcus aureus* infection?	Intravenous nafcillin 2 g every 4 hours
What is the treatment for a gram-negative organism?	Third-generation cephalosporin (ceftriaxone)
When is surgical debridement necessary?	Failed medical treatment, undrained pus, or septic arthritis

SERONEGATIVE SPONDYLOARTHROPATHIES

Name the four spondyloarthropathies.	Ankylosing spondylitis, Reiter syndrome, colitic arthritis, psoriatic arthritis
What do they have in common?	Spondylitis, sacroiliitis, inflammation at the tendon insertion points (enthesopathy), asymmetric oligoarthritis, extraarticular findings (e.g., inflammatory eye disease, urethritis, mucocutaneous lesions), and HLA-B27 association

Ankylosing Spondylitis

How does ankylosing spondylitis present?

Inflammation and ossification of joints and ligaments of the spine and sacroiliac joints (most commonly hips and shoulder)

What disease is associated with it?

Inflammatory bowel disease (10% of patients)

What is the diagnostic radiographic finding?

"Bamboo-spine" with fusion of the sacroiliac joints

What lab test supports the diagnosis?

HLA-B27 positive

What is the goal of treatment?

Because fusion of the spine cannot be prevented, the goal of treatment is to increase the likelihood that it will occur in a straight line.

What is the treatment?

NSAIDs (e.g., indomethacin) for symptom relief.
Methotrexate and sulfasalazine may benefit some patients.
Use glucocorticoids only after other medications have failed.
Sleep on a firm bed without a pillow.
No cigarette smoking.
Refer to ophthalmologist if anterior uveitis is present.

Reiter Syndrome

How does Reiter syndrome (reactive arthritis) present?

Usually seen in young men with the clinical tetrad of conjunctivitis, urethritis, mucocutaneous lesions, and asymmetric oligoarthritis

What joints are commonly affected?

Knee and ankle

When is Reiter syndrome considered reactive?

When it develops days or weeks after a dysenteric infection (*Salmonella*, *Shigella*, or *Yersinia*) or sexually transmitted infection

How is reactive Reiter syndrome distinguished from gonococcal arthritis?	Gonococcal arthritis markedly improves after 24–48 hours of antibiotics. The culture result often reveals organism.
How is the diagnosis made?	Clinical history and presentation
What lab test is often positive?	HLA-B27
What is the treatment for Reiter syndrome?	NSAIDs (e.g., indomethacin) for pain and inflammation. Sulfasalazine or methotrexate may provide symptomatic relief in some patients not responding to NSAIDs. If joint disease is severe, consider glucocorticoids. Refer to ophthalmologist for uveitis.

Colitic Arthritis

What disease is associated with colitic arthritis?	Inflammatory bowel disease [IBD (20% of patients)]
Where does the arthritis typically present?	In the peripheral joints of the knee or ankle
What disease features may be correlated with IBD activity?	Peripheral arthritis (not spinal disease)
What extraintestinal features of IBD may be found?	Pyodermic gangrenosum, uveitis, erythema nodosum
Should joint aspiration be considered?	Yes, it will help rule out septic arthritis.
How is the diagnosis made?	Clinical presentation and a negative HLA-B27 lab test
What is the treatment strategy?	Sulfasalazine for intestinal inflammation NSAIDs for peripheral arthritis Local injection of glucocorticoids and physical therapy as needed

Psoriatic Arthritis

How does psoriatic arthritis present?	With asymmetric oligoarthritis or symmetric polyarthritis
What joint is typically involved in asymmetric oligoarthritis?	Distal interphalangeal (DIP) joints in the hand (sausage appearance)
What is a classic radiographic finding?	Pencil and cup deformity of the phalanx
How is the diagnosis made?	Clinical presentation with associated psoriatic findings on skin, nails, and hair
How is it distinguished from rheumatoid arthritis?	Rheumatoid factor is negative in psoriatic arthritis
What is the treatment?	NSAIDs (e.g., indomethacin) Intra-articular steroids if oligoarticular form of the disease Consider low-dose methotrexate if severe skin and joint disease present

OSTEOARTHRITIS AND ARTHROPATHIES

OSTEOARTHRITIS

Define osteoarthritis.	The most common form of arthritis; characterized by deterioration of the articular cartilage and formation of reactive new bone at the articular surface in one or more joints
What two types of joints are affected most commonly?	Joints under chronic use; weightbearing joints
What is the main risk factor?	Age (most often after 40)
How does it commonly present?	With short-lived morning stiffness (often <30 minutes), pain, and crepitus with movement

What are common physical exam findings?	Decreased range of joint motion, pain with movement, small effusions, crepitus, Heberden nodes (bony deformity at DIP common), Bouchard nodes [bony deformity at posterior interphalangeal (PIP) joints less common]
How is it diagnosed?	Clinical exam and radiographic findings (joint space narrowing with osteophytes)
What are the associated lab findings?	Normal WBC count and ESR; straw-colored joint fluid with few WBCs
What is the treatment strategy?	NSAIDs or aspirin Weight reduction, exercise, physical therapy Total joint replacement if disabled

ACUTE GOUTY ARTHRITIS

Define acute gouty arthritis.	An arthritic condition in which an inborn error in uric acid metabolism leads to crystal deposition in the peripheral joints
What are the five risk factors?	Surgery, dehydration, fasting, binge eating (meat), and high alcohol intake
How does it commonly present?	Acute attack of excruciating pain in a single joint of the foot or ankle, most commonly the big toe (podagra)
How is the diagnosis made?	By aspirated joint fluid: finding needle-shaped negatively birefringent crystals within polymorphonuclear neutrophils (PMNs) under a polarized light microscope
Is hyperuricemia required to make the diagnosis?	No, one third of patients have normal serum uric acid levels during an acute attack.
What is the first line of treatment?	High-dose oral NSAIDs

Name two common contraindications to NSAID use.	History of NSAID-related bleeding and advanced renal insufficiency
What is the next therapy?	Intravenous (IV) or high-dose oral colchicine
What are the side effects of oral compared to IV colchicine?	High-dose oral colchicine often has severe GI toxicity. IV colchicine frequently causes severe myelosuppression.
Give two situations when steroids are indicated.	1. Intra-articular injection for rapid relief 2. When colchicine and NSAIDs are contraindicated
What medication can be used prophylactically between attacks?	Colchicine
What medication can be used to treat patients with consistent hyperuricemia due to uric acid overproduction?	Allopurinol 300 mg/day
When should the dose of allopurinol be decreased?	Kidney or liver disease
What drug can be used to treat chronic underexcretion of uric acid (<700 mg/24 hours)?	Uricosuric drugs (probenecid or sulfinpyrazone)

PSEUDOGOUT

What is pseudogout?	An inflammatory arthritic disease caused by the accumulation of calcium pyrophosphate crystals in the peripheral joint space
What are the risk factors?	Old age, trauma, advanced osteoarthritis, gout, hyperparathyroidism, hemochromatosis, diabetes, hypothyroidism, and amyloidosis

Name two ways it can present.	As an acute monoarthritis (like gout), or as a chronic polyarthritis (mimics rheumatoid arthritis or osteoarthritis)
How is acute monoarthritis different from gout?	Acute monoarthritis has a similar presentation but less severe symptoms
What are the signs and symptoms?	Joint pain with regional warmth and tenderness
What joint is most commonly affected?	Knee
How is the diagnosis made?	Examination of aspirated joint fluid under a polarized light microscope shows positively birefringent rhomboid-shaped crystals.
What is the treatment strategy?	Brief course of high-dose NSAIDs (e.g., indomethacin) as first-line treatment NSAIDs are followed by IV or oral colchicine (may decrease recurrent attacks) as tolerated Aspiration of joint space and intra-articular injection of glucocorticoids may be beneficial

RHEUMATOID ARTHRITIS

What is rheumatoid arthritis?	A chronic systemic inflammatory disease of unknown etiology causing symmetric joint inflammation, deformation, and bone erosion due to chronic synovial inflammation
Who is at greater risk for rheumatoid arthritis?	Women 20–50 years old
What are the common symptoms?	Significant morning stiffness lasting >1 hour with fatigue, weakness, and joint pain

What are the musculoskeletal physical exam findings?	Symmetrical joint pain, tenderness, swelling, warmth, and decreased range of motion most commonly involving the hands [PIP and metacarpophalangeal (MCP) joints very common, DIP spared], wrists, elbows, ankles, and feet
What are four common extra-articular exam findings?	Rheumatoid nodules, pulmonary fibrosis, pericarditis, and vasculitis
Describe two syndromes associated with rheumatoid arthritis (RA).	Felty syndrome (triad of RA, splenomegaly, and granulocytopenia) and Sjögren syndrome (dry eyes, dry mouth, and parotid gland enlargement)
What two clinical finding strongly suggest the diagnosis?	Significant morning stiffness lasting >1 hour and symmetric polyarthritis
What lab tests support the diagnosis?	A positive rheumatoid factor with an elevated ESR
What is the first line of treatment?	NSAIDs to reduce pain and swelling
What is a common concern with NSAID use in RA patients?	Chronic use of high doses may lead to renal, liver, and GI toxicity
What is the next therapy?	Short-term steroid use
What additional drugs may be helpful?	Gold, methotrexate, hydroxychloroquine, penicillamine, sulfasalazine, azathioprine, and cyclophosphamide
When are they helpful?	As steroid-sparing agents and as aggressive treatment to decrease the progression of joint and bone destruction
What additional nonmedical treatment may be helpful?	Physical therapy

When is surgery warranted?	When other therapies have failed to reduce chronic pain and improve joint function
Name two common surgical procedures.	Synovectomy and total joint replacement (hip and knee most common)

SEPTIC ARTHRITIS

What is septic arthritis?	An infection of the joint, usually caused by gonococci or staphylococci
When is septic arthritis considered chronic?	Cases lasting >6 weeks are generally considered chronic.
What are common risk factors for acute and chronic conditions?	Acute: IV drug abuse, trauma, surgery, arthroscopy, and immunosuppressive conditions Chronic: Lyme disease, syphilis, tuberculosis, and fungal infections
How does the patient usually present?	With fever and painful, warm, erythematous, and swollen joints with limited range of motion
What is the differential for septic arthritis?	Gout, pseudogout, spondyloarthropathy, juvenile rheumatoid arthritis, foreign body synovitis, rheumatoid arthritis, rheumatic fever, AIDS, cellulitis, Lyme arthritis, neuropathic arthropathy, and sarcoidosis
What joints are commonly affected?	Large joints (knee or hip most commonly)
What is the presentation of gonococcal septic arthritis?	Gonococcal cases often begin as a migratory polyarthralgia that becomes a monoarthritis, with tenosynovitis of the wrists, fingers, knees, and ankles, and a maculopapular or vesicular dermatitis of the lower extremities or trunk. Patient also has a sexually active social history.

What is the diagnostic approach?

Aspirate joint fluid for WBC count, culture, and gram stain; blood cultures; all orifices cultured for *Neisseria gonorrhoeae* in Thayer-Martin medium

If gonorrhea is suspected, what additional test should be ordered?

Syphilis serology

What are the characteristics of septic synovial fluid?

Turbid appearance, WBC count greater than 50,000 cells/μL, PMNs greater than 90%

What is the treatment for septic arthritis?

Hospitalize for administration of intravenous antibiotics
Aspirate joint space
Immobilize joint
Replace infected prosthetic joints after antibiotic therapy

What dictates antibiotic selection?

Gram stain and culture results

What is the antibiotic treatment for staphylococcal infections?

Intravenous nafcillin or vancomycin followed by an oral antibiotic (dicloxacillin) for a total of 3–6 weeks

What is the antibiotic treatment for gonococcal infections?

Ceftriaxone 1 g/day for 14 days (but for at least 7 days after symptoms resolve)

When should surgery be considered?

Septic hip, inadequate needle drainage, no response to therapy after 5–7 days, coexistent osteomyelitis, prosthetic joint infection

15

Surgery

GASTROINTESTINAL SYSTEM

ABDOMINAL INJURY

What is the first priority in the management of any patient presenting with acute abdominal trauma?

Establish an adequate airway.

Beyond physical exam, what three diagnostic modalities are most useful in assessing blunt abdominal trauma (BAT)?

Ultrasound scan, computed tomography (CT) scan, diagnostic peritoneal lavage (DPL)

What are the criteria for a positive DPL in BAT?

Aspiration of 10 mL of gross blood, red blood cell (RBC) count = 100,000/mm^3, white blood cell (WBC) count = 500/mm^3, amylase > serum, presence of bile or food fibers

What two intra-abdominal organs are most commonly injured in BAT?

Spleen (first) and liver (second)

What is the initial therapy for a hemodynamically stable patient with a splenic or liver injury?

Observe in the intensive care unit and closely monitor blood pressure and hemoglobin.

What are two principal indications for laparotomy?

Persistent bleeding or hemodynamic instability

What are the options for intraoperative management of splenic injuries?

Total or partial splenectomy, splenorrhaphy, topical hemostatic agents

Name two potential complications of splenectomy.

Thrombocytosis and overwhelming postsplenectomy infection

Although all penetrating trauma can cause abdominal organ damage, what are the usual boundaries chosen to evaluate for wounds involving the abdominal cavity?

From nipple line to gluteal crease

What intra-abdominal organ is most commonly injured in penetrating trauma?

Small intestine

What diagnostic tests are helpful in a stable patient with an abdominal stab wound but without peritoneal signs?

Local wound exploration (rule out penetration of the fascia), DPL, CT scan, diagnostic laparoscopy

What is the best initial management for a gunshot wound to the abdomen? Why?

Exploratory laparotomy, because about 80% cause significant injury

What is the most common cause of bladder injuries?

Pelvic fractures

What is the best diagnostic test to evaluate the genitourinary system of patients with pelvic fractures combined with gross hematuria?

Retrograde urethrocystography

What is the preferred initial treatment for extraperitoneal bladder injuries?

Foley catheterization

Which diagnostic tests are helpful in evaluating renal trauma?

Urinalysis may replace intravenous pyelography to look for hematuria, CT scan

APPENDICITIS

What is the most common cause of appendicitis?	Luminal obstruction from lymphoid hyperplasia (fecalith is second)
The diagnosis of acute appendicitis is made primarily on the basis of what?	History and physical exam
What is the classic presenting triad of symptoms?	Abdominal pain, nausea, and fever
Which symptom typically occurs first, nausea or pain?	Abdominal pain, followed by nausea and anorexia
Where does the abdominal pain localize after initially being perceived in the periumbilical region?	McBurney's point, about one-third the distance from the right anterior superior iliac spine to the umbilicus
What is the cardinal physical finding?	Localized tenderness, usually at McBurney's point, but varies with the location of the appendix
What is the Rovsing sign?	Pain in the right lower quadrant of the abdomen when applying pressure in the left lower quadrant
What is the psoas sign?	Right lower quadrant abdominal pain with the patient lying on the left side and with passive extension of the right thigh
What is the obturator sign?	Hypogastric pain while the patient is supine with passive rotation of the flexed right thigh
Which lab test results are helpful in the diagnosis?	Elevated leukocyte count or left shift in the differential, a few red cells in the urinalysis, elevated C-reactive protein

If the diagnosis is in doubt, what studies may be helpful?	Abdominal x-rays, ultrasound scan, CT scan, or diagnostic laparoscopy
What is the differential diagnosis?	Gastroenteritis, cholecystitis, pyelonephritis, salpingitis, tubo-ovarian abscess, ruptured ovarian cyst, perforated peptic ulcer, ectopic pregnancy, regional enteritis, ureteral stones, cystitis
Once the diagnosis of acute appendicitis is made, what is the appropriate therapy?	Intravenous (IV) fluids, IV antibiotics covering both aerobic and anaerobic organisms, and urgent appendectomy
What is the acceptable percentage of patients who are diagnosed clinically with appendicitis but actually have a normal appendix at operation?	10–15%
Why is this false-positive diagnostic rate accepted?	To prevent the increased morbidity and mortality of appendiceal perforation
If a normal appendix is encountered during operation, what should be done?	Explore to eliminate other possible causes, such as enteric inflammatory or neoplastic lesions, Meckel diverticulum, tubo-ovarian disease, and gallbladder or duodenal disease. If no other cause is identified, proceed with appendectomy.
What are the common early complications after appendectomy?	Wound infection and intra-abdominal abscess

BLEEDING

What are the five most common causes of upper gastrointestinal bleeding (UGIB)?	Gastritis, peptic ulcer disease, Mallory-Weiss tear, esophageal varices, gastric neoplasm

What are some of the major risk factors for UGIB?	Alcohol abuse, cirrhosis, nonsteroidal anti-inflammatory drugs, *Helicobacter pylori*, hyperemesis, gastric stasis, and acid hypersecretory states
How does UGIB present?	Hematemesis or melena; hematochezia if profuse bleeding
What lab tests should be performed?	Hemoglobin, hematocrit, platelets, prothrombin time (PT), partial thromboplastin time (PTT), type and crossmatch
What is the best diagnostic test?	Esophagogastroduodenoscopy
In adults, what is the most common cause of blood in stools?	Anorectal disease, usually hemorrhoids or anal fissure
Name the two most common causes of profuse lower gastrointestinal bleeding (LGIB)?	Diverticulosis and angiodysplasia
What are other common causes of LGIB?	Neoplasms, inflammatory bowel disease, ischemic and infective colitis, radiation proctitis, Meckel diverticulum, intussusception
What diagnostic investigations are useful in identifying the source of LGIB?	Colonoscopy, technetium-labeled RBC scan, angiography
What is the medical treatment of gastrointestinal bleeding?	Resuscitate with IV fluids and blood transfusions. Correct coagulopathy. Discontinue exacerbating medications (e.g., heparin, Coumadin). Identify the source.
What is the usual outcome in patients whose LGIB is managed medically?	Most will stop bleeding spontaneously.

What are the indications for surgery in patients with LGIB?	Transfusion of four or more units of blood, hemodynamic instability, rebleeding episode
Surgical treatment by segmental resection of a LGIB source requires what?	Localization of the actual bleeding site
What is the best operation for a patient who requires emergent surgery for massive LGIB that has not been localized?	Total abdominal colectomy

GALLBLADDER DISEASE

Acute Calculous Cholecystitis

What is acute calculous cholecystitis?	Gallbladder (GB) inflammation caused by gallstone obstruction of the cystic duct or impaction in Hartmann pouch
What are the presenting symptoms and signs?	Right upper quadrant (RUQ) abdominal pain, nausea, vomiting, fever
What is the Murphy sign?	Inspiratory arrest during RUQ palpation
What is the differential diagnosis?	Acute appendicitis, peptic ulcer disease, acute pancreatitis
What are the best diagnostic tests?	Abdominal ultrasound (AUS) scan or radionuclide scan with hepatobiliary iminodiacetic acid (HIDA scan)
What are the important findings on AUS?	Cholelithiasis, thickened GB wall, pericholecystic fluid
Which other lab or x-ray findings may be helpful?	Leukocytosis, hyperbilirubinemia, radiopaque gallstones on abdominal x-ray
What is the medical treatment?	Antibiotics, fluids, bowel rest, and analgesics
What is the surgical treatment?	Cholecystectomy

Acute Acalculous Cholecystitis

What two factors are involved in the etiology?	GB stasis and ischemia
Who is most at risk to develop acalculous cholecystitis?	1. Septic patients 2. Posttraumatic patients 3. Postoperative critically ill patients 4. Patients with diabetes
What is the best diagnostic test?	HIDA scan that demonstrates nonfilling GB
If the patient's condition prevents cholecystectomy, what is the treatment of choice?	Emergent cholecystostomy
What is the major complication if untreated?	GB gangrene with perforation

Chronic Cholecystitis

What is the cause?	Transient obstruction of the GB outlet by a stone
What are the symptoms?	Intermittent RUQ or epigastric abdominal pain and nausea
What triggers these symptoms?	Eating, especially fried or fatty foods
What are the physical findings between attacks?	None
What is the best diagnostic test?	AUS, revealing cholelithiasis
What is the optimal treatment?	Cholecystectomy

HERNIA

What is hernia?	Protrusion of intra-abdominal contents though a defect in the abdominal wall

What are the risk factors?	Obesity, pregnancy, chronic cough, ascites, and excessive straining
What is the most common type of hernia?	Inguinal; femoral and ventral hernias are less common.
How do most inguinal hernias present?	Often asymptomatic. Most are found on routine physical exam by palpating a mass or bulge in the inguinal canal as the patient coughs.
How do incarcerated hernias present?	As a firm, nonreducible red mass that is tender to palpation
What are the dreaded complications of incarcerated hernias?	Strangulation and infarction
How are hernias diagnosed?	Physical exam
How are reducible hernias treated?	Elective surgical repair
How are nonreducible hernias treated?	Immediate surgical repair

VASCULAR SURGERY

ABDOMINAL AORTIC ANEURYSM (AAA)

What is an AAA?	A localized dilatation of the abdominal aorta
What are the risk factors?	Atherosclerosis (most common), hypertension, smoking, family history of AAA, trauma, vasculitis, and Marfan syndrome
How does it present?	Often asymptomatic, but may present with a deep boring pain in the low back or flank
How does a ruptured AAA present?	Severe abdominal pain with hypotension, shock, or myocardial ischemia

What sign may be present on physical exam?	A palpable, pulsating, tender mass
What is the most useful radiographic screening test?	Ultrasound scan (to locate and determine size of AAA)
What is the most useful diagnostic radiographic test?	CT with IV contrast
What are the associated abdominal x-ray findings?	Aortic calcifications
What additional radiographic test may be helpful?	Aortography or magnetic resonance (MR) imaging
How is AAA diagnosed?	Presentation and CT scan
What is the treatment for	
AAA < 5 cm?	Outpatient management with periodic ultrasound scans to assess growth and current size
AAA > 5 cm?	Elective surgical resection of aneurysm and synthetic graft replacement
A ruptured AAA?	IV fluids, transfusion with packed RBCs as needed, and urgent surgery

UROLOGY

BENIGN PROSTATIC HYPERTROPHY

What is benign prostatic hypertrophy (BPH)?	Nonmalignant enlargement (benign adenomatous hyperplasia) of the prostate secondary to increased cellular growth
What effect does BPH have on the urethra?	The enlarging prostate compresses the prostatic urethra, resulting in decreased urine flow
Who is at risk?	Men >50 years old

How does BPH present?

Lower urinary tract symptoms (hesitancy, decreased stream strength, dribbling, urinary retention, and sense of incomplete emptying)

What additional symptoms may occur?

Irritable bladder symptoms (increased frequency, urgency, nocturia, and urge incontinence)

What causes irritative symptoms?

Overdistended bladder or urinary tract infection (UTI)

What are patients with BPH at increased risk for?

UTI, hydronephrosis, nephrolithiasis, bladder stones, and renal failure

What is often revealed on the rectal exam?

An enlarged prostate

What lab tests should be included in the workup, and how do they help narrow the differential?

Urinalysis (nonspecific—microhematuria and UTI), blood urea nitrogen and creatinine (nonspecific—renal failure can be present), prostate-specific antigen (PSA; may be elevated in either BPH or prostate cancer), postvoid residual volume (present in BPH or neurogenic bladder)

What diagnostic study may be helpful?

Transrectal ultrasound (increased sensitivity)

What is the initial treatment of BPH?

α-Blockers (e.g., prazosin, terazosin, doxazosin, tamsulosin) to inhibit urinary bladder sphincter contractions and hormone therapy (5α-reductase) to inhibit prostatic conversion of testosterone to dihydrotestosterone, which reduces prostate size. The drugs must be taken for the rest of the patient's life.

What medications are contraindicated? Why?

Alcohol, caffeine, and nonprescription cold medicines because of α-adrenergic or anticholinergic effects

What is the next step if medical intervention fails?

Surgery with transurethral prostatectomy (TURP) is the gold standard (either spinal/regional or general anesthesia). Alternative therapies that are less invasive can be performed under local anesthesia.

CYSTITIS

What is cystitis?	Inflammation of the bladder, or a clinical syndrome usually accompanied by an abrupt onset of dysuria, increased urinary frequency and urgency, and suprapubic pain
What is the most common causative organism?	Gram-negative bacteria (e.g., *Escherichia coli*)
Who is at greatest risk?	Sexually active women
What condition places men at increased risk?	Prostatitis, BPH, urethral stricture, prior UTI
What additional medical conditions place patients at risk?	Diabetes mellitus, pregnancy, congenital urologic abnormalities, and immunocompromised states
What are the presenting symptoms of cystitis?	Increased urinary frequency, urgency, dysuria, nocturia, suprapubic pain, hematuria
What findings are often appreciated on physical exam?	Fever and suprapubic pain
What is the initial lab test in the workup?	Urinalysis
What are the diagnostic values?	Positive leukocyte esterase, increased nitrates, increased pH
What is the next test if the urinalysis is positive?	Urine culture with sensitivities
What bacterial count is diagnostic of a UTI?	A single species with >100,000 bacteria/mL
What is the first-line treatment?	Trimethoprim-sulfamethoxazole orally for 3–7 days

What additional antibiotics are commonly used?	Amoxicillin and ciprofloxacin
Should asymptomatic bacteriuria be treated during pregnancy?	Yes
Why should asymptomatic bacteriuria be treated during pregnancy?	Because of the increased risk of developing acute pyelonephritis and sepsis, with resultant increased risk of prematurity and perinatal mortality
What two groups of antibiotics are considered the safest in pregnant women?	Penicillins and cephalosporins
What other two antibiotics can be used during pregnancy? What are their limitations?	Sulfonamides—only in the first two trimesters, because the fetus in utero handles excess unconjugated bilirubin through the placenta Nitrofurantoin—only in first two trimesters. Contraindicated in third trimester; can cause hemolytic anemia in neonates with an immature enzyme system.

PROSTATE CANCER

What are the risk factors for prostate cancer?	Men >60 years old, African American race, and family history
What is the most common histologic type?	Adenocarcinoma
How does it present early in the disease course?	Often asymptomatic
How does it present late in the disease course?	Bladder outlet obstruction symptoms (decreased stream strength, increased urinary frequency, sense of incomplete voiding) with or without UTI/pyuria, bone pain, hematuria, lymphadenopathy, and weight loss

What metastatic symptoms may be present?

Back pain (bone metastasis), weight loss, hematuria, and lymphadenopathy

What are common findings on rectal exam?

Firm, nodular, or irregular prostate

What are the associated lab findings?

Increased PSA and serum acid phosphatase

Does a normal PSA value rule out prostate cancer?

No, but it makes the diagnosis less likely

What increase in PSA is strongly correlated with prostate cancer?

A level 2.5–4.0 times the normal value (PSA > 10 ng/mL)

How is the diagnosis confirmed?

Needle biopsy

What additional tests should be ordered if metastasis is suspected?

Bone scan (bone metastasis) and CT scan or MR imaging (metastatic lymphadenopathy)

What is the treatment strategy for men >70 years old? Why?

Conservative or palliative therapy (hormonal ablation) and radiation therapy. Patients >70 years old have an increased incidence of side effects (incontinence, erectile dysfunction) after radical prostatectomy.

What is the treatment for men <70 years old?

Radical prostatectomy and radiation (external beam or interstitial seed radiation therapy)

What additional therapy may be beneficial in late-stage disease with progression of metastatic disease?

Antiandrogen therapy or castration

What tumor marker test should be ordered periodically to screen for cancer recurrence?

PSA

Does an elevated PSA level indicate recurrence

After radical prostatectomy?

Yes. PSA level should be nondetectable (<0.2 ng/mL).

After radiation therapy?

Possibly could indicate a recurrence, but can be elevated with BPH.

PROSTATITIS

What is prostatitis?

An acute (90% of cases) or chronic bacterial (or nonbacterial) infection of the prostate

What organisms frequently cause it?

Gram-negative organisms (e.g., *E. coli*)

What causes nonbacterial prostatitis?

Etiology unknown

Who is at increased risk

For bacterial prostatitis?   Older men

For nonbacterial prostatitis?   Younger men

What symptoms are common to both acute and chronic prostatitis?

Increased urinary frequency, urgency, dysuria, low back pain, and perineal pain

What additional symptoms may present with acute prostatitis?

High fever and chills

Chronic bacterial prostatitis patients are at increased risk for what?

UTI

What are the associated findings on rectal exam?

Warm, tender, swollen prostate. Rectal exam of prostate to obtain prostatic secretion (i.e., prostatic message) is contraindicated in acute prostatitis. It can cause bacterial sepsis.

What laboratory test should be included in the workup?

Urinalysis, urine culture, and culture of prostatic secretions from prostatic massage

How is bacterial prostatitis diagnosed?	Positive bacterial counts from prostate specimens
How is nonbacterial prostatitis diagnosed?	Presentation, increased white blood cell (WBC) count, and negative culture from prostatic secretions
What is the treatment for bacterial prostatitis?	Trimethoprim-sulfamethoxazole (Bactrim) or fluoroquinolones (ciprofloxacin) for 6 weeks
What additional therapy is required for sepsis (may occur in acute prostatitis)?	IV ampicillin and gentamicin for 4 weeks
How is nonbacterial prostatitis treated?	As an outpatient, with nonsteroidal anti-inflammatory drugs, α-blockers, Sitz baths (to relieve pain and spasm), hydration, and stool softeners

PYELONEPHRITIS

What is pyelonephritis?	Infection of the renal parenchyma
What organism usually causes it?	*E. coli* (often ascends from the lower urinary tract)
What are the risk factors?	Urinary tract obstruction, stasis, indwelling catheter, diabetes mellitus, immunocompromised state, vesicoureteral reflux nephrolithiasis
How does it present?	Sudden onset of fever, chills, nausea, vomiting, and flank pain with or without concomitant UTI symptoms
What does the physical exam reveal?	Costovertebral tenderness on the affected side
What is the diagnostic test of choice?	Urinalysis and microscopic analysis
What are the diagnostic lab findings?	Urinalysis: dipstick—elevated leukocyte esterase, and nitrates; microscopic—WBC casts, RBCs, WBCs, and bacteria (rods or chains of cocci)

What tests should be considered if obstruction is suspected?	CT scan, ultrasound scan, or intravenous pyelogram (IVP)
What is the treatment for pyelonephritis and	
Ureteral obstruction?	Percutaneous nephrostomy or cystoscopy with indwelling ureteral stent placement
Bladder outlet obstruction?	Urethral Foley catheter or suprapubic catheter placement
What additional test should be ordered? Why?	Urinalysis culture and sensitivity, to select antibiotic
What is the treatment?	IV fluoroquinolone (Ciprofloxacin) or third-generation cephalosporin (ceftriaxone) for 1 to 2 days, followed by oral ciprofloxacin for 2 weeks

URETHRITIS

What is urethritis?	Inflammation of the urethra
What are the risk factors?	New sexual partner; history of other sexually transmitted disease (STD)
How is urethritis classified?	Gonococcal (GC) or nongonococcal (NGC)
What causes GC urethritis?	*Neisseria gonorrhoeae*
What causes NGC urethritis?	*Chlamydia trachomatis* and *Ureaplasma urealyticum*
What symptoms may occur in both?	UTI symptoms (increased frequency, urgency, and dysuria)
How is the urethral discharge characterized in GC urethritis?	Purulent

How is the urethral discharge characterized in NGC urethritis?	Thin, clear to white, scanty discharge
What lab tests are included in the workup?	Culture and Gram stain of urethral discharge (or cervical mucus in women), urinalysis
How is GC urethritis diagnosed?	History, presentation, and gram-negative intracellular diplococci in WBCs or positive Thayer-Martin culture
How is NGC diagnosed?	History, presentation, and a negative Gram stain
What is the treatment strategy?	Treat both GC and NGC because of high incidence of coinfection
What is the treatment?	Ceftriaxone (for GC) and doxycycline, tetracycline, or Zithromax (for NGC)
What are patients at risk for without treatment?	Urinary strictures, pelvic inflammatory disease, and infertility

Index

AAA (abdominal aortic aneurysm), 113, 441–442
AAT supplementation, 362
ABC drugs (Avonex, Betaseron, Copaxone), 205
ABCD (**A**symmetry, **B**order irregularity, **C**olor variation, **D**iameter), 52
ABCs (**A**irway, **B**reathing and ventilation, **C**irculation with hemorrhage control, **D**isability, **E**xposure), 74, 79, 90, 96
Abdominal aortic aneurysm, 113, 441–442
Abdominal aortic grafts, 113
Abdominal injury, surgery, 434–435
Abdominal paracentesis, 154
Abdominal ultrasound (AUS) scan, 439
ABG (arterial blood gas)
  altered mental status and, 109
  for asthma, 358
  cardiogenic shock and, 92
  ILD (interstitial lung disease), 364
  pneumonia, 352
  preoperative evaluation, 383
  pulmonary edema and, 24
  pulmonary embolism and, 37
  during septic shock, 98
  sickle cell disease and, 172
  status epilepticus and, 236
ABO incompatibility, 95
Abortion, 284–287
ABRS (acute bacterial rhinosinusitis), 178
Acalculous cholecystitis, 440
Acarbose, 57
Accelerated idioventricular rhythm (AIVR), 102
ACE (angiotensin-converting enzyme) inhibitors, 5, 23, 33, 367, 403, 419
Acetaminophen toxicity, 137, 138
Acetazolamide, 168
Acetoacetate, 395
Acetyl-CoA dehydrogenase, 216
Acetylcholine, 35

Acetylcholine release, 211
Achalasia, 158
AChE (acetylcholinesterase) inhibitor, 209
Achondroplasia, 280
ACI_1 receptor antibodies, 208–209
Acid-base disorders, 384–389
Acid maltase, 216, 217
Acidemia, 384, 388, 389
Acidosis, 95, 100, 384
ACLS (advanced cardiac life support), 42, 43, 101
Acne keratosis, 45–46
Acne vulgaris, 44–45
ACOG (*see* American College of Obstetricians and Gynecologists)
Acoustic neuroma, 202
Acrocyanosis, 98
Acromegaly, 68, 216
ACTH (adrenocorticotropic hormone), 2, 65–66, 67, 68, 382
Actinobacillus, 184
Actinomyces, 266
Activated charcoal, 107, 138
Acute acalculous cholecystitis, 440
Acute bacterial rhinosinusitis (ABRS), 178
Acute calculous cholecystitis, 439
Acute chest syndrome, 172
Acute cholecystitis, 134
Acute gouty arthritis, 428–429
Acute leukemia, 159–160
Acute lower back pain, 421–422
Acute monoarthritis, 430
Acute myocardial infarction, 32–34
Acute noninflammatory diarrhea, 131–132
Acute otitis media, 176–177
Acute pancreatitis, 154–156, 439
Acute pericarditis, 25–26
Acute pneumothorax, 26–28
Acute pyelonephritis, 445
Acute sinusitis, 178–179
Acute vasoocclusive crisis, 172
Acyclovir, 48, 116, 188

Addison disease, 65, 216
Adenocarcinoma, 119, 156, 247, 381, 382, 445
Adenomatous villous polyps, 125
Adenosine, 41
Adenovirus, 72, 178, 180, 217, 299, 306, 317
ADH (antidiuretic hormone), 397, 399, 400
ADHD (attention deficit hyperactivity disorder), 330–331
Adjustment disorder with depressed mood, 336
Adnexal cysts, 240
Adrenal glands, hyperplasia, 5
Adrenal overproduction, 2
β-Adrenergic agonists, 20, 277
α-Adrenergic blocker, 10
β-Adrenergic blockers, 20
Adrenocortical insufficiency, 65–66
Adult hemoglobin molecule, 170
Adult respiratory distress syndrome, 191 (see ARDS)
Adult thalassemia, 171
AEIOU TIPS, 108
AFB (acid-fast bacillus), 355, 376
AFP (α-fetoprotein), 280
Agitation, 199
β₂-Agonist bronchodilators, 359, 362
β₂-Agonist effect, 405
Agoraphobia, 333
Agranulocytosis, 63, 330
AIDP (acute inflammatory demyelinating polyneuropathy), 192, 206 (see also Guillain-Barré syndrome)
AIDS (see also HIV/AIDS)
    adrenocortical insufficiency, 66
    non-Hodgkin lymphoma and, 164
    PCP (Pneumocystis carinii pneumonia), 26, 356
    septic arthritis and, 432
Airway
    acute abdominal trauma and, 434
    assessing, 74
    diseases, 373
    edema, 105
    obstruction, 89
    septic shock and, 99
AIVR (accelerated idioventricular rhythm), 102
Albumin, 94, 141, 152
Albuterol, 90, 359

Alcohol consumption
    acute pancreatitis and, 154
    altered mental status, 109
    benign prostatic hypertrophy and, 443
    cardioembolic stroke and, 223
    contraindication to liver transplantation, 143
    GERD and, 31
    hepatic encephalopathy and, 153
    hepatitis and, 137, 153
    hypertension and, 3, 4
    liver disease, 134–136
    OSAHS (obstructive sleep apnea-hypopnea syndrome) and, 377
    osteoporosis and, 256
    peptic ulcer disease and, 122
    subarachnoid hemorrhage and, 231
    upper GI bleeding and, 438
Alendronate, 71
Alkalemia, 389
Alkaline phosphatase, 64, 139, 140, 142, 144, 148, 149, 157
Alkalosis, 153
ALL (acute lymphoblastic leukemia), 159
Allopurinol, 429
Alport syndrome, 280
Alprazolam, 333
ALS (amyotrophic lateral sclerosis, 194–196, 370
ALT (alanine aminotransferase), 134, 138–144, 149, 157
Altered mental status, 107–110, 152
Alveolar hemorrhage, 371, 373
Alveolar-oxygen equation, 368
Alzheimer's disease, 196–199, 348
Amanita muscaria poisoning, 106
Amaurosis fugax, 220
Amenorrhea, 68, 249–252
American Burn Association, 105
American College of Obstetricians and Gynecologists, 243
American Heart Association, 184
Amiloride, 400
Aminoglycosides, 210, 395
Aminophylline, 90
Amiodarone, 101, 216
Amitriptyline, 339
AML (acute myelogenous leukemia), 159
Ammonia, 152, 326
Amnestic disorder, 346
Amniocentesis, 279

Amoebic colitis, 124
Amoxicillin, 123, 177, 179, 318, 320, 415, 445
Amoxicillin-clavulanic acid, 179
Amphetamines, 110
Amphotericin, 402
Ampicillin, 130, 267, 315, 448
Amylase, 155
Amyloid angiopathy, 229
β-Amyloid plaques, 197, 348
Amyloidosis, 429
Amyotrophic lateral sclerosis (ALS), 194–196, 370
ANA (antinuclear antibody), 374, 376, 412, 420
Anaerobic antibiotics, 47
Anaerobic bacteria, 352
Anal fissure, 438
Analgesics (narcotics)
　for hemorrhoids, 155
　for herpes zoster, 48
　hyponatremia and, 398
　for kidney stones, 410
　for pharyngitis, 318
　for sickle cell crisis, 173
Anaphylactic shock, 88–91
ANCA (antineutrophil cytoplasmic antibody), 374, 409
Androgenic steroids, 66
Androgens, 44
Anemia (see also Sickle cell disease)
　anorexia nervosa and, 344
　aplastic, 168–169
　of chronic disease, 173–174
　chronic renal failure and, 393
　CLL (chronic lymphocytic leukemia) and, 162, 163
　with elevated ESR, 417
　hemolytic, 278
　hemorrhagic gastritis and, 120
　hypertension, 3
　hypochromic microcytic, 166
　iron deficiency anemia, 119, 165–168
　megaloblastic, 167–168
　multifactorial, 166
　normochromic normocytic, 173
　pernicious, 150, 208
　sickle cell disease, 171–173
　sideroblastic, 169–170
　syncope and, 111
　thalassemia, 170–171
Aneurysm, 15, 50, 113, 221, 228, 230, 231, 233, 373

Angioaccess, 396
Angiodysplasia, 113–114, 125, 438
Angioedema, 5, 89
Angiography, 438
Angiotensin receptor blockers, 403
Angular stomatitis, 166
Anion gap, 58, 385, 387
Anisocoria, 78
Ankylosing spondylitis, 424, 425
Anorexia nervosa (AN), 65, 73, 343
Anosmia, 78
Anterior pituitary diseases, 67–68
Anterograde amnesia, 346
Anti–double-stranded DNA, 420
Anti–glomerular basement membrane antibody, 374
Anti-GM1 titer, 196
Anti-HBe, 141
Anti-HCV test, 142
Anti–intrinsic factor antibody, 168
Anti–liver-kidney microsomal antibody, 137
Anti–parietal cell antibody, 168
Anti–Smith antibodies, 420
Anti–smooth muscle antibody, 137
Antiandrogen therapy, 446
Antiarrhythmic drugs, 42, 43, 102
Antibiotic therapy (see also names of specific antibiotics)
　for acute pericarditis, 155
　after hemothorax, 86
　for aortic regurgitation, 16
　for aortic stenosis, 19
　for bacterial meningitis, 191, 315
　for brain abscess, 187
　broad-spectrum, 160
　for diabetes mellitus, 47
　empiric, 100, 134
　for endocarditis, 18
　for GABHS, 181
　for infectious colitis, 128
　for mitral regurgitation, 23
　for pelvic inflammatory disease, 267
　for pneumonia, 320, 353
　for sickle cell crisis, 173
　for spontaneous bacterial peritonitis, 154
　for toxic megacolon, 130
Anticardiolipin, 221, 223, 227
Anticholinergic syndrome, 106
Anticholinergic toxicity, 110
Anticholinergics, 129, 201
Anticoagulant drugs, 222–223

Anticoagulant hemorrhage, 81
Anticoagulant syndrome, 227
Anticoagulants, 25
Anticoagulation, 39, 40, 413
Anticonvulsants, 188, 236, 237
Antidepressants, 337, 345, 350
Antidiarrheal drugs, 129
Antidiarrheal medications, 301
Antidiuretic hormone, 69
Antifungal drugs, 321
Antihistamines, 106
Antihypertensive drugs, side effects, 5
Antineoplastic anthracenedione, 205
Antinuclear antibodies, 223
Antiphospholipid syndrome, 223, 227
Antipsychotic medications, 330, 335, 350
Antipyretics, 318
Antisecretory therapy, 120
Antisocial personality disorder, 349
Antispasmodics, 205
Antithrombin III studies, 36, 221, 223
Antithyroid drugs, 63
α_1-Antitrypsin deficiency, 136
Antituberculosis agents, 321
Antral biopsy, 123
Anxiety (*see* Psychiatry)
Anxiolytic medications, 332
AOM (acute otitis media), 176–177
Aortic aneurysms, 15, 50
Aortic dissection, 28–30, 91, 92, 110
Aortic insufficiency, 3
Aortic regurgitation, 14–17
Aortic stenosis, 17–19
Aortoenteric fistula, 113
Aplastic anemia, 168–169
Apolipoprotein E-4 allele, on
 chromosome 19, 197
Appendicitis, 436–437, 439
AR (*see* Aorta, aortic regurgitation)
Arachidonic acid, 89
Arcanobacterium haemolyticum, 180
ARDS (adult respiratory distress
 syndrome), 80, 98, 368, 369, 370–373
ARF (acute renal failure), 389–392, 411
Arnold-Chiari malformation, 307
Arrhythmias (*see* Cardiology)
Arterial blood gas (*see* ABG)
Arterial CO_2 tension, 386
Arterial stenotic stroke, 220–221
Arterial vasospasm (*see* Vasospasm)
Arteriolosclerosis, 228, 229
Arteriovenous malformation (*see* AVM)
Arteritis, 28

Arthralgias, 323
Arthritis, 323, 426–433 (*see also*
 Rheumatology)
Artificial heart valves, 187, 221
Arylsulfatase A, 196
AS (*see* Aortic stenosis)
Asbestosis, 365
"Ascending neuropathy", 206
Ascites, 151–152
Ascitic fluid PMN count, 154
Aseptic meningitis, 190
Asherman syndrome, 262
Aspergilloma, 379
Aspiration pneumonia, 351–352
Aspirin
 for arterial stenotic stroke, 221
 for cardioembolic stroke, 223
 for cardiogenic shock, 92
 for hemoptysis, 373
 hemorrhagic gastritis and, 120
 for lacunar strokes, 224
 peptic ulcer disease and, 122
 for pleurisy, 35
 for prevention of MI, 33, 92
 for Prinzmetal angina, 26
 Reye syndrome and, 325
 for thrombosis, 227
Aspirin plus dipyridamole, 221, 223
Asplenia, 172
AST (aspartate aminotransferase), 134,
 138–144, 157
Asthma, 90, 116, 320, 357–360, 369, 385
Astrocytoma, 202
Asystole, 100
Atelectasis, 320
Atherosclerosis, 220, 224, 230, 256, 441
Atherosclerotic coronary artery disease,
 32, 35
Atherosclerotic disease, 130, 255
Atrial fibrillation, 38–40, 221, 222
Atrial flutter, 40–41
Atrioventricular malformation, 228
Atrioventricular node disease, 110
Atropine, 106
"Atypical" pneumonia, 351
Auditory hallucinations, 108
AUS (abdominal ultrasound) scan, 439
Austin Flint murmur, 15
Autoimmune destruction, 65
Autoimmune diseases, 150, 227
Autoimmune hepatitis, 136–137
Autoimmune multifocal motor
 neuropathy, 195

Autoimmune myositis, 218, 219–220
Autosplenectomy, 172
Autotransfusion, 86
AV nodal blocking agent, 41
AV nodal re-entrant tachycardia, 41
AVM (arteriovenous malformation), 113–114, 125, 232–233
Avoidant personality disorder, 350
AVPU (**A**lert, **V**ocal stimuli, **P**ainful stimuli, **U**nresponsive), 75
Azathioprine, 137, 219, 364, 431
Azithromycin, 318, 353
Azoospermia, 295
AZT (zidovudine), 186

B cells, 163
Bacillus cereus, 131
Back pain, 421–422
Baclofen, 205
Bacteremia, 177, 183
Bacterial endocarditis, 221, 228
Bacterial meningitis, 99, 190, 315, 316
Bacterial prostatitis, 447, 448
Bacteriuria, 445
Bacteroides, 266
Bactrim, 300
BAER (brainstem auditory-evoked response), 204
Band ligation, 118
Bariatric surgery, 378, 379
Barium studies, 31, 129, 130, 242, 248, 302
Barotrauma, 86
Barrett esophagus, 31, 114, 115, 116
Barrier methods of contraception, 281–282
Bartter syndrome, 387, 402
Basal body temperature, 262
Basal cell carcinoma (BCC), 51
Basal nucleus of Meynert, 197
Basilar skull fracture, 79
Basophil kallikreins, 89
Basophilic stippling, 171
BAT (blunt abdominal trauma), 434
Battle sign, 78
BBC casts, 406
BCC (basal cell carcinoma), 51
BCLS (basic cardiac life support), 42
Beck triad, 81
Becker dystrophy, 213, 215
Beclomethasone, 307
Bell (seventh nerve) palsy, 366
Bence-Jones protein, 411

Benign breast disease, 283
Benign prostatic hypertrophy, 442–443
Benzathine penicillin G, 51, 318
Benzodiazepines, 205, 332, 333, 335, 336, 369
Benzoyl peroxide, 44
Bereavement, 336–337
Berger disease, 408
Beriberi, 3
Bicarbonate therapy, 60
Bile duct cancers, 149
Biliary bypass, 157
Biliary colic, 146–147
Biliary tract disease, 71
Bilirubin, 134, 138–142, 144, 148, 149, 157, 172, 326
Bilirubinuria, 148
Billroth II surgery, 119
Bismuth, 123
Bisphosphonate treatment, 71
Bladder outlet obstruction, 449
Bladder stones, 443
Blast crisis, 162
Blastomycosis, 379
Blighted ovum, 285
Blindness, premature birth, 277
β-Blockers, 29, 30, 33, 39, 41, 57, 63, 117, 210, 403
Blood alcohol, 109
Blood cultures, 222, 352, 376
Blood glucose, 58, 60, 111, 198, 235, 236, 326, 331–332, 376
Blood pressure (*see* BP)
Blumer shelf, 156
Blunt abdominal trauma (BAT), 434
BMI (body mass index), 71
Body dysmorphic disorder, 341
Bone biopsy, 423
Bone marrow
    aspiration, 159, 160, 164, 165
    biopsy, 159, 164, 166, 168
    ringed sideroblasts, 169, 170
    stem cells, 168
    transplant, 160, 161, 162, 169
Bone mineral density, 71
Bone scan, 382, 446
Borderline personality disorder, 349
Borrelia burgdorferi, 414
Botulism, 209, 211–212, 289
Bouchard nodes, 428
BP (blood pressure)
    acute hemorrhage and, 94
    in hypertension, 3

BP—*continued*
in pheochromocytoma, 8
widened pulse pressure, 15
BPH (benign prostatic hypertrophy),
442–443
Bradyarrhythmias, 110
Bradycardia, 61, 62
Brain abscess, 179, 187, 315
Brain aneurysms, 373
"Brain concussion", 78
Brain edema, 77, 78, 79
Brain imaging, 79
Brain injury, in closed head trauma, 77
Brain stem, structural pressure, 110
Brain tumor, 202–203
Brainstem auditory-evoked response
(BAER), 204
Brainstem infarction, 212
Brainstem raphe nuclei, 197
Brancher enzymes, 216
BRCA1 gene, 245, 259
BRCA2 gene, 245, 259
Breast cancer, 259–260, 295
Breast-feeding, contraindications, 340
Breathing, assessing, 74
Brenner carcinoma, 245
Bromocriptine, 68, 201
Bronchial arteriography, 374
Bronchiectasis, 397
Bronchitis, 360–363
Bronchodilators, 359
Bronchoscopy, 364, 373, 374
Brudzinski sign, 315
Bulimia nervosa (BN), 343, 345
BUN (blood urea nitrogen), 198, 237,
391, 410, 443
Burn shock, 104
Burns, 102–105
Buspirone, 332

C-ANCA (cytoplasmic antineutrophil
cytoplasmic antibody), 408, 409
C-reactive protein, 227, 423
C282Y (Hfe) gene mutation, 138
C_3 test, 412
C_4 test, 412
CA 19-9 tumor marker, 157
CA125 tumor marker, 246
Cabergoline, 68
Cachexia, 361
CAD (*see* coronary artery disease)
Caffeine, 39, 256, 443
Calcinosis, 150

Calcitriol, 393
Calcium, 109, 235, 331–332
Calcium acetate, 393
Calcium channel antagonists, 277
Calcium-channel blockers, 39, 41
Calcium channel mutations, 216
Calcium gluconate, 404
Calcium oxalate kidney stones, 409
Calcium pyrophosphate, 429
Calcium supplementation, 71
Calculous cholecystitis, 439
Campylobacter jejuni, 206
Campylobacter species, 128, 133, 134, 299
Candida albicans, 46, 182
Candida infection, 116
Candidiasis (thrush), 46, 317
Captopril renogram, 13
Carbamazepine, 70, 236, 336, 398
Carbohydrates, 59, 60
Carbon monoxide, 200
Carbon tetrachloride, 137
Carboxyhemoglobin, 109
Carcinoembryonic antigen (CEA), 119,
126, 157
Carcinomatous meningitis, 207
Cardiac arrest, 100–102
Cardiac lesion, 183
Cardiac syncope, 111
Cardiac tamponade, 80–82, 94 (*see also*
Cardiology)
Cardiac thromboembolic events (stroke),
39, 40
Cardiobacterium, 184
Cardioembolic stroke, 221–223
Cardiogenic shock, 91–93
Cardiology
arrhythmias and conduction disorders
anorexia nervosa and, 344
atrial fibrillation, 38–40, 221, 222
atrial flutter, 40–41
AV nodal re-entrant tachycardia, 41
bulimia nervosa and, 345
complications of resuscitation, 95
obesity and, 73
sarcoidosis and, 366
torsades de pointes, 41–42
ventricular fibrillation, 42–43
ventricular tachycardia, 43
chest pain
acute myocardial infarction, 32–34
acute pericarditis, 25–26
acute pneumothorax, 26–28
aortic dissection, 28–30

GERD (gastroesophageal reflux disease), 30–31, 115–116
mediastinal emphysema, 31–32
pleurisy, 34–35
Prinzmetal angina, 35–36
pulmonary embolism, 36–38
CHF (congestive heart failure)
aortic dissection and, 28–30, 91, 92, 110
aortic regurgitation, 14–17
aortic stenosis, 17–19
HCM (hypertrophic cardiomyopathy), 19–21
hyponatremia and, 397
mitral regurgitation, 21–23, 92
pulmonary edema, 23–25
respiratory alkalosis and, 384
respiratory failure, 368, 369
risk for stroke, 40
spironolactone therapy, 402
torsades de pointes and, 42
Down syndrome and, 294
hypertension
acute renal failure and, 390
arterial stenotic stroke and, 220
cardioembolic stroke and, 223
chronic renal failure and, 392
coarctation of the aorta, 1
Cushing syndrome, 2, 72
essential hypertension, 2–5
hyperaldosteronism, 5–7, 387, 402
intracerebral hemorrhage and, 229
lacunar strokes and, 224
obesity and, 71
pheochromocytoma, 7–10
pulmonary, 89
renal parenchymal hypertension, 10–12
renovascular disease, 12–14
subarachnoid hemorrhage and, 231
hypoestrogenic symptoms, 255
Kawasaki disease, 312–313
MI (myocardial infarction), 32–34, 43, 58, 100, 110
OSAHS (obstructive sleep apnea-hypopnea syndrome) and, 377
Turner syndrome, 28, 250, 296
Cardiomyopathies, 21, 43, 91, 371 (*see also* HCM)
Cardioversion, 39, 40, 42, 43
Carnitine deficiency, 216
Carnitine palmitoyltransferase deficiency, 216

Carotid artery stenosis, 224
Carotid endarterectomy, 221, 224
Carotid sinus massage, 41, 111
Carotid stenosis, 220
Castration, 446
Catatonic schizophrenia, 329
Catechol-*o*-methyltransferase (COMT) inhibitors, 201
Catecholamine hypersecretion, on the cardiovascular system, 8
Caudal cranial nerves, 211
CBC (complete blood cell) counts
for abruptio placentae, 273
for acute leukemia, 159
for altered mental status, 109
for Alzheimer's disease, 198
for diarrhea/gastroenteritis, 300
for diverticulosis, 127
for epilepsy, 235, 236
for FUO (fever of unknown origin), 309
for GAD (generalized anxiety disorder), 331
for hemoptysis, 374
for lung cancer, 382
for major depressive disorder, 338
for myositis, 219
for peptic ulcer disease, 123
for pneumonia, 352
for RSV (respiratory syncytial virus), 304
for syncope, 111
CD4$^+$ T lymphocytes, 184, 185, 186
CEA (carcinoembryonic antigen), 119, 126, 157
Cefepime, 353
Cefotaxime, 154, 190, 315
Cefoxitin, 395
Cefpodoxime, 179
Ceftazidime, 353
Ceftriaxone, 190, 353, 424, 433, 449, 450
Cefuroxime axetil, 179
Celiac blocks, 157
β-Cells of the pancreas, 55
Cellulitis, 46–47, 99, 432
Central core disease, 216
Central pontine myelinolysis, 207
Central zone of coagulation, 103
Cephalosporin, 154, 190, 318, 320, 353, 424, 445, 449
Cephazolin, 47
Cerebellar hemorrhage, 228, 229
Cerebral edema, 191

Cerebral palsy, 277
Cerebritis, 187
Cerebrospinal fluid (*see* CSF)
Cerebrovascular accident (*see* CVA)
Cerebrovascular disease, 256
Ceruloplasmin level, 201
Cervical carcinoma, 286
Cervical lymphadenitis, 321
Cervical polyps, 286
Cervical stenosis, 195
β-Chain mutation, 171
Charcot-Bouchard aneurysm, 228
Charcot triad, 148
Chem 7 panel, 109
Chemical burns, 102
Chemistry panel, 236
Chemoembolization, 149
Chemotherapy
   for acute leukemia, 160, 162
   for CLL, 163
   for non-Hodgkin lymphoma, 165
   for small cell lung cancer, 383
Chest CT scan, 209
Chest pain (*see* Cardiology)
Chest tube (tube thoracostomy), 84, 88
Chest x-ray, 374
   for acute leukemia, 160
   for asbestosis, 365
   for asthma, 358
   for cardioembolic stroke, 222
   for cervical cancer, 248
   for Kawasaki disease, 313
   for metastasis, 244
   for ovarian cancer, 246
   for pneumonia, 187, 320, 352
   for RSV (respiratory syncytial
     virus), 304
   for sickle cell disease, 172
CHF (*see* Cardiology)
CHF (congestive heart failure), 368,
   369, 397, 402
Chickenpox (herpes varicella), 48,
   305–306
Child abuse, 326–328
Chlamydia pneumoniae, 180
Chlamydia species, 319, 351
Chlamydia trachomatis, 266, 449
Chlorambucil, 163, 165
Chloramphenicol, 168, 169
Chloroquine, 210, 216
Chlorpromazine, 330, 344
Chlorpropamide, 70, 398
Cholangiocarcinoma, 149, 151

Cholangitis, 99, 134, 148
Cholecystectomy, 439
Cholecystitis, 147, 437, 440
Cholestatic diseases, 146–151
Cholesteatoma, 177
Cholesterol, 412
Cholesterol-lowering agents, 218
Cholestyramine, 150
Cholinergic crisis, 110, 210
Cholinergic syndrome, 106
Cholinesterase inhibitors, 199, 348
Chordae tendineae rupture, 92
Chorioangioma, 278
Chorioangiomas, 280
Chromogranin A, 9
Chromogranin B, 9
Chromosome 1, 197, 348
Chromosome 13q, 245
Chromosome 14, 197, 348
Chromosome 19, 197, 348
Chromosome 21, 293, 348
Chronic alcoholism, 169
Chronic bronchitis, 360–363
Chronic cholecystitis, 440
Chronic hepatitis, 408
Chronic hypercapnic failure, 370
Chronic inflammation, 169
Chronic interstitial nephritis, 404
Chronic lymphocytic leukemia, 162–163
Chronic myelogenous leukemia,
   160–162
Chronic obstructive pulmonary disease
   (*see* COPD)
Chronic pancreatitis, 146
Chronic pulmonary disease, 277
Chronic stool retention, 324
Churg-Strauss disease, 409
Cigarette smoking
   abdominal aortic aneurysm and, 441
   abruptio placentae and, 272
   acute MI and, 32
   arterial stenotic stroke and, 220
   cardioembolic stroke and, 223
   cervical cancer and, 247
   coronary artery disease and, 32
   deep venous thrombosis and, 37
   emphysema and, 361
   hemoptysis and, 373
   lacunar strokes and, 224
   leiomyomas and, 241
   lung cancer and, 381
   oral contraceptives and, 283
   osteoporosis and, 256

peptic ulcer disease and, 122
subarachnoid hemorrhage and, 231
Cimetidine, 90, 123, 218, 395
Circle of Willis, 221
Circulation, assessing, 75
Cirrhosis, 134, 136, 139, 140, 143,
149–150, 402, 438 (see also
Hepatocellular carcinoma)
Cisplatin, 402
CK (creatinine kinase), 92
CK-MB (creatine kinase, myocardial
bound), 92
Cl⁻ (urinary chloride), 386–387
Clarithromycin, 124
Clavulanate, 353
Clear cell carcinoma, 244, 245
Climacteric, 254–259
Clindamycin, 44, 47, 267, 318, 353
CLL (chronic lymphocytic leukemia),
162–163
Clofibrate, 216, 398
Clomiphene, 263
Clomiphene citrate, 264
Clomipramine, 332
Clopidogrel, 221, 223, 224
Clostridium botulinum, 211, 212
Clostridium difficile, 133, 134, 299
Clostridium perfringens, 131
Clotting factors, 412
Clozapine, 330
Clubbing, 183
Cluster A personality disorder, 349
Cluster B personality disorder, 349
Cluster C personality disorder, 350
CMAP (compound muscle action
potentials), 207
CML (chronic myelogenous leukemia,
160–162
CMV (cytomegalovirus), 168
CNS (central nervous system)
brain tumor, 202–203
degenerative and hereditary diseases
ALS (amyotrophic lateral sclerosis,
194–196
Alzheimer's disease, 196–199
motor neuron disease, 194–196
Parkinson's disease, 199–201
demyelinating diseases
Guillain-Barré syndrome, 206–207
multiple sclerosis, 203–205
embolic events, 183
episodic disorders
epilepsy, 234–237

postictal state, 237–238
infectious diseases
brain abscess, 179, 187
herpes simplex virus encephalitis,
188–189
meningitis, 79–80, 99, 177, 179,
189–191
poliomyelitis, 191–194
neuromuscular junction and muscle
botulism, 211–212
muscular dystrophy, 212–215
myasthenia gravis, 208–211
myopathy, 215–217
myositis, 217–220
respiratory alkalosis and, 385
septic shock and, 98, 99
SLE (systemic lupus erythematosus)
and, 421
vascular diseases
antiphospholipid syndrome, 227
arterial stenotic stroke, 220–221
cardioembolic stroke, 221–223
intracranial hemorrhage, 77, 78, 79,
109, 228–230
lacunar strokes, 224
MELAS syndrome, 228
subarachnoid hemorrhage, 230–233
vertebral basilar system strokes,
224–226
CO₂ carbon dioxide, 358
CO₂ renal angiography, 11, 13–14
Coagulase-negative staphylococci, 423
Coagulopathy, 191
Coarctation of the aorta, 1
"Coca-Cola urine", 407
Cocaine, 39, 211, 272
Coccidioides, 352
Coccidioidomycosis, 379
Cognitive/behavioral abnormalities, 191
Cognitive-behavioral therapy, 333
Cognitive function screening test, 348
Cognitive skills, toddlers, 291
Cognitive therapy, 335
Colchicine, 216, 429
Cold pressor test, 35
Colic, 297–299
Colitic arthritis, 424, 426
Collagen vascular diseases, 14, 25, 315
Colonoscopy, 125, 127, 128, 129, 131, 438
Color flow mapping, 280
Colorectal cancer, 125–126
Colposcopic biopsy, 248
Columnar epithelium, 177

Coma
aneurysms and, 231
diabetes mellitus and, 58, 59
elevated ammonia and, 326
lacunar strokes and, 226
nonketotic hyperosmolar, 59–60
prognosis, 80
Common bile duct stone, 148
Communication skills
infants, 289, 290
preschoolers, 292
toddlers, 290, 291
Community-acquired pneumonia, 353
Complete abortion, 284
Complete blood cell count (*see* CBC)
COMT (catechol-*o*-methyltransferase)
inhibitors, 201
Conduction disorders (*see* Cardiology,
arrhythmias and conduction disorders)
Conduction system disease, 110
Cone biopsy, 248
Confabulation, 346
Congenital aneurysm, 228
Congenital heart defects, 187, 228
Congenital myopathy, 216
Congestive heart failure, 73, 320
Conjugated estrogen, 254, 258
Conn syndrome (hyperaldosteronism,
5–7, 387 (*see also* GRA)
Connective tissue diseases, 15, 34
Contact burns, 102
Contact dermatitis, 47–48
Contaminated needles, 233
Contraception, 281–284
"Contrecoup" injuries, 77
Conus medullaris, 422
Conversion disorder, 341
Cooley anemia, 171
COPD (chronic obstructive pulmonary
disease), 26, 86, 360–363, 368,
369, 370
Copper metabolism, 145
Coronary artery disease (CAD), 42, 71, 73
Coronavirus, 178
Corpus luteum, 257, 270
Corrigan pulse, 15
Corticosteroids, 49, 207, 362, 364
Cortisol, 2, 66, 109, 344
Corynebacterium diphtheriae, 180
Cosyntropin, 66
"Coup" injuries, 77
Courvoisier gallbladder, 156
Couvelaire uterus, 275

Coxsackie A & B, 25, 217, 317
CPAP (continuous positive airway
pressure), 378, 379
CPK (creatine phosphokinase), 214, 217,
218, 219
Cranial nerve III, 110
Cranial nerve VI palsy, 203
Creatine phosphokinase, 92
Creatinine, 198, 237, 391, 395, 410, 443
Creatinine kinase (*see* CK)
Creatinine urine catecholamines, 9
CREST (**C**alcinosis, **R**aynaud
phenomenon, **E**sophageal
dysmotility, **S**clerodactyly,
Telangiectasia) syndrome, 150, 419
Creutzfeldt-Jakob disease, 198
CRF (chronic renal failure), 392–396
(*see also* Nephrology)
Critical care management, 74–77
Crohn's disease, 128, 129, 130
Croup, 306–307
Cryoprecipitate, 175
Cryosurgery, 46
Cryptococcal antigen, 190
Cryptococcosis, 379
Cryptococcus neoformans, 189
CSF 14-3-3-protein level, 198
CSF (cerebrospinal fluid), 77, 79, 109,
188, 190, 196, 314, 315
CSF rhinorrhea, 78
CT scans
abdominal, 113, 146, 155, 157, 434
for acute lower back pain, 422
for aortic dissection, 29
brain imaging, 79, 111, 187, 188, 202,
203, 222, 224, 229, 230, 238
for cancer staging, 115, 141
chest, 209
for Hodgkin lymphoma, 164
for hyperaldosteronism, 6
with IV contrast, 442
for neurologic abnormalities, 382
for non-Hodgkin lymphoma, 165
for osteomyelitis, 423
for parenchymal hypertension, 11
of pelvis and abdomen, 246
for pheochromocytoma, 9
for prostate cancer, 446
for pulmonary embolism, 38
for pyelonephritis, 449
for renovascular hypertension, 13
for retropharyngeal abscess, 322
for secondary survey, 77

CTT (computed transaxial tomography), 410

Culdocentesis, 270

Cullen sign, 155

Curare, 210

Cushing syndrome, 2, 66–67, 68, 72, 216, 387

Cutaneous gumma, 50

CVA (cerebrovascular accident), 28, 29, 58, 111

CVP (central venous pressure), 93, 100

Cyclic antidepressants, 106

Cyclophosphamide, 165, 364, 398, 407, 431

Cycloserine, 169

Cyclosporine, 220, 403

Cyclothymic disorder, 337

Cyproheptadine, 344

Cystic fibrosis, 26, 86, 280, 320

Cysticercosis, 218

Cystitis, 437, 444–445

Cystoscopy, 248

Cytomegalovirus, 116, 132, 133, 134, 206

Cytomegalovirus (CMV), 168

Cytoscopy, 449

Cytosine arabinoside, 161

Cytotoxic therapy, 364

D₅ solution, 60

Danazol, 240

DDAVP (desamino-8-D-arginine vasopressin), 69, 175, 400

De Musset sign, 15

Deafness, premature birth, 277 (see also Hearing loss)

Debrancher enzymes, 216

Decerebrate posturing, 109

Decorticate posturing, 109

Deep venous thrombosis, 36, 37, 411

Degenerative and hereditary diseases (see CNS)

Dehydration, 59, 69, 153, 172, 300

Delirium, 108, 346–347

Delta hepatitis (see Hepatitis D)

Demeclocycline, 70, 398

Dementia, 108, 197–198, 347–349

Demyelinating diseases (see CNS)

Dental erosions, 31

Dental procedures, 187

Dependent personality disorder, 350

Depression (see also Psychiatry)
    anorexia nervosa and, 344
    diabetes mellitus and, 55

treatment, 199
Wilson's disease and, 145

Depression screening, 198

Dermatology
    erythematous dermatitis, 218
    lumps and tumors of the skin
        BCC (basal cell carcinoma), 51
        malignant melanoma, 52–53
        SCC (squamous cell carcinoma), 53
    septic shock and, 98–99
    skin eruptions
        acne keratosis, 45–46
        acne vulgaris, 44–45
        candidiasis, 46
        cellulitis, 46–47
        contact dermatitis, 47–48
        herpes zoster ("shingles"), 48–49
        keloids, 54
        psoriasis, 49
        scabies, 49–50
        syphilis, 50–51
        viral warts, 53–54

Dermatomyositis, 218, 417–418

Desferrioxamine, 139

"Designer drugs", 200

Desipramine, 339

Desmopressin, 69

Dexamethasone suppression test, 2, 67, 307

Dextrose, 58

DI (see Diabetes insipidus)

Diabetes insipidus (DI), 69, 398, 399–401

Diabetes mellitus (DM) (see also Endocrine disorders)
    CRF (chronic renal failure) and, 392
    cystitis and, 444
    diagnosis and treatment, 55–57
    endometrial cancer and, 244
    enuresis and, 324
    foot disease, 55
    habitual abortion and, 284
    hyperkalemia and, 404
    hypertension and, 3
    MI (myocardial infarction) and, 223
    nephrotic syndrome and, 412
    pseudogout and, 429
    pyelonephritis and, 448
    stroke and, 40, 220, 224

Diabetic autonomic neuropathy, 405

Diabetic hypoglycemia (see Hypoglycemia)

Diabetic ketoacidosis (DKA), 57–59

Diagnostic peritoneal lavage (DPL), 434, 435

Dialysis, 392–393, 395
Diaphragmatic disease, 31, 385
Diarrhea
    acidosis and, 388
    acute noninflammatory, 131–132
    infectious inflammatory, 136
    pediatrics and, 299
DIC (disseminated intravascular
    coagulation), 159
Diclofenac, 137
Dicloxacillin, 433
Diffuse esophageal spasms, 158
Digitalis, 20
Digoxin, 41
Dilated pupils, 110
Diltiazem, 20, 41
DIP (distal interphalangeal) joints, 427,
    428, 431
Diphenhydramine, 90
Diphtheria, 212, 317
Disability, assessing, 75
Disopyramide, 20, 102
Disorganized schizophrenia, 329
Disseminated intravascular coagulation
    (DIC), 159, 275
Diuretics, 20, 24, 70, 152, 153, 401, 402
Diverticulosis, 126–127, 438
DKA (diabetic ketoacidosis), 57–59, 386,
    388, 389, 395, 405
DLCO (decreased carbon monoxide
    diffusion capacity), 364, 367
DM (see Diabetes mellitus)
DNA, anti–double-stranded, 420
DNA repair genes, 244
Dobutamine, 24, 93
Donepezil, 199, 348
Dopa-sparing medications, 201
Dopamine, 90, 93, 100
Dopamine agonists, 68, 201
Dopamine receptor antagonists, 330
Dopaminergic neurons, 199
Doppler velocimetry, 280
Dose-dependent hepatotoxins, 137
Down syndrome, 280
Doxazosin, 443
Doxepin, 339
Doxercalciferol, 393
Doxorubicin, 165, 216
Doxycycline, 179, 415, 450
DPL (diagnostic peritoneal lavage),
    434, 435
Drug abuse, 200, 233, 369
Drug-induced hepatitis, 137–138

Drug-induced lupus syndrome, 63, 227
Drug-induced myasthenia, 209
Drug-induced myositis, 218
Drug-induced parkinsonism, 200
Drug screen, 338
DSM-IV-R, 197
DTaP (diphtheria, tetanus, and acellular
    pertussis) vaccine, 310
Duchenne dystrophy, 213, 214, 215, 280
Duodenal ulcers, 122
DXA (dual-energy x-ray absorptiometry),
    71
Dysenteric infection, 425
Dysfunctional uterine bleeding, 252–254
Dysmenorrhea, 239, 414
Dyspareunia, 239
Dysphagia, 31
Dysrhythmia, 89
Dysrhythmias, 91
Dysthymic disorder, 337
Dystrophin gene, 213

Eating disorders, 343–345
EBV serology, 318
Ecchymosis, 78
ECF (eosinophilic chemotactic factor of
    anaphylaxis), 89
ECG (electrocardiogram)
    for acute pericarditis, 25
    for aortic regurgitation, 16
    for arrhythmias and conduction
        disorders, 42
    for atrial flutter, 40
    for cardiac tamponade, 81
    for coarctation of the aorta, 1
    for HCM, 20
    pulmonary edema and, 24
    for pulmonary embolism, 37
    for syncope, 111
Echocardiogram
    for acute pericarditis, 26
    for aortic stenosis, 18
    for HCM, 20
    for hemoptysis, 374
    for infective endocarditis, 183
    for syncope, 111
    two-dimensional, 222
Echovirus, 217
Eclampsia, 274
Ectopic pregnancy, 267–272, 286, 437
Efavirenz, 186
Egg allergy, 311
EHEC (enteroinvasive E. coli), 132, 133

Ehlers-Danlos syndrome, 28
Eikenella, 184
Electrical burns, 102
Electrical cardioversion (*see* Cardioversion)
Electrocautery, 46
Electroconvulsive therapy, 339, 340
Electrolytes, 58, 59, 60, 198, 235, 237, 331–332, 338, 345
Electromyography, 195, 196, 212, 370
Electrophysiologic studies, 111
Electrophysiologic tests, 204
ELISA (enzyme-linked immunosorbent assay), 185, 300, 314, 415
Embolic events, 183
Embolism, 221
Embryonic cell rests, 202
Emergency contraception, 283
Emergency medicine
    altered mental status, 107–110
    burns, 102–105
    cardiac arrest, 100–102
    chest trauma
        cardiac tamponade, 80–82
        flail chest, 82–83
        hemothorax, 82, 83
        pneumothorax, 26–28, 34, 86–88
    critical care, 74–77
    head trauma, 77–80
    poisoning, 105–107
    shock
        anaphylactic, 88–91
        cardiogenic, 91–93
        hemorrhagic, 93–95
        hypovolemic, 96–97, 104
        septic, 97–100
    syncope, 110–112
Emesis, 106, 303
Emphysema, 360–363
Empiric antibiotic therapy, 100, 134
Empyema, 99, 375
Empyema of gallbladder, 353
Encapsulated organisms, 172
Encephalitis, 315, 397
Encephalopathy, 310, 325
End-stage liver disease, 136, 150
Endocarditis, 14, 18, 221, 222, 228
Endocrine disorders
    adrenocortical insufficiency, 65–66
    anterior pituitary diseases, 67–68
    Cushing syndrome, 2, 66–67, 68, 72, 216, 387
    diabetes mellitus, 3, 40, 55–57

DKA (diabetic ketoacidosis), 57–59, 220, 223, 224, 386, 388, 389, 395
    hypoglycemia, 60, 65, 66, 68, 107, 111, 112, 234, 236
    hypothyroidism, 3, 61–62, 72, 216, 220, 223, 284, 429
    nonketotic hyperosmolar coma, 59–60
    obesity, 71–73
    osteoporosis, 67, 70–71, 255, 256
    posterior pituitary diseases, 69–70
    primary hyperparathyroidism, 64–65
Endocrine myopathy, 216, 217
Endocrinopathies, 215
Endogenous benzodiazepines, 152
Endometrial adenocarcinoma, 244
Endometrial biopsy, 243, 244
Endometrial cancer, 243
Endometriosis, 239–240, 265
Endotracheal intubation, 97
Entamoeba histolytica, 124, 134
Enteric gram-negative bacilli, 352
Enterohemorrhagic *Escherichia coli,* 128
Enteroviral pharyngitis, 318
Enterovirus, 178, 190, 299
Enthesopathy, 424
Ependymomas, 202
Epidural abscess, 315
Epidural hemorrhages, 79
Epiglottitis, 308–309, 321
Epilepsy, 234, 234–237
Epilepticus, 236
Epinephrine, 90–91, 101
Episodic disorders (*see* CNS)
Epithelial cells, 353
Epstein-Barr virus, 168, 180, 206, 313, 317, 318
EPV (*see* Epstein-Barr virus)
ERCP (endoscopic retrograde cholangiopancreatography), 148, 151
Ergonovine, 35
Erosive esophagitis, 31
ERT (estrogen replacement therapy), 240, 256, 258 (*see also* HRT)
Erysipelas, 99
Erythema, 176
Erythema chronicum migrans, 415
Erythema nodosum, 366
Erythematous dermatitis, 218
Erythroblasts, 173
Erythromycin, 42, 44, 45, 181, 318, 353
Erythropoietin, 170, 173
Escherichia coli, 128, 299, 314, 444, 447, 448

Escherichia histolytica, 132, 133, 190
Esophageal cancer, 114–115
Esophageal dysmotility, 157–158
Esophageal manometry, 31, 158
Esophageal motility disorders, 150
Esophageal spasms, 158
Esophageal tears, 345
Esophageal ulcers, 115–117
Esophageal varices, 117–119, 437
Esophagitis, 115–117
Esophagogastroduodenoscopy, 438
ESR (erythrocyte sedimentation rate), 219, 223, 376, 417, 423, 431
ESRD (end-stage renal disease), 392, 394, 396, 413 (*see also* Nephrology)
Essential hypertension, 2–5
Estradiol, 344
Estrogen replacement therapy (*see* ERT)
Estrogens, 257
ETEC (enterotoxigenic *E. coli*), 131
Ethanol, 39, 216
Ethosuximide, 236
Ethylene glycol, 388
Exercise-induced anaphylaxis, 90
Exercise-induced asthma, 90
Exercise-induced rhabdomyolysis, 401
Exogenous estrogen use, 244
Exophthalmos, 62
"Exposure and environmental control", 76
Exposure therapy, 333
Exudative pharyngitis, 180–181
Exudative pleural effusion, 375

Facioscapulohumeral dystrophy, 213–214, 215
Factitious fever, 310
Factitious disorder, 342
Factor V Leiden, 36, 221, 223, 227
Factor VII deficiency, 227
Familial ALS, 195
Fasciitis, 99
Fasting serum transferrin saturation, 138
Fatty acid oxidation, 216
Fatty liver, 134
FDA (Food and Drug Administration)
    drug approved for acute leukemia, 162
    drugs approved for obesity, 72
Fecal leukocytes, 133
Fecalith, 436
Female infertility, 260–265
Femoral hernia, 441
FENa (fractional excretion of sodium), 390

Ferritin levels, 171
Fetal congestive heart failure, 278
Fetal hemoglobin, 171
Fetal thrombocytopenia, 278
FEV/FVC (forced expiratory volume/forced vital capacity) ratio, 358, 362
FEV_1 value, 359, 362, 367, 383
Fiberoptic bronchoscopy, 380
Fibrinolytic agent, 34
Fibroids (*see* Leiomyoma)
Fibroma, 379 (*see* Leiomyoma)
Fibromyalgia (fibrositis, fibromyositis), 414
57,XXY form of X chromosome, 295
FIGO (International Federation of Gynecology and Obstetrics), 245, 246, 247
Filariasis, 379
Fine needle aspiration, 63, 382
Finger-stick blood sugar, 109
Finger stick for glucose, 236
FIO_2, 387
First-degree (superficial) burns, 102, 103, 104
Five Cs (**C**oma, **C**onvulsions, **C**austics, **C**yclic antidepressants, and hydro**C**arbons), 106
Five Hs (hypovolemia, hypoxia, hydrogen ion, hypothermia/ hyperthermia, and hypokalemia/ hyperkalemia), 100
Five Ts (toxins, tamponade, tension pneumothorax, thrombosis coronary, thrombosis pulmonary), 100
Flail chest, 82–83, 385
Flecainide, 40
Flexible sigmoidoscopy, 130
Fluconazole, 116, 182
Fludrocortisone, 66
Fluid resuscitation, 94, 97, 118, 123
Fluorescent treponemal antibody absorption test (FTA-ABS), 51
Fluoroquinolone, 128, 134, 154, 300, 353, 445, 448, 449
5-Fluorouracil, 46, 157
Fluoxetine, 333, 334, 344
Fluvoxamine, 332
Focal infection, 109
Focal segmental glomerulosclerosis, 413
Folate deficiency, 167, 168
Folate supplements, 173
Foley catheter, 155, 435

Folic acid, 280
Foreign body aspiration, 320
Foreign body synovitis, 432
Formula allergy, in infants, 298
Foscarnet, 116
Fosphenytoin, 189, 236
14q11.2-q13 gene, 214
Fourth-degree burns, 103
Free air x-ray series, 123
French-Canadian genetic factors, oculopharyngeal dystrophy, 214
Fresh frozen plasma, 94
Frontal lobe, 197
Frontotemporal dementia, 198
FSH (follicle-stimulating hormone), 67, 242, 251, 252, 254, 255, 297
FTA-ABS (Fluorescent treponemal antibody absorption test), 51
Functional asplenia, 172
Functional esophageal dysmotility, 158
Fungal cultures, 190
Fungal infections, 432
FUO (fever of unknown origin), 309–310
Furosemide, 24, 152
FVC (forced vital capacity), 367

G-banded chromosome study, 297
GABHS (Group A β-hemolytic streptococci), 46, 180–181, 317, 318–319, 406
GAD (generalized anxiety disorder), 331–332
Galactorrhea, 68
Galanthamine, 199
Gallbladder
    appendicitis and, 437
    calculous cholecystitis, 439
    cancer, 149
    Courvoisier gallbladder, 156
    empyema of, 99
    scarring, 147
    surgery, 439–441
Gallop, 390
Gallstones, 121, 146, 154
Gamma globulin, 210
Ganciclovir, 134, 321
Gastric lavage, 107, 138
Gastrin level, 123
Gastritis, 119–121, 437
Gastroenterology
    acute pancreatitis, 154–156
    cholestatic disease

biliary colic, 146–147
cholangitis, 99, 148
cholecystitis, 147, 437, 440
chronic pancreatitis, 146
Gilbert syndrome, 148
hepatocellular carcinoma (hepatoma), 148–149
primary biliary cirrhosis, 149–150
PSC (primary sclerosis cholangitis), 150–151
complications of portal hypertension
ascites, 151–152
hepatic coagulopathy, 152
hepatic encephalopathy, 152–153
hepatorenal syndrome, 153
SBP (spontaneous bacterial peritonitis), 153–154
diarrhea
acute noninflammatory diarrhea, 131–132
infectious inflammatory diarrhea, 132–134
drug-induced hepatitis, 137–138
esophageal dysmotility, 157–158
gastric neoplasm, 437
gastric stasis, 438
gastroenteritis, 437
gastrointestinal bleeding, 373, 437–439
hepatic inflammation
alcoholic liver disease, 134–136
α_1-antitrypsin deficiency, 136
autoimmune hepatitis, 136–137
hemochromatosis, 138–139
hepatitis A, 139–140
hepatitis B, 95, 140–141
hepatitis C, 142–143
hepatitis D, 143
hepatitis E, 144
ischemic hepatitis, 144
Wilson's disease, 145–146, 200, 201
lower GI bleeding
amoebic colitis, 124
angiodysplasia, 113–114, 125
colorectal cancer, 125–126
diverticulosis, 126–127
hemorrhoids, 127–128
infectious colitis, 128
inflammatory bowel disease, 128–130, 149, 438
ischemic bowel disease, 130–131
radiation enteritis, 131
pancreatic cancer, 156–157
pediatrics, 297–303

Gastroenterology—*continued*
  surgery
    abdominal injury, 434–435
    appendicitis, 436–437
    cystitis, 444–445
    gallbladder disease, 439–441
  upper GI bleeding
    angiodysplasia, 113–114, 438
    aortoenteric fistula, 113
    causes, 437–438
    diverticulosis, 438
    esophageal cancer, 114–115
    esophageal varices, 117–119
    esophagitis and esophageal ulcers,
      115–117
    hematobilia, 121
    hemorrhagic gastritis, 119–121
    Mallory-Weiss tears, 121–122, 437
    peptic ulcer disease, 122–124, 437
    peptic ulcer disease and, 439
Gastrointestinal swelling, 89
Gastroplasty, 73
GBM (anti-glomerular basement
  membrane) antibody, 374
GC (gonococcal) urethritis, 449, 450
GCS (*see* Glasgow Coma Scale)
Genetic factors (*see also* Hereditary
  conditions)
  African Americans
    angioedema, 5
    gastric cancer, 119
    hypertension, 3
    prostate cancer, 445
    sarcoidosis, 366
    sarcoma carcinoma, 114
  ALS (amyotrophic lateral sclerosis, 194
  Alzheimer's disease, 197
  Becker dystrophy, 213
  brain tumors, 202
  diabetes mellitus, 55
  Down syndrome, 294–296
  Duchenne dystrophy, 213
  epilepsy, 234
  facioscapulohumeral dystrophy, 213
  GRA (glucocorticoid remedial
    aldosteronism), 7
  HCM (hypertrophic cardiomyopathy),
    19, 21
  hemochromatosis, 139
  Kawasaki disease, 312–313
  Klinefelter syndrome, 294–296
  mitochondrial diseases, 217
  muscular dystrophy, 212
  myotonic dystrophy, 213, 214
  oculopharyngeal dystrophy, 214
  ovarian cancer, 245
  Parkinson's disease, 199
  premature ovarian failure, 255
  prenatal testing, 280
  pyloric stenosis, 303
  SMA (spinal muscle atrophy), 194
  spontaneous abortion, 284
  thalassemia, 170
  Turner syndrome, 28, 250, 296–297
Genital system infection, 284
Genital tract abnormality, 252 (*see also*
  Gynecology)
Gentamicin, 130, 267, 315, 448
Genus *Morbillivirus*, 313–314
GERD (gastroesophageal reflux disease),
  30–31, 115–116
German measles, 322–324
Gestational trophoblastic disease, 286
GFR (glomerular filtration rate), 11,
  397, 413
GH (growth hormone), 67, 68
Ghon lesion, 355
Giant bands, 167
Giant cell arteritis (temporal arteritis),
  416–417
Giardia species, 132, 134
Gigantism, 68
Gilbert syndrome, 148
Gingivitis, 116
Gitelman syndrome, 402
Glasgow Coma Scale (GCS), 75, 79,
  108, 109
Glatiramer, 205
Glial tumors, 202
Glioblastoma, 202
Global disorientation, 107
α-Globin genes, 170
β-Globin genes, 170
Glomerulonephritis, 406
Glossitis, 166
Glucagon, 60, 90
Glucocorticoid therapy, 65, 71, 130, 426
Glucocorticoids, 66
Glucose (*see* Blood glucose)
Glucose challenge test, 68
Glucose intolerance test, 279
Glycogen, 216
Glycogenoses, 216, 217
Glycosylated hemoglobin A_{1c}, 56
GnRH (gonadotropin-releasing
  hormone) agonists, 242

GnRH analogs, 240
GnRH stimulation test, 250
Gold therapy, 431
Gonadal dysgenesis (Turner syndrome), 28, 250
Gonadectomy, 250
Gonadotropin therapy, 263
Gonococcal septic arthritis, 432–433
Gonococcal urethritis, 449
Goodpasture syndrome, 407
Gout, 428–430, 432
GRA (glucocorticoid remedial aldosteronism), 6–7 (*see also* Hyperaldosteronism)
Gram-negative bacteria, 444, 447
Gram stain, 190, 266, 300, 433
Graves disease, 62, 63
Grey Turner sign, 155
Group C streptococci, 317
Group G streptococci, 317
Growth and development (*see* Pediatrics)
Growth hormone (*see* GH)
Guaiac test, 120, 125, 126
Guglielmi coils, 232
Guillain-Barré syndrome, 206–207, 212 (*see also* AIDP)
Gynecology (*see also* Obstetrics)
  breast cancer, 259–260
  cervical cancer, 247–249
  climacteric, 254–259
  endometriosis, 239–240
  menopause, 254–259
  menstrual disorders
    amenorrhea, 68, 249–252
    dysfunctional uterine bleeding, 252–254
  ovarian cancer, 245–247
  PID (pelvic inflammatory disease), 265–267
  uterus
    endometriosis, 239–240
    leiomyoma, 240–243
    uterine cancer, 243–245
Gynecomastia, 295, 296

H^+ concentration, 386
H_2 blockers, 155
H_2-receptor antagonist, 31, 120, 121, 123
Habitual abortion, 284
"HACEK" group (*Haemophilus, Actinobacillus, Cardiobacterium, Eikenella, Kingella*), 184

Haemophilus influenzae
  ABRS (acute bacterial rhinosinusitis) and, 178
  acute otitis media and, 176
  epiglottitis and, 308
  functional asplenia and, 172
  HIV and, 352
  infective endocarditis and, 184
  meningitis and, 314
  pneumonia and, 319, 351
  preventive strategies, 316
  septic shock and, 99
Hallucinations, 108
Haloperidol, 330
Halothane, 137
Hampton hump, 37
Hartmann pouch, 439
Hashimoto thyroiditis, 61
"Hatchet face" appearance, 214
HAV (hepatitis A virus), 139–140
HAV IgM serum, 139
HbA_{1c}, 196
HBC (hepatitis C virus), 95, 142–143
HBeAg test, 141
HBIG (hepatitis B immunoglobulin), 141, 310
HBsAg test, 140
HbSS (homozygous S) patients, 171
HBV (hepatitis B virus), 95, 140–141, 412
HBV vaccine, 310
HCC (*see* Hepatocellular carcinoma)
hCG (human chorionic gonadotropin), 268–269, 286
β-hCG level, 253, 268–269, 270, 279
HCM (hypertrophic cardiomyopathy), 19–21
HCV (hepatitis C virus), 142–143
Head trauma, 77–80, 228, 230 (*see also* Stroke)
Hearing loss, 176, 191
Heart (*see* Aortic aneurysms; Cardiology; Coronary artery disease)
Heart block, 91
Heart murmur, 183
Heberden nodes, 428
Heimlich valve, 87–88
Heinz bodies, 170
Helical CT scanning, 11, 13
Helicobacter pylori gastritis, 119, 120, 123, 438
Helium and oxygen, for croup, 307
HELLP (hemolysis elevated liver enzymes, and low platelet count), 275

Hemartoma, 379
Hematobilia, 121
Hematocrit, 120, 438
Hematology and oncology
  anemia
    aplastic, 168–169
    of chronic disease, 173–174
    iron deficiency anemia, 119,
      165–168
    sickle cell disease, 171–173
    sideroblastic, 169–170
    thalassemia, 170–171
  hemophilia, 174–175
  malignant neoplasms
    acute leukemia, 159–160
    chronic lymphocytic leukemia,
      162–163
    chronic myelogenous leukemia,
      160–162
    Hodgkin lymphoma, 163–164
    non-Hodgkin lymphoma, 164–165
  von Willebrand disease, 175
Hematuria, 406
Hemiparesis, 228, 237
Hemiplegic migraine, 228
Hemochromatosis, 138–139, 429
Hemodynamic compromise, 80
Hemodynamic instability, 86
Hemodynamic monitoring, 96
Hemoglobin, 166, 438
Hemoglobin A₂, 171
Hemoglobin electrophoresis, 171, 172
Hemoglobin genes, 170
Hemoglobin H disease, 171
Hemolysis, 170
Hemolytic anemia, 278
Hemolytic reaction, 95
β-Hemolytic streptococcus (see also
  GABHS), 270, 321
Hemophilia, 174–175
Hemophilias, 280
Hemopoietic cells, 168
Hemoptysis, 373–375
Hemorrhage
  anticoagulant, 81
  controlling, 75
  epidural, 79
  intracranial, 77, 78, 79, 109, 397
Hemorrhagic adrenal infarction, 65
Hemorrhagic gastritis, 119–121
Hemorrhagic shock, 93–95
Hemorrhagic stroke, 228
Hemorrhagic telangiectasia, 373

Hemorrhoids, 127–128, 438
Hemothorax, 82, 83, 86
Hemotympanum, 78
Henoch-Schönlein purpura, 301, 408
Heparin, 38, 223, 403
Hepatic coagulopathy, 152
Hepatic encephalopathy, 152–153, 235
Hepatitis, 63, 134, 136, 356, 408
Hepatitis A, 139–140
Hepatitis A vaccine, 186
Hepatitis B, 95, 140–141
Hepatitis B vaccine, 143, 186
Hepatitis C, 95, 142–143, 412
Hepatitis D, 143
Hepatitis E, 144
Hepatitis E serum antibody test, 144
Hepatobiliary ultrasound, 134
Hepatocellular carcinoma (hepatoma),
  136, 139, 140, 143, 148–149 (see also
  Cirrhosis)
Hepatorenal syndrome, 153
Heptoglobin, 172
Hereditary conditions (see also Genetic
  factors)
  angiodysplasia, 113
  facioscapulohumeral dystrophy, 213
  HCM (hypertrophic cardiomyopathy),
    19
  hemophilia, 174
  obesity, 72
  ovarian cancer, 245
  renal parenchymal hypertension, 10
  sideroblastic anemia, 169, 170
Hernia, 440–441
Herpes simplex, 116, 180
Herpes simplex virus encephalitis,
  188–189
Herpes varicella (chickenpox), 48,
  305–306
Herpes zoster ("shingles"), 48–49
Heterophile antibodies, 180
Heterotopic pregnancy, 268,
  269–270, 271
Hexosaminidase A, 196
Hiatal hernia, 31, 122
HIB (Haemophilus influenzae type B)
  vaccine, 310, 311, 314
HIDA (hepatoiminodiacetic acid) scan,
  134, 148, 439, 440
High-power fields, 242
Hip joint, septic arthritis, 432, 433
Hippocampus, 197
Hirsutism, 67

Histamine, 89
Histoplasma, 352
Histoplasmosis, 379
Histrionic personality disorder, 349
HIV/AIDS, 26, 184–186, 189, 228, 247
  (*see also* AIDS)
HLA-B27 test, 424, 426
Hodgkin lymphoma, 163–164
Holter monitor, 111
Homozygous S patients (HbSS), 171
Hormone replacement therapy (*see*
  HRT)
Horner syndrome, 225, 226, 381
Howell-Jolly bodies, 172
HPFs (high-power fields), 242
HPIV-1 (human parainfluenza type 1
  virus), 306
HPV (human papillomavirus), 53,
  95, 247
HRT (hormone replacement therapy),
  71, 252, 256, 258–259
HSG (hysterosalpingogram), 262–263
HTLV (Human T-cell lymphotrophic
  virus), 95
Human chorionic gonadotropin (hCG),
  268–269
Human immunodeficiency virus (*see*
  HIV/AIDS)
Human papillomavirus (*see* HPV)
Humoral immunity defects, 189
Huntington's disease, 200, 280
Hydatid cyst, 379
Hydralazine, 25
Hydramnios, 278
Hydration, 130
Hydrocephalus, 109, 191, 198, 348
Hydrocortisone, 62, 66
Hydrogen ion (acidosis), 95, 100
Hydronephrosis, 443
Hydrops fetalis, 171, 323
Hydroxychloroquine, 216, 421, 431
Hymenoptera, 89
Hyperaldosteronism, 5–7, 387, 402 (*see*
  also GRA)
Hyperbilirubinemia, 439
Hypercalcemia, 64, 400
Hypercalciuria, 64
Hypercapnia, 24, 362, 370
Hypercapnic respiratory failure, 369–370
Hypercholesterolemia, 220, 344
Hypercoagulable states, 130
Hyperemia, 103, 438
Hypergammaglobulinemia, 367

Hyperglucagonemia, 57
Hyperglycemia, 2, 57, 58, 59, 72, 157, 405
Hyperglyceridemia, 220
Hyperkalemia, 65, 66, 95, 100, 403–405
Hyperkalemic periodic paralyses, 216
Hyperketonemia, 58
Hyperlipidemia, 71, 223, 396, 411 (*see*
  also Nephrology)
Hypernatremia, 5, 399–401 (*see also*
  Hyponatremia; Nephrology)
Hyperparathyroidism, 71, 393, 409, 429
Hyperpigmentation, 65, 66
Hyperplasia, 64
Hyperprolactinemia, 68
Hyperproteinemia, 396 (*see also*
  Nephrology)
Hypersegmented neutrophils, 167
Hypersensitivity pneumonitis, 365
Hypertension (*see* Cardiology,
  hypertension)
Hypertensive retinopathy, 4
Hyperthermia, 102
Hyperthyroidism, 3, 39, 62–64, 71
Hypertonic saline, 70
Hypertrophic cardiomyopathy, 20, 110
Hyperuricemia, 220, 223
Hyperventilation, 35, 58, 102
Hypoalbuminemia, 344
Hypocalcemia, 95, 234
Hypocapnia, 27
Hypochloremic metabolic alkalosis, 344
Hypochondriasis, 342
Hypochromic microcytic anemia, 166
Hypoestrogenic amenorrhea, 251
Hypoglycemia, 60, 65, 66, 68, 107, 111,
  112, 234, 326
Hypoglycemic agents, 57
Hypokalemia, 2, 5, 59, 95, 100, 102, 153,
  344, 401–402
Hypomagnesemia, 5, 95, 401
Hypomania, 335
Hyponatremia, 62, 66, 70, 396–399
Hypoparathyroidism, 216
Hypoperfusion, 95
Hypophosphatemia, 59, 64
Hypopituitarism, 68, 216
Hyporeflexia, 62
Hypotension, 62, 86, 93, 339
Hypothalamic disease, 67, 250, 251
Hypothalamus, 69
Hypothermia, 61, 62, 76, 95, 102
Hypothyroidism, 3, 61–62, 72, 216, 220,
  223, 284, 429

Hypoventilation, 62, 369
Hypovolemia, 69, 96, 100, 111
Hypovolemic shock, 96–97, 104
Hypoxemia, 27, 83, 362
Hypoxemic respiratory failure, 368–370
Hypoxia, 100, 307, 384, 387
Hysterectomy, 243

IABP (intra-aortic balloon pump), 93
ICD (implantable cardioverter
    defibrillator), 20, 43
ICP (intracranial pressure), 187,
    188, 229
Idiopathic ALS, 195
Idiopathic epilepsy, 234
Idiopathic nephrotic syndrome, 413
Idiosyncratic hepatotoxins, 137
IE (infective endocarditis), 14, 21,
    182–184
IFN-a, 61, 141, 142
IgA nephropathy, 408, 409
IgG (antinuclear antibody
    hypergammaglobulinemia), 137, 139,
    143, 204
IgM anti-HBcAb, 140, 143
ILD (interstitial lung disease), 363–365
Ileostomy, 130
Imipramine therapy, 325, 339
Immune system dysregulation, 203
Immunizations, 310–312
Immunoglobulins, 162, 207, 220
Immunosuppressive therapy, 220
Impetigo, 406
Implantable cardioverter-defibrillator
    (see ICD)
In vitro fertilization (see IVF)
[111]In-octreotide scintigraphy, 9
Inactivated (Salk) poliovirus vaccine, 192
Incentive spirometry, 83
Inclusion-body myositis, 218
Incomplete abortion, 284, 286–287
Incontinentia pigmenti, 280
Indinavir, 186
Indomethacin, 277
Inevitable abortion, 284, 286
Infants, growth and development,
    288–290
Infectious disease (see also CNS;
    Pediatrics; Pulmonary disorders)
    altered mental status and, 107
    head and neck
        acute otitis media, 176–177
        acute sinusitis, 178–179

exudative pharyngitis, 180–181
    oral thrush, 182
HIV/AIDS, 184–186
infectious colitis, 128
infective endocarditis, 182–184
inflammatory diarrhea, 132–134
mononucleosis, 180
sickle cell disease and, 172
Infectious mononucleosis, 318
Infectious mononucleosis viral
    pharyngitis, 318
Infectious myositis, 217–218
Infective carditis, 182–184
Infective colitis, 438
Infective endocarditis, 14, 21, 182–184
Inferior vena cava filter, 38
Infertility, 260–265, 295
Inflammatory bowel disease, 128–130,
    149, 438
Inflammatory myopathies, 215
Influenza, 178, 217–218, 306, 317, 325,
    351 (see also Haemophilus
    influenzae)
Influenza vaccine, 186
Inguinal hernia, 441
Injection drug users, 183
Inorganic dust ILD, 365
Inotropes, 22
Inotropic agents, 24
Inotropic support, 100
Insect stings, 89
Insulin clearance, 394
Insulin resistance, 72
Insulin sensitizers, 57
Insulin therapy, 56–57, 60, 405
Intercostal nerve block, 83
Interferon, 161
Interferon alfa, 61, 141, 142
Interferon beta, 205
Interferon gamma, 364
Interleukin-2, 61
International Federation of Gynecology
    and Obstetrics (see FIGO)
Internuclear ophthalmoplegia, 203
Interstitial lung disease, 320
Intra-aortic balloon counterpulsation, 22
Intra-aortic balloon pump (see IABP)
Intracranial hemorrhage, 77, 78, 79, 109,
    228–230, 328, 397
Intracytoplasmic sperm injection, 263
Intraesophageal pH monitoring, 116
Intramuscular (IM) vitamin B_{12}, 168
Intrathecal antibodies, 203

Intrauterine cardiac death, 278
Intrauterine growth failure, 278
Intravenous pyelogram, 410
Intravenous pyelography, 242, 248, 449
Intussusception, 301–302, 438
Iodine, 61
Ionizing radiation, 114
Ipecac, 216, 345
IPF (idiopathic pulmonary fibrosis, 363–364
Ipratropium, 362
Ipsilateral Horner syndrome, 225
IPV (inactivated poliovirus vaccine), 192
Iron deficiency anemia, 119, 165–168, 171
Iron overload, 170
Irritable bowel syndrome, 414
Ischemia, 39, 43
Ischemic bowel disease, 130–131
Ischemic exercise testing, 217
Ischemic heart disease, 111
Ischemic hepatitis, 144
Isocarboxazid, 339
Isoniazid, 137, 169, 355
Isotonic saline, 59
Isotretinoin, 45
"Itch mite" (*Sarcoptes scabiei*), 49
IUD (intrauterine device), 281
IUDs (injection drug users), 183
IV hydration for sickle cell crisis, 173
IVF (in vitro fertilization), 263, 264, 265, 268
IVP (intravenous pyelogram), 242, 248, 449

J points, in acute pericarditis, 25
Jaffe (picric acid) reaction, 395
Janeway lesions, 183
Jaundice, 157
Jimsonweed, 106
Juvenile rheumatoid arthritis, 313, 432
JVD (jugular venous distention), 81, 92, 390

K distribution, 387–388, 401, 403–405
K-sparing diuretics, 402
Karyotype analysis, 250, 280, 295
Kawasaki disease, 312–313, 315
Kayser-Fleischer rings, 145, 201
KCl supplements, 402
Keloids, 54
Kerley B lines, 24
Kerning sign, 315
Ketoacidosis, 58
Ketoconazole, 46, 137

Ketone body production, 57
Kidney stones, 409
Kidneys, 3, 11–12, 394, 408, 429 (*see also* Nephrology)
Kingella, 184
Klebsiella pneumoniae, 190
Knee joint
  pseudogout, 430
  septic arthritis, 432
Koilonychia ("spoon nail"), 166
Koplik spots, 313–314
KUB (kidneys, ureter, and bladder), 410
Kussmaul sign, 58
Kyphoscoliosis, 370

L5-S1 disk, 422
β-Lactamase inhibitor, 353
Lactate dehydrogenase, 138, 161, 216
Lactic acidosis, 388, 389
Lactic dehydrogenase levels, 326
Lacunar strokes, 224
Lambert-Eaton syndrome, 209
Lamivudine, 141
Lamivudine (3TC), 186
Language skills
  preschoolers, 292
  toddlers, 291
Laparoscopic cholecystectomy, 121, 147, 148
Laparoscopy, 157, 240, 262, 263, 264, 266, 271
Laparotomy, 240, 264, 271, 434, 435
Laryngeal edema, 89
Laryngitis, 116
Laryngospasm, 308
Lateral medullary syndrome, 225
Lateral neck x-ray, 309, 322
Laxative abuse, 345
LDH (lactate dehydrogenase), 138, 161, 172, 376
Lead poisoning, 169, 290
Left ventricular infarction, 33, 91
Legionella influenza, 351
Legionella pneumophila, 99, 319, 351
Leiomyoma, 240–243
Leiomyosarcoma, 119
Leptin, 72
Leptospirosis, 313
Leukapheresis, 160, 162
Leukocytosis, 161, 439
Leukopenia, 344
Leukostasis, 160
Leukotrienes, 89

Levodopa/carbidopa, 201
Levofloxacin, 353
Lewy bodies, 198, 200, 348
LH (luteinizing hormone), 67, 242, 297
Licorice ingestion, 402
Lidocaine, 210
Life-table analysis, 281
Life-threatening conditions, 74, 84, 130
Lifelong copper-chelating agents, 145
Lindane cream, 50
Linear salpingostomy, 271
Lipase, 155
Lipid metabolism, 216
Lipoma, 379
Listeria monocytogenes, 190, 314
Lithium, 61, 210, 335, 340, 400
Liver biopsy, 136, 137
Liver diseases, 136, 429
Liver enzyme tests, 134
Liver function studies, 109, 198, 237, 338, 374, 382
Liver, injury, 434
Liver transplant, 143, 145–146
Lobar hemorrhage, 228, 229
LOC (loss of consciousness), 80
Locked-in syndrome, 226
Locus ceruleus, 197
Long-acting contraceptives, 282
Loperamide, 132
Loratadine, 42
Lower back pain, 421–422
Lumbar puncture, 187, 190, 198, 235, 315
Lung abscess, 351
Lung cancer, 2, 66, 70, 202, 381–383, 397
Lung/chest wall abscess, 34
Lupus anticoagulant syndrome, 227
Lupus syndrome, drug-induced, 63
LV infarction (*see* Left ventricular infarction)
LVEDP (left ventricular end-diastolic pressure), 15
Lye ingestion, 114
Lyme disease, 414–416, 432
Lymph node status, 157
Lymphadenopathy, 163
Lymphocyte count, 163
Lymphoid hyperplasia, 436
Lymphoma, 202
Lynch II syndrome, 259

Macroglossia, 377
Macrolides, 179, 320, 321, 353

Macrovascular disease, 55
Magnesium, 235
Magnesium sulfate, 42, 102, 210, 277
Magnetic resonance angiography, 11, 13
Male-factor infertility, 261, 263
Malignancy, 34, 169
Malignant melanoma, 52–53
Malignant neoplasms, 159–165
Mallory hyaline, 134
Mallory-Weiss tears, 121–122, 437
Mammography, 260
Mandibular osteotomy-hyoid myotomy), 378
Manganese, 200
Mania, 335
MAO-B inhibitors, 199
MAO (monoamine oxidase inhibitor), 73
MAOIs (monoamine oxidase inhibitors), 333, 334, 338, 339
Marfan syndrome, 15, 28, 280, 441
Massive transfusion, 95
Mastoiditis, 177
Maternal serum α-fetoprotein, 279
McBurney's point, 436
MCP (metacarpophalangeal) joints, 431
MCV (mean cell volume), 126, 134, 166, 168
MDR-TB (multiple drug-resistant TB), 354, 356
Mean arterial pressure, 92
Mean cell volume (*see* MCV)
Measles (rubeola), 313–314
Mechanical dysphagia, 157
Meckel diverticulum, 301, 437, 438
Mediastinal emphysema, 31–32
Mediastinal germ cell tumors, 295
Medroxyprogesterone acetate, 253, 258
Megaloblastic anemia, 167–168
MELAS syndrome, 227–228
Membrane active agents, 41
Membranoproliferative glomerulonephritis, 413
Membranous glomerulopathy, 413
MEN (multiple endocrine neoplasia), 8 (*see also* Pheochromocytoma)
Meningioma, 202, 203
Meningitides, 317
Meningitis
  acute otitis media and, 177, 179
  aseptic, 190
  bacterial, 99, 190
  carcinomatous, 207

diagnosis and treatment, 79–80, 189–191
epilepsy and, 235
hyponatremia and, 397
pediatrics and, 314–316
pneumonia and, 353
preventing, 79–80
Menopause, 254–259
Mental development, 295, 297 (*see also* Pediatrics)
Mental retardation, 277, 295
Mental status, altered, 107–110, 152
Mental status exam, 109
Meperidine, 210, 395
Mesalamine, 131
Metabolic abnormalities, 72
Metabolic acidosis, 58, 345, 385
Metabolic alkalosis, 5, 345, 384, 387
Metabolic encephalopathy, 107
Metabolic enzyme deficiencies, 215
Metabolic myopathy, 216, 217
Metabolic syncope, 110
Metastatic bone disease, 422
Metformin, 57
Methacholine, 31
Methacholine challenge test, 358
Methanol, 388
Methimazole, 63
Methotrexate, 220, 271, 417
3-methoxy-4-hydroxymandelic acid, 9
Methyldopa, 137
Methylphenidate, 331
Methylprednisolone, 90, 205
Methysergide, 25
Metronidazole, 47, 123, 124, 134, 216
MHA-TP (microhemagglutination-*Treponema pallidum*), 51
MI (myocardial infarction), 32–34, 43, 58, 100, 110, 221 (*see also* Stroke)
MIBG (^{123}I- or ^{131}I-metaiodobenzylguanidine), 9
Microcytic hypochromic BBCs, 171
Microemboli, 98
Micrognathia, 377
Microhemagglutination-*Treponema pallidum* (MHA-TP), 51
Microinvasive carcinoma, 248–249
Middle ear, columnar epithelium, 177
Migraines, 228
Miller-Fisher variant, 212 (*see also* Guillain-Barré syndrome)
Mineralocorticoids, 66
Mini-mental state examination (MMSE), 348

Minimal change (nil) disease, 413
Minnesota Multiphasic Personality Inventory, 350
Misoprostol, 124
Mitochondrial cytopathies, 215
Mitochondrial disease, 216
Mitoxantrone, 205
Mitral annular calcification, 21 (*see also* MI)
Mitral regurgitation, 21–23, 92 (*see also* MI)
Mitral stenosis, 23
Mitral valve disease, 228
Mitral valve insufficiency, 91
Mitral valve prolapse, 21 (*see also* MI)
MLH1 gene, 244
MMO (maxillary and mandibular advancement), 378
MMR (polio, measles, mumps, rubella) vaccine, 310, 311, 323
MMSE (mini-mental state examination), 348
MOHM (mandibular osteotomy-hyoid myotomy), 378
Monoarthritis, 430
Monospot (heterophil antibodies), 318
Mood disorders (*see* Psychiatry)
Mood stabilizers, 350
Moraxella catarrhalis, 176, 178
Morbilliform rash, 313–314
Morphine, 210
Morphine sulfate, 24
Mosaicism, 295
Motility disorder, 157
Motor neuron disease, 194–196
Motor neuropathies, 195
Motor skills
infants, 288
preschoolers, 292
toddlers, 290, 291
MPTP, 200
MR (*see* Mitral regurgitation)
MRI (magnetic resonance imaging)
for aortic dissection, 29
brain imaging, 79, 187, 188, 201, 202, 230, 238
of cervical and thoracic spine, 196
for coarctation of the aorta, 1
for hyperaldosteronism, 6
for osteomyelitis, 423
for pericardial fluid, 26
for pheochromocytoma, 9
for prostate cancer, 446

MRI—*continued*
  for retropharyngeal abscess, 322
  T2-weighted, 204
MSH2 gene, 244
MTB (*Mycobacterium tuberculosis*), 354
Mucocutaneous bleeding, 175
Multifactorial anemia, 166
Multiple endocrine neoplasia (*see* MEN)
Multiple myeloma, 71, 422
Multiple sclerosis, 203–205
Mumps, 316–317
Munchausen syndrome, 327, 342
Murphy sign, 147, 439
Muscular dystrophy, 212–215, 370
MVP, 21 (*see also* Mitral valve
  prolapse)
Myasthenia gravis, 208–211, 212, 370
Mycobacteria, 379
Mycobacterial infection, 189, 190
Mycobacterium tuberculosis, 352
Mycoplasma, 306
Mycoplasma pneumoniae, 180, 206,
  319, 351
Mycoplasma species, 319
Mycotic aneurysm, 233
Myectomy, 21
Myelodysplastic syndrome, 169
Myocardial contusion, 91
Myocardial infarction (*see* MI)
Myocardial ischemia, 89, 371
Myoglobinuria, 219
Myoma (*see* Leiomyoma)
Myomectomy, 243, 264
Myometritis, 99
Myopathy, 215–217
Myositis, 217–220
Myotomy, 21
Myotonic dystrophy, 214, 215, 280
Myotubular myopathy, 216
Myxedema crisis, 61

N-acetylcysteine, 13, 138
Nafcillin, 424, 433
Nailbed infarcts, 218
Narcissistic personality disorder, 349
Narcotic overdose, 110
Narcotics (*see* Analgesics)
Nasal congestion, 89
Natural family planning, 283–284
NCA (neutrophil chemotactic activity), 89
Nebulized racemic epinephrine, 307
Necrosis, 98
Needle biopsy, 446

Negative inotropic calcium channel
  blocker, 29–30
Neisseria gonorrhoeae, 180, 266, 317, 449
Neisseria meningitidis, 190, 191, 314, 316
Nemaline rod myopathy, 216
Neoplasms, 202–203
Nephrogenic DI, 69, 70
Nephrology
  acid-base disorders, 384–389
  ARF (acute renal failure), 389–392, 411
  CRF (chronic renal failure), 392–396
  hyperkalemia, 65, 66, 95, 100,
    403–405
  hypernatremia, 399–401
  hypokalemia, 2, 5, 59, 95, 100, 102,
    153, 344, 401–402
  hyponatremia, 62, 66, 70, 396–399
  nephritic edema, 407
  nephritic syndrome, 406–409
  nephrolithiasis, 409–411, 443
  nephropathy, 55
  nephrotic syndrome, 411–413
  pediatrics and, 324–326
  pyelonephritis, 448–449
  renal insufficiency, 59, 64, 275, 443
  renal parenchyma infection, 448
Nephrotoxins, 395
Nerve conduction studies, 195, 206, 370
Neurofibromatosis, 8, 202, 280 (*see also*
  Pheochromocytoma)
Neurogenic bladder, 205
Neuroimaging, 198
Neurologic syncope, 110, 112
Neurologic testing, 111
Neuromuscular junction and muscle
  (*see* CNS)
Neuropathic arthropathy, 432
Neuropathy, 55
Neurotic (β-amyloid) plaques, 348
Neurotransmitters, 338
Neutropenia, 98, 162, 163
Neutrophil chemotaxis, 371
Neutrophilia, 98
Neutrophils, hypersegmented, 167
Newborns (*see* Infants)
NFH gene, 194
NGC (nongonococcal) urethritis,
  449, 450
NHL (non-Hodgkin lymphoma),
  164–165
Nifedipine, 277
Night terrors, 293
Nil disease, 413

NIPPV (noninvasive positive-pressure ventilation), 370
Nissen fundoplication, 116
Nitrates, 20
Nitrofurantoin, 137, 445
Nitroglycerin, 24, 118
Nitroprusside, 22, 24, 30
Nocardia species, 352
Non-Hodgkin lymphoma, 164–165
Non-nucleoside analog reverse transcriptase inhibitor, 186
Non–small cell carcinoma, 382
Nonbacterial prostatitis, 447, 448
Nonglial tumors, 202
Nongonococcal urethritis, 449, 450
Noninfectious inflammatory disorders, 109
Noninflammatory diarrhea, 131–132
Nonketotic hyperosmolar coma, 59–60
Nonparalytic poliomyelitis, 192
Noonan syndrome, 28
Norepinephrine, 100, 338
Norfloxacin, 154
Normochromic normocytic anemia, 173
Nortriptyline, 339
Norwalk virus, 131, 299
Nosocomial pneumonia, 352, 353
NSAIDs (nonsteroidal anti-inflammatory drugs), 400
  for acute gouty arthritis, 428
  for acute pericarditis, 26
  chronic renal failure and, 395
  for colitic arthritis, 426
  contraindication for hemophilia, 174
  contraindications, 429
  for hemoptysis, 373
  hemorrhagic gastritis and, 120
  hyponatremia and, 398
  for kidney stones, 410
  Misoprostol and, 124
  peptic ulcer disease and, 122
  for pleurisy, 35
  for PMR and TA, 417
  for pseudogout, 430
  for psoriatic arthritis, 427
  for rheumatoid arthritis, 431
  for SLE (systemic lupus erythematosus), 421
  upper GI bleeding and, 438
Nulliparity, 244, 256
Nuts, 89
NYHA (New York Heart Association), 16, 23

Nystatin, 46
Nystatin clotrimazole troches, 182

Oat-cell (small cell) lung cancer, 2, 66, 70
Obesity, 71–73, 223, 244
Obesity-hypoventilation syndrome, 370
Obsessive-compulsive personality disorder, 332, 350
Obstetrics (*see also* Gynecology)
  abortion, 284–287
  contraception, 281–284
  female infertility, 260–265
  pregnancy
    abruptio placentae, 272–273
    cystitis and, 444
    drugs contraindicated, 45, 63, 124
    ectopic pregnancy, 267–272, 286, 437
    HIV/AIDS and, 186
    placenta previa, 273–274
    pregnancy-induced hypertension, 274–275
    premature labor, 276–277
    prenatal testing, 277–280
    respiratory alkalosis and, 384
    septic shock and, 99
    sickle cell disease and, 172
Obturator sign, 436
Occult blood in stool, 120
Occupational lung diseases, 364–365
OCD (obsessive-compulsive disorder, 332, 350
Octreotide infusion, 118
Oculopharyngeal dystrophy, 214, 215
Oligoarthritis, 424
Oligoclonal bands, 203
Oligodendrogliomas, 202
Oliguria, 59
Omeprazole and amoxicillin, 123
Open-lung biopsy, 364, 380
Opsonins, 412
Optic nerve dysfunction, 366
Optic neuritis, 203
OPV (oral polio vaccine), 192
Oral azole antifungals, 182
Oral contraceptives, 253, 254, 282–283
Oral hypoglycemic agents, 57
Oral ribavirin, 142
Oral thrush, 182
Organic disease, 108
Organic dust ILD, 365
Organophosphates, 216
Orientation, in altered mental status, 107
Orlistat, 72, 73

Orthostatic hypotension, 110, 111, 112
Orthostatic test, 127
OSAHS (obstructive sleep apnea-hypopnea syndrome), 377–379
Osler nodes, 183
Osteoarthritis, 71, 427–428
Osteomalacia, 71
Osteomyelitis, 423–424
Osteoporosis, 67, 70–71, 255, 256, 422
Otitis media, acute, 176–177
Outer zone of hyperemia, 103
Ovarian cancer, 245–247
Ovarian cyst, 437
Ovulatory dysfunction, 263–264, 284
Oxacillin, 47
Oxygen
    for cardiogenic shock, 92
    consumption, 96
    extraction, 97
    for hypoxia, 307
    for ILD (interstitial lung disease), 365
Oxygen saturation, 304
Oxytocin, 69

P-ANCA levels, 409
P-wave, 81
P_2 heart sound, 361
p53 tumor suppressor gene, 243, 245
Pacemaker (*see* Ventricular pacemaker)
Packed red blood cells, 123
$PaCO_2$ value, 369
PAF (platelet-activating factor), 89
Paget disease, 3, 422
Pain disorder, 342–343
Palivizumab, 304
Pallidotomy, 201
Pan cultures, 160
Pancoast tumor, 381
Pancreas
    acute pancreatitis, 154–156, 439
    chronic pancreatitis, 146
    pancreatic cancer, 156–157
Pancytopenia, 168
Panic disorder, 333
PaO_2 (partial pressure of oxygen), 357, 364, 368 (*see also* Oxygen)
PAOP (pulmonary artery occlusion pressure), 24, 371
Pap smear, 244, 248
Papaverine, 232
Papillary muscle dysfunction, 92
Papillary serous adenocarcinoma, 244
Papilledema, 231

Paracentesis, 152
Paradoxical chest wall motion, 82
Parainfluenza, 178, 317
Parainfluenza type 3, 306
Parainfluenza virus, 217
Paralytic poliomyelitis, 192
Paramyxovirus, 313–314, 316
Paranasal sinus infections, 187
Paranoid personality disorder, 349
Paranoid schizophrenia, 329
Parapneumonic effusions, 353, 375, 376
Paraprotein, 411
Parathyroid adenoma, 64
Parathyroid gland (*see* Endocrine disorders)
Parathyroid hormone (*see* PTH)
Parathyroidectomy, 65
Parenchymal disease, 368, 373
Parenteral iron replacement, 166
Parenteral penicillin, 89
Paresthesias, 61
Parietal lobe, 197
Parkinson's disease, 199–201
Parkland formula, 104
Paroxysm, 298
Partial salpingectomy, 271
Partial thromboplastin time (*see* PTT)
Pauci-immune RPGN, 409
pCO_2 level, 386
PCP (*Pneumocystis carinii* pneumonia), 26, 356–360
PCR (polymerase chain reaction), 142
PE (*see* Pulmonary embolism)
PEA (pulseless electrical activity), 100
Peak capacity flow, 359
Pearl Index, 281
Pediatrics
    child abuse, 326–328
    gastroenterology
        colic, 297–299
        diarrhea/gastroenteritis, 299–301
        intussusception, 301–302
        pyloric stenosis, 302–303
    genetic disorders
        Down syndrome, 293–294
        Klinefelter syndrome, 294–296
        Turner syndrome, 28, 250, 296–297
    growth and development
        infants, 288–290
        preschoolers, 292–293
        toddlers, 290–292
    infectious diseases
        chickenpox, 48, 305–306

croup, 306–307
epiglottitis, 308–309
FUO (fever of unknown origin), 309–310
immunizations, 310–312
Kawasaki disease, 312–313, 315
measles (rubeola), 313–314
meningitis, 314–316
mumps, 316–317
pharyngitis, 317–319, 321
pneumonia, 319–321
retropharyngeal abscess, 321–322
Reye syndrome, 315
RSV (respiratory syncytial virus), 304–305
rubella, 322–324
nephrology, 324–326
PEEP (positive end-respiratory pressure), 371, 372
Pelvic adhesions, 264
Pelvic exenteration, 249
Pelvic fractures, 435
Pelvic sonography, 240
Penicillamine, 168, 208, 431
D-Penicillamine, 145, 218
Penicillin, 181, 318, 320, 353, 445
Peptic strictures, 116
Peptic ulcer disease, 122–124, 437, 439
Peptostreptococci, 266
Percutaneous needle aspiration, 380
Percutaneous nephrostomy, 449
Pergolide, 201
Pericardial effusion, 25, 26
Pericardial tamponade, 91, 92, 110
Pericardiocentesis, 81, 82
Pericarditis, 25–26, 39, 81, 431
Perimenopause, 254
Periorbital edema, 61, 218
Peripheral blood smear, 159
Peripheral neuropathy, 356
Peripheral vascular disease, 55, 130
Peristalsis, 301
Peritoneal carcinoma, 246
Peritoneal invasion, 157
Peritonsillar abscess, 321
Periumbilical node, 156
Permethrin cream, 50
Pernicious anemia, 150, 208
Personality disorders, 349–350
Personality test, 350
Pertussis vaccine, 310
PET (position emission tomography), 164, 380

Petechiae, 183
PFT (pulmonary function tests), 358, 359, 383
pH monitoring, 116, 386, 410
Pharyngitis, 180–181, 317–319, 321, 406
Phenelzine, 339
Phenothiazine, 102, 227, 398
Phenothiazines, 210
Phentolamine, 10
Phenylketonuria, 234, 280
Phenytoin, 25, 137, 189, 210, 236
Pheochromocytoma, 7–10
Philadelphia chromosome, 161
Phlebotomy, 139
Phosphate binders, 393
Phosphodiesterase inhibitors, 24
Phosphoglycerate mutase, 216
Phosphorus, 137
Phosphorylase, 216
Physical therapy, for rheumatoid arthritis, 431
Physiologic stress, 122
Pick's disease, 198
Picric acid (Jaffe) reaction, 395
PID (pelvic inflammatory disease), 265–267
Pinpoint pupils, 110
PIO$_2$ (partial pressure of inspired oxygen), 368 (see also Oxygen)
Pioglitazone, 57
PIP (posterior interphalangeal) joints, 428, 431
Pituitary adenoma, 67, 202
Pituitary diseases, 61, 67–70, 250
Pituitary dysfunction, 250
Pituitary irradiation, 67
Plaquenil, 367
Plasma cortisol levels, 344
Plasma D-dimer, 37
Plasma estradiol levels, 344
Plasma free-fatty acid levels, 72
Plasma, fresh frozen, 94
Plasma glucose level, 60
Plasma metanephrine:creatinine ratio, 9
Plasmapheresis, 207, 210, 220, 407
Plasminogen deficiency, 36
Platelet count, 143, 275
Platelet transfusion, 160
Platelets, 169
Pleocytosis, 187, 204
Pleural effusion, 24, 375–377
Pleurisy, 34–35
Plummer-Vinson syndrome, 114

PMN (polymorphonuclear leukocyte), 300
PMN (polymorphonuclear neutrophils), 134, 190, 353, 428
PMR (polymyalgia rheumatica), 416–417
Pneumatic dilatation, 158
Pneumococcal polysaccharide vaccine, 191
Pneumococcal vaccine, 186, 310, 311–312
Pneumococci, 172
Pneumocystis, 379
Pneumocystis carinii, 86, 186, 319, 321, 352
Pneumonia, 34, 187, 228, 319–321, 351–353, 368
Pneumothorax, 82
Pneumothorax, 26–28, 34, 86–88, 356
PO_4 level, 393
Podagra, 428
Poisoning, 105–107
Polio vaccine, 311
Poliomyelitis, 191–194, 207, 212, 218
Poliovirus, 191
Polyarthralgia, 418
Polyarthritis, 430
Polycystic ovary syndrome, 244
Polycythemia, 241
Polydipsia, 58
Polyhydramnios, 272
Polymerizes ("sickles"), 171
Polymyositis, 417–418
Polymyxins, 210
Polyuria, 58
Pontine hemorrhage, 228, 229
Pontine infarct, 110
Porphyria, 207
Portal hypertension, 151–154
Portosystemic shunt surgery, 153
Post-radiation, 81
Postcoital test, 262
Posterior pituitary diseases, 69–70
Postgastrectomy patients, with hypoglycemia, 60
Postictal states, 236, 237–238
Postovulatory endometrial biopsy, 262
Postpartum depression, 340–341
Postpartum endometritis, 99
Poststreptococcal GN, 407
Potassium hydroxide, 46
Potassium supplementation, 59, 60, 152
PPD (purified protein derivative) skin test, 355, 376
Pramipexole, 201
Prazosin, 443
Precancerous lesion, 45

Prednisone, 48, 116, 134, 137, 163, 165, 219, 367, 407, 417
Pregnancy (*see* Obstetrics)
Premature labor, 276–277
Premature ovarian failure, 255–256
Presenilin-2, 197
Pretibial myxedema, 62
Primary biliary cirrhosis, 149–150
Primary hyperparathyroidism, 64–65
Primary sclerosing cholangitis, 149
Prinzmetal angina, 35–36
PRL (prolactin), 67
Probenecid, 415
Procainamide, 25, 42, 102, 210, 218, 395
Procaine, 210
Proctosigmoidoscopy, 127, 128, 129, 131
Progestational agent, 253
Progesterone, 270
Progestin challenge test, 251
Progestins, 240, 258, 282
Progestogens, 257
Prokinetic agent, 31, 116
Propafenone, 41
Propionibacterium acnes, 44
Propranolol, 334
Prostacyclin, 36, 89
Prostaglandin inhibitors, 277
Prostaglandins, 89
Prostate cancer, 445–447
Prostatectomy, 446
Prostatitis, 444, 447–448
Prosthetic valve endocarditis (PVE), 184
Protein C levels, 36, 221, 223, 227
Protein S levels, 36, 221, 223, 227
Proteinuria, 406
Prothrombin time (*see* PT)
Proton pump inhibitors, 116, 120
Protozoans, 132
PSA (prostate-specific antigen), 443, 446, 447
PSC (primary sclerosis cholangitis), 150–151
Pseudodementia, 237, 348 (*see also* Depression; Psychiatry)
Pseudogout, 429–430, 432
Pseudohyperkalemia, 403
Pseudomonas aeruginosa, 352
Psoas sign, 436
Psoriasis, 49
Psoriatic arthritis, 424, 427
Psychiatry
  ADHD, 330–331
  altered mental status and, 108

anxiety
  GAD (generalized anxiety disorder), 331–332
  OCD (obsessive-compulsive disorder), 332
  panic disorder, 333
  PTSD (posttraumatic stress disorder), 334
  social phobia, 334
cognitive disorders
  amnestic disorder, 346
  delirium, 108, 346–347
  dementia, 108, 347–349
eating disorders, 343–345
mood disorders
  adjustment disorder with depressed mood, 336
  bipolar disorder, 335–336
  complicated bereavement, 336–337
  cyclothymic disorder, 337
  dysthymic disorder, 337
  major depressive disorder, 337–339
  postpartum depression, 340–341
  puerperal psychosis, 340
personality disorders, 349–350
psychiatric syncope, 110, 112
psychiatric testing, 111
psychosis
  auditory hallucinations, 108
  puerperal, 340
  schizophrenia, 329–330
  treatment, 199
  Wilson's disease and, 145
somatoform disorders
  body dysmorphic disorder, 341
  conversion disorder, 341
  factitious disorder, 342
  hypochondriasis, 342
  pain disorder, 342–343
  somatization, 343
Psychogenic polydipsia, 398
Psychosocial learning, 295
Psychostimulants, 331
Psychotherapy, 335, 337, 338, 340, 341, 344, 345, 350
PT (prothrombin time), 134, 138, 140, 141, 157, 229, 374, 382, 438 (*see* PTT)
PTEN gene, 243
PTH (parathyroid hormone), 64, 382, 393
PTSD (posttraumatic stress disorder), 334
PTT (partial thromboplastin time), 223, 229, 374, 382, 438

PTU (propylthiouracil), 63
Puerperal psychosis, 340
Pulmonary diseases, 70, 277
Pulmonary disorders
  ARDS (adult respiratory distress syndrome), 80, 98, 368, 369, 370–373
  hemoptysis, 373–375
  infectious diseases
    PCP (*Pneumocystis carinii* pneumonia), 26, 356–360
    pneumonia, 34, 187, 228, 319–321, 351–353
    tuberculosis (TB), 70, 354–356, 365, 397, 432
  lung cancer, 2, 66, 70, 202, 381–383
  obstructive and restrictive diseases
    asthma, 90, 116, 320, 357–360, 369, 385
    COPD (chronic obstructive pulmonary disease), 26, 86, 360–363, 368, 369, 370
    ILD (interstitial lung disease), 363–365
    sarcoidosis, 366–368, 380, 432
  OSAHS (obstructive sleep apnea-hypopnea syndrome), 377–379
  pleural effusion, 24, 375–377
  pulmonary contusion, 82
  pulmonary edema, 23–25, 92, 100, 371
  pulmonary embolism, 36–38, 91, 100, 110, 373, 384, 411
  pulmonary fibrosis, 431
  pulmonary hemosiderosis, 320
  pulmonary hypertension, 89, 363
  pulmonary infarction, 34
  pulmonary parenchymal disease, 368
  respiratory failure, 368–373
  solitary pulmonary nodule, 379–381
Pulseless electrical activity), 100
Pulsus paradoxus, 81
Purified protein factor, 94
Purulent otorrhea, 176
PVE (prosthetic valve endocarditis), 184
Pyelonephritis, 437, 445, 448–449
Pyloric stenosis, 302–303
Pylorotomy, 303
Pyrazinamide, 169
Pyridostigmine, 209
Pyridoxine, 170, 356
Pyridoxine antagonists, 169

Q-waves, 20, 26
QRS complexes, 41
QT interval, 102, 344
QT syndromes, 43
Quadriplegia, 226
Qualitative HCV RNA, 143
Quinidine, 42, 102, 210

R-wave, 81
RA (see Rheumatoid arthritis)
Radiation, 168, 202 (see also CT scans; X-rays)
Radiation burns, 102
Radiation enteritis, 131
Radiation proctitis, 438
Radical prostatectomy, 446
Radiocontrast drugs, 395
Radiofrequency ablation, 41, 43, 149
Radiographic studies, 79, 155
Radiolucent stones, 410
Radionucleotide bone scanning, 423
Radionuclide scan, 439
RADTs (rapid streptococcal antigen detection tests), 318
RAI (radioactive iodine), 63
Rales, 390
Ranitidine, 123
Ranson's criteria, 156
Ranitidine, 218
Rapid antigen detection tests, 181
Rapid plasma reagin (RPR), 51
Raynaud phenomenon, 150, 418
RBC (red blood cells)
    Heinz bodies, 170
    nucleus, 169
    packed, 123
    ringed sideroblasts, 170
    for sickle cell crisis, 173
    sickle-shaped, 172
    transfusion, 95, 169
Reactive arthritis, 425
Rectal exam, 248
Rectosigmoidoscopy, 248
Red blood cells (see RBC)
Reed-Sternberg cells, 163
Regional enteritis, 437
Reiter syndrome, 424, 425–426
Renal function studies, 374
Renal insufficiency, 59, 64, 275, 443
Renal parenchymal hypertension, 10–12
Renal replacement therapy, 396
Renal tubular acidosis, 401 (see RTA)
Renal ultrasound, 410

Renal vein thrombosis, 411
Renovascular disease, 12–14
Repolarization, 102
Reset osmostat, 398
Residual schizophrenia, 330
Respiratory acidosis, 387
Respiratory alkalosis, 384–385
Respiratory chain (mitochondria), 216
Respiratory failure, 368–370
Respiratory syncytial virus, 178
Resuscitation, 76, 97
Reticulocyte count, 166
Retinal hemorrhage, 327
Retinal lesions, 183
Retinoic acid, 44
Retinopathy, 4, 55
Retrognathia, 377
Retrograde amnesia, 346
Retrograde urethrocystography, 435
Retropharyngeal abscess, 321–322
Reye syndrome, 315, 325–326
Rh-negative patients, 279, 286–287
Rhabdomyolysis, 401
Rheumatology
    arthropathies
        acute gouty arthritis, 428–429
        pseudogout, 429–430
        rheumatoid arthritis, 430–432
        septic arthritis, 432–433
    disorders of the back, spine, and bone
        acute lower back pain, 421–422
        osteomyelitis, 423–424
        seronegative spondyloarthropathies, 424–427
    musculoskeletal problems
        dermatomyositis, 218, 417–418
        fibromyalgia (fibrositis, fibromyositis), 414
        Lyme disease, 414–416, 432
        PMR (polymyalgia rheumatica), 416–417
        polymyositis, 417–418
        scleroderma, 150, 418–419
        SLE (systemic lupus erythematosus), 81, 208, 227, 420–421
        TA (temporal arteritis), 416–417
    osteoarthritis, 71, 427–428
    rheumatic fever, 180, 221, 432
    rheumatic heart disease, 14, 17, 19, 21
    rheumatoid arthritis, 34, 150, 208, 227, 432
    rheumatoid nodule, 380

Rhinovirus, 178, 317
Rho(D) immune globulin, 287
Ribavirin, 142
Rickettsia species, 319
Rifampin, 191, 316, 355
Right ventricular infarction, 33, 92
Riluzole, 196
Ringed sideroblasts, 169, 170
Ringer lactate, 94, 99, 104
Risedronate, 71
Risperidone, 330
Ristocetin cofactor activity, 175
Ristocetin-induced platelet
    aggregation, 175
Ritodrine, 277
Rivastigmine, 199
Rocky Mountain spotted fever, 313
Ropinirole, 201
Rorschach test, 350
Rosiglitazone, 57
Rotavirus, 131
Rotavirus, 299
Rotazyme assay, 300
Roth spots, 183
Rovsing sign, 436
RPGN, pauci-immune, 409
RPR (rapid plasma reagin), 51
RSV-IGIV (RSV Immune Globulin
    Intravenous), 304
RSV (respiratory syncytial virus),
    304–305, 306
RTA (renal tubular acidosis), 385,
    387–388
Rubella, 322–324
Rule of nines, 104
RUQ (right upper quadrant) pain, 439, 440
RV infarction (*see* Right ventricular
    infarction)

Saccular (berry) aneurysm, 230
Salicylates, 385
Saline, 94
Salk vaccine, 192
Salmeterol, 362
Salmonella species, 133, 134, 299, 425
Salmonellae, 172
Salpingitis, 266, 437
Salpingostomy, 271
SaO$_2$ (oxygen saturation) in arterial
    blood, 359
Sarcoidosis, 366–368, 380, 432
Sarcoptes scabiei ("itch mite"), 49
Sevelamer, 393

SBP (spontaneous bacterial peritonitis),
    153–154
Scabies, 49–50
Scalds, 102
Scarlet fever, 313
SCC (squamous cell carcinoma), 46, 53,
    114, 381, 382
SCD (sudden cardiac death), 42
Schilling test, 168
Schizoid personality disorder, 349
Schizophrenia, 329–330
Schizotypal personality disorder, 349
Sclerodactyly, 150
Scleroderma, 150, 418–419
Sclerosant injection, 118
Sclerosing cholangitis, 149
Scopolamine, 106
Second-degree (partial thickness) burns,
    103, 104
Secondary survey, emergency
    medicine, 76
Sedatives, 153, 377
Seizure activity
    after closed head injury, 78–79
    brain abscess and, 189, 191
    preterm birth and, 277
Semen analysis, 262
Sengstaken-Blakemore tube, 118
Senile degenerative disease, 14, 17
Sepsis, 97–98, 353, 387, 445
Septic abortion, 99, 285
Septic arthritis, 432–433
Septic embolus, 379
Septic shock, 98–100
Septic synovial fluid, 433
Seronegative spondyloarthropathies,
    424–427
Serotonin, 338
Serotonin reuptake inhibitors, 199
Serum aminotransferase, 137, 326
Serum β-hCG, 253
Serum bicarbonate, 92, 386
Serum calcium, 410
Serum ceruloplasmin level, 145
Serum copper level, 145
Serum creatinine, 11, 219, 326
Serum cystatin C, 11
Serum glucose, 58
Serum homocysteine, 221, 223
Serum iron, 171
Serum kinase, 326
Serum lactate, 92
Serum lead, 196

Serum lipid levels, 231
Serum osmolality, 69, 109
Serum osmolar gap, 388
Serum potassium, 152
Serum screens, 109
Serum sodium, 396
Serum toxicology screens, 106
Serum transaminases, 275
Serum uric acid, 398
7-valient protein conjugate vaccine, 311–312
Sexual abuse, 327–328
Sexually transmitted infection, 425
Shaken baby syndrome, 327
Shellfish, 89
Shigella species, 128, 132, 134, 299, 300, 425
"Shingles" (herpes zoster), 48–49
Shock
   anaphylactic, 88–91
   bacterial meningitis and, 191
   cardiogenic, 91–93
   diabetes mellitus and, 58, 59
   due to MI, 33, 91
   hypovolemic, 96–97, 104
   septic, 98–100
SIADH (syndrome of inappropriate antidiuretic hormone secretion), 69, 70, 80, 382, 397–398
Sibutramine, 72, 73
Sicca syndrome, 150
Sick sinus syndrome, 110
Sickle cell disease, 171–173, 221, 227, 280, 324, 404
Sideroblastic anemia, 169–170
SIDS (sudden infant death syndrome), 288
Sigmoid colon, 126
Sigmoidoscopy, 125, 133
Silicosis, 365
Sinus puncture, 179
Sinusitis, acute, 178–179
Sister Mary Joseph node, 156
Situational syncope, 112
Sjögren syndrome, 150, 227
Skin (*see also* Dermatology)
   changes during hemorrhage, 94
   septic shock and, 98
Skin grafting, 104
Skull depression, 78
Skull fracture, 77, 79
SLE (systemic lupus erythematosus), 81, 208, 227, 404, 413, 420–421

Sleep apnea, 71, 385
Sleeping position, for newborns, 288
Slitlamp exam, 201
SLUDGE (**S**alivation, **L**acrimation, **U**rination, **D**efecation, **G**astrointestinal cramps, and **E**mesis), 106
SMA (spinal muscle atrophy), 194–195
Small cell carcinoma, 382
Small cell lung cancer, 2, 66, 70
Smooth muscle malignoma, 244
SNARE proteins, 211
Social phobia, 334
Social skills
   infants, 288, 289
   preschoolers, 292, 293
   toddlers, 290, 291
SOD1 gene, 194
Sodium bicarbonate, 59
Sodium succinate, 90
Sodium retention, 412
Soft tissue, and septic shock, 98
Solid foods, for infants, 288–289
Solitary pulmonary nodule, 379–381
Somatization, 343
Somatosensory evoked potentials (SSEP), 204
Sonohysterogram, 262–263
Spinal cord diseases, 195
Spinal cord injury, 94
Spiral CT, 38
Spironolactone, 152, 402, 403
Spleen, 434
Splenectomy, 435
Splenomegaly, 163, 180, 183
Splinter hemorrhages, 183
Spondyloarthropathy, 432
Spontaneous abortion, 284, 285
Spontaneous arterial dissection, 228
"Spoon nail", 166
Sporadic oncogenes, 243
"Spot" test (Monospot), 180
Squamous cell carcinoma (SCC), 46, 53, 114, 247, 381, 382
SSEP (somatosensory evoked potentials), 204
SSRI (selective serotonin reuptake inhibitors), 332, 333, 334, 338, 339, 340, 398
ST elevation, 25, 26, 32
Staphylococcus aureus, 46, 99, 131, 132, 176, 178, 218, 321, 352, 423, 424
Staphylococcus species, 299, 300

Stasis, 448
Statins, 218
Sterilization, 283
Steroids
    for acute gouty arthritis, 429
    androgenic, 66
    for ARDS, 372
    for asthma, 359
    for brain abscess, 188
    chronic use, 422
    for edema in brain tumors, 203
    for endocrine myopathy, 216
    nebulized, 307
    for PMR and TA, 417
    for sarcoidosis, 367
    systemic, 48
    topical, 131
    for toxic megacolon, 130
    for Wegener granulomatosis, 408
Stevens-Johnson syndrome, 313
STI571, 161, 162
Stomatitis, angular, 166
Stool culture, 128, 129, 133, 300
Streptococcal pharyngitis, 318
Streptococcus agalactiae (group B
    streptococcus), 314
Streptococcus pneumoniae, 99, 176, 178,
    190, 312, 314, 319, 351, 352, 353
Streptococcus pyrogenes, 176, 180, 218,
    317, 318
Stress
    diabetes mellitus and, 58
    nonketotic hyperosmolar coma and, 59
    physiologic, 122
Striatum, 199
Stroke (*see also* CNS; MI)
    aortic stenosis and, 17
    arterial stenotic, 220–221
    atrial fibrillation and, 39, 40
    cardioembolic, 221–223
    drugs contraindicated, 73
    hemorrhagic, 34, 228
    hyperaldosteronism and, 6
    hypercapnic failure, 369
    hypertension and, 3, 33
    hypertrophic cardiomyopathy and, 20
    lacunar, 224
    nonketotic hyperosmolar coma and, 59
    preeclampsia and, 275
    pulmonary embolism and, 36
    SIADH and, 70
    vertebral basilar system, 224–226
Stromal malignoma, 244

Struvite kidney stones, 410
Sturge-Weber disease, 228
Subarachnoid hemorrhage, 228, 230–233
Subcortical nuclei, 197
Subdural abscess, 315
Subdural hematoma, 228, 348
Subhyoid hemorrhages, 231
Substantia nigra pars compacta, 199, 200
Succinylcholine, 210
Sucralfate, 124
Sulfasalazine, 131, 426, 431
Sulfonamides, 445
Sulfonylureas, 60
Supine hypotension, 96
Supine tachycardia, 96
Suppurative cholangitis, 99
Supraclavicular node, 156
Surgery
    gastrointestinal system
        AAA (abdominal aortic aneurysm),
            441–442
        abdominal injury, 434–435
        appendicitis, 436–437
        bleeding, 437–439
        gallbladder disease, 439–440
        hernia, 440–441
    urology
        benign prostatic hypertrophy,
            442–443
        prostate cancer, 445–447
        prostatitis, 447–448
        pyelonephritis, 448–449
        urethritis, 449–450
Surgical resection, 157
SVC (superior vena cava) syndrome, 381
Sympathomimetic overdose, 110
Sympathomimetic syndrome, 106
Synovectomy, 432
Synthetic dopamine agonists, 201
α-Synuclein, 200
Syphilis, 15, 50–51, 198, 219, 223,
    348, 432
Systemic embolic phenomenon, 183
Systemic lupus erythematosus (*see* SLE)
Systemic steroids, 48

T cells, 164
T-helper lymphocyte immune
    response, 366
T-score, bone mineral density, 71
T waves, 25, 26, 402
T_4 (thyroxine), 61, 62, 71
TA (temporal arteritis), 416–417

Tachyarrhythmia, 43, 110
Tachycardia, 96 (*see also* Cardiology)
Tacrolimus, 403
TAH-BSO (total abdominal hysterectomy and bilateral salpingo-oophorectomy), 240
Tamponade (*see* Cardiac tamponade; Pericardial tamponade)
Tamsulosin, 443
Tar, topical, 49
Tay-Sachs disease, 280
TB (*see* Tuberculosis)
TBSA (total body surface area), 104, 105
3TC (lamivudine), 186
TCAs (tricyclic antidepressants), 42, 102, 199, 332, 333, 338, 339, 340
Td vaccine, 311
Technetium-labeled RBC scan, 438
TEE (transesophageal echocardiography), 29, 39, 183, 220–221, 222
Tegmentum of the pons, 226
Telangiectasia, 51, 150, 373
Temper tantrums, 291
Temporal arteritis, 416–417
Tension headache, 414
Tension pneumothorax, 87, 88, 94
Terazosin, 443
Terbutaline, 277
Terfenadine, 42
Testosterone, 296
Tetanus, diphtheria without pertussis (Td) vaccine, 311
Tetracycline, 45, 124, 210, 450
Tetralogy of Fallot, 294
Thalassemia, 170–171
α-Thalassemia syndromes, 171
β-Thalassemia syndromes, 171
Thalidomide, 116
Thematic apperception test, 350
Theophylline, 39, 360, 362
Thiamine deficiency, 348
Thiazides, 400
Third-degree (full thickness) burns, 103, 104
Thoracentesis, 376, 382
Thoracostomy, 85
Thoracotomy, 81, 382
Threatened abortion, 284, 285, 286
Throat culture, 181
Thrombocytopenia, 98, 163
Thrombolytic agent, 34, 38
Thromboxane, 89

Thrush (*see* Candidiasis)
Thymoma, 208, 209
Thyroid disorders, 109, 150, 294, 338, 348 (*see also* Endocrine disorders)
Thyroid function tests, 198
Thyroid storm, 64
Thyroiditis, 62
Thyrotoxicity, 216
Thyroxine (*see* T_4)
TIA (transient ischemic attack), 220 (*see also* Stroke)
TIBC (total iron-binding capacity), 166
Tic paralysis, 212
Ticarcillin, 353
Tick bites, 414–415
Ticlopidine, 223
Tilt-table testing, 111
Timed urine collections for metanephrine, 9
Tinnitus, 176
Tissue biopsy, 165
Tissue diseases, 15
Tizanidine, 205
TLC (total lung capacity), 367
TM (tympanic membrane), 176, 177
TMP-SMZ (*see* Trimethoprim-sulfamethoxazole)
TNF (tumor necrosis factor), 371
TNM (Tumor, Node, Metastasis) staging, 115
Tobacco abuse (*see* Cigarette smoking)
Tocolytic therapy, 276
Todd's paralysis, 237
Togavirus, 323
Toilet training, 292
TONG therapies, 108–109
Tonsillectomy, 378, 379
Topical tar, 49
Torsades de pointes, 41–42, 101–102
Total abdominal colectomy, 439
Total body surface area (TBSA), 104, 105
Total colectomy, 130
Total iron-binding capacity (TIBC), 166
Total proctocolectomy, 130
Total protein, 376
Tourette syndrome, 332
Toxic ingestions, 107
Toxic megacolon, 130
Toxic myositis/myopathy, 218
Toxic neuropathies, 195
Toxic shock syndrome, 99, 313
Toxicology screen, 235, 236, 237
Toxin exposures, 215

Toxoplasmosis, 218
Tracheostomy, 378
Transbronchial biopsy, 382
Transcranial Doppler studies, 221
Transdermal estrogens, 257–258
Transesophageal echocardiography, 29, 39, 183
Transfusion of red blood cells, 95
Transient cerebral hypoxia, 110
Transient ischemic attack, 220 (*see also* Stroke)
Transluminal balloon angioplasty, 232
Transphenoidal microadenomectomy, 2, 67
Transrectal ultrasound, 443
Transthoracic echocardiogram, 81
Transudate, 375
Transvaginal sonography, 280
Tranylcypromine, 339
Trendelenburg position, 97
Treponema pallidum spirochete, 50
Treponema pallidum spirochete, 317
Trichinosis, 218
Tricyclic antidepressants, 398 (*see* TCAs)
Triglycerides, 376
Trimethoprim, 403
Trimethoprim-sulfamethoxazole (TMP-SMZ), 134, 177, 179, 186, 321, 357, 395, 444, 448
Triple-antibiotic therapy, 267
Trisomy, 293
Troponin, 92
TSH (thyroid-stimulating hormone), 61, 62, 67, 143
TTKG (transtubular K gradient), 404
Tubal disease, 262
Tube thoracostomy, 84, 85–86, 88
Tubercular pericarditis, 81
Tuberculosis, 70, 354–356, 365, 397, 432
Tuberous sclerosis, 202
Tubo-ovarian abscess, 437
Tuboplasty, 264
Tubular polyps, 125
Tubulointerstitial renal disease, 401
Tularemia, 317
Tumor suppressor genes, in endometrial cancer, 243
Turner syndrome, 28, 250, 296–297
TURP (transurethral prostatectomy), 443
24-hour intraesophageal pH monitoring, 116
24-hour urinary copper levels, 145, 201
24-hour urinary free cortisol, 2, 67

Tylosis, 114
Tympanic membrane (TM), 176
Type 1 diabetes (insulin-dependent), 55
Type 2 diabetes (non-insulin-dependent), 55, 59, 71
Tyramine hypertensive crisis, 339
Tyrosine kinase inhibitor, 161
Tzanck smear, 48

U waves, 402
UGIB (upper gastrointestinal bleeding), 437–438 (*see also* Gastroenterology)
Ulcerative colitis, 128, 130
Ultrafast magnetic resonance imaging, 280
Ultrasonography, 280
Ultraviolet light, 49
Undifferentiated schizophrenia, 330
Unopposed estrogen, 244
Upper endoscopy, 123
Upper GI bleeding (*see* Gastroenterology)
UPPP (uvulopalatopharyngoplasty), 378, 379
Uremia, 81, 235, 395 (*see also* Nephrology)
Ureaplasma urealyticum, 449
Ureteral obstruction, 449
Ureteral stones, 437
Urethritis, 449–450
Uric acid stones, 410
Urinalysis
    for acute renal failure, 390
    for altered mental status, 109
    for benign prostatic hypertrophy, 443
    for cystitis, 444
    for enuresis, 324
    for major depressive disorder, 338
    for nephrolithiasis, 410
    for preeclampsia, 275
    for prostatitis, 447
    for pyelonephritis, 448
    for renal trauma, 435
Urinary anion gap (*see* Anion gap)
Urinary chloride (Cl⁻), 386–387
Urinary pH, 410
Urinary protein, 411
Urinary sediment, 411
Urinary sodium (UNa), 390
Urine culture, 444, 447
Urine drug screens, 109
Urine microscopy, 374
Urine screens, 106

Urology
    benign prostatic hypertrophy, 442–443
    cystitis, 444–445
    prostate cancer, 445–447
    prostatitis, 444, 447–448
    pyelonephritis, 448–449
    urethritis, 449–450
    urinary tract obstruction, 448
    UTI (urinary tract infections), 324, 443
Urticaria, 89
US (ultrasound) scan, abdominal, 155
Uterine fibroids, 262
Uterus (*see* Obstetrics)
UTI (urinary tract infections), 324,
    443, 447
Uveitis, 366

V/Q (ventilation/perfusion) scan, 374
Vaccinations, for sickle cell crisis, 173
Vaccines (*see* Immunizations)
Vagal maneuvers, 41
Vaginitis, 286
Valproic acid, 137, 236, 336
Valsalva maneuver, 41, 111
Valvular disease, 39, 70, 111
Valvular stenosis, 110
Valvuloplasty, 18
Vancomycin, 134, 190, 433
Vanillylmandelic acid, 9
VAPP (vaccine-associated paralytic
    polio), 192
Variceal bleeding (*see* Esophageal
    varices)
Varicella vaccine, 310, 311
Varicella viruses, 325
Varicella-zoster virus, 48
Vascular dementia, 198
Vascular diseases (*see* CNS)
Vascular ectasias, 113–114, 125
Vascular surgery, 441–442
Vasculitis, 63, 98, 431, 441
Vasoconstriction, 89
Vasoconstrictors, 125
Vasodilation, 89
Vasopressin, 69, 101, 125
Vasopressor therapy, 97
Vasospasm, 36, 232
Vasovagal syncope, 110, 111, 112
VDRL (Venereal Disease Research
    Laboratory), 51, 190, 420–421
Venous lactate levels, 217
Venous thromboembolism, 283
Venous thrombosis, 411

Ventilation, assessing, 74
Ventral hernia, 441
Ventricular aneurysm, 221
Ventricular drain, 187
Ventricular fibrillation, 42–43, 100
Ventricular pacemaker, 102, 110
Ventricular septal defects, 14
Ventricular septal wall rupture, 91
Ventricular tachycardia, 41, 43
VEP (visual evoked potentials), 204
Verapamil, 20
Verbal skills, 295
Vertebral basilar system strokes, 224–226
Vertebral fractures, 422
Vertigo, 176
Vesicoureteral reflux nephrolithiasis, 448
VF/VT (ventricular fibrillation/pulseless
    ventricular tachycardia), 100, 101
Vibrio cholerae, 131, 132
Villous polyps, 125
Vincristine, 165, 216, 398
Viral bronchiolitis, 304
Viral encephalitis, 228
Viral illness, 34, 168
Viral pharyngitis, 318
Viral rhinosinusitis, 178
Viral warts, 53–54
Virchow node, 156
Visual hallucinations, 108
Vital functions, 74 (*see also* ABCs)
Vitamin B_{12} deficiency, 167, 234, 348
Vitamin B_{12} levels, 198
Vitamin D
    hydroxylation, 64
    for hyperparathyroidism, 393
    for infants, 288
    supplementation, 71
Vitamin D-resistant rickets, 280
Vitamin K
    malabsorption, 157
    for Reye syndrome, 326
    supplementation, 59, 60, 152
Vitiligo, 150
VMA (vanillylmandelic acid), 9
Volume depletion, 96
Von Hippel-Lindau, 8 (*see also*
    Pheochromocytoma)
Von Willebrand disease, 175
VRS (viral rhinosinusitis), 178

Warfarin, 38
Water deprivation test, 69
Wegener granulomatosis, 380, 408, 409

Weight loss, 378
Western blot, 185
White blood cell (WBC) count, 134, 190
Wilson's disease, 145–146, 200, 201
Wolf-Parkinson-White syndrome, 101

X chromosome, 295
X-linked pattern, 174
X-rays
    abdominal, 155
    barium, 129
    chest, 160, 172, 187, 222, 244, 246,
        248, 304, 313, 320, 352, 358,
        365, 374

free air series, 123
KUB (kidneys, ureter, and bladder), 410
neck, 309, 322
in secondary survey, 76
stages of sarcoidosis, 367
upper GI, 303
Xp21 gene, 213

Y chromosome, 250
Yersinia species, 299, 425

Z-score, bone mineral density, 71
Zidovudine (AZT), 186, 216
ZZ genotype test, 136